THE DOG CARE
HANDBOOK

THE DOG CARE HANDBOOK

Things I Wish My Vet Had Told Me

CHRISTOPHER LITTLE

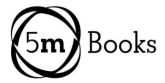

First published 2024

Published by
5M Books Ltd,
Lings, Great Easton,
Essex CM6 2HH, UK,
Tel: +44 (0)1371 870897
www.5mbooks.com

Follow us on
Twitter @5m_Books
Instagram 5m_books
Facebook @5mBooks
LinkedIn @5mbooks

A Catalogue record for this book is available from the British Library
ISBN 9781789182385
eISBN 9781789182705
DOI 10.52517/9781789182705

Book layout by Cheshire Typesetting Ltd, Cuddington, Cheshire
Printed by Short Run Press, Exeter
Photos by the author unless otherwise indicated
Illustrations by Elaine Leggett
Cover image: AdobeStock_347612143

CONTENTS

PART III   FREQUENTLY ASKED QUESTIONS AND RELATED ISSUES

'Outside of a dog, a book is a man's best friend. Inside of a dog it's too dark to read.'
Groucho Marx

'I PROMISE AND SOLEMNLY DECLARE that I will pursue the work of my profession with integrity and accept my responsibilities to the public, my clients, the profession and the Royal College of Veterinary Surgeons and that ABOVE ALL my constant endeavour will be to ensure the health and welfare of the animals committed to my care.'
Royal College of Veterinary Surgeons Oath on entry to the profession

'Without good evidence we are all just muddling around in the darkness.'
Dr Dan O'Neill (Veterinary Epidemiologist and former practitioner)

'I'll know my song well before I start singing.'
Bob Dylan

PREFACE

This is a book about partnerships; between you, your dog and your vet.

A visit to the vet can be extremely stressful for dog owners and their dogs. Dogs are worried that vets can be evil. Clients are concerned about their dog's health, their ability to explain their dog's clinical problems and health needs, how serious a problem the dog might have, the costs involved, and many other practical issues, such as how easy, or difficult, it will be to medicate their dog. From the veterinarian's perspective there are issues too; vets worry that clients often don't fully appreciate how best to maintain and enhance the health and welfare of their dog. We perceive our clients are anxious, but find it is virtually impossible to allay their fears under the constraints of a short consultation because veterinary medicine is complex and uncertain. For instance, accurate diagnosis of disease from examination of a dog, even when very thorough, may be impossible, so that to reach this goal certain tests – such as radiographs, blood or urine tests – may be needed. Such tests are often expensive and the findings themselves may be equivocal. It is no wonder that both clients and their vets sometimes feel the process has been frustrating, or worse! This book aims to deliver exactly what the title says. I want to provide all the information you need, to get the maximum satisfaction from visiting a vet from the first time that you enter their practice and meet them.

I have been a practising vet for 40 years and a dog owner for most of my life. I know different people may want dogs for different reasons, but also that people often acquire a dog that is unsuitable for them or unhealthy, perhaps because they don't know how to choose the right dog. A basic grasp of some fundamental concepts and a grounding in dog behaviour can help a great deal in choosing a dog and managing the first few weeks of their life with you.

Vets appreciate well-informed clients. Dog owners benefit most from their vets when they feel they can trust and understand them. Vets differ in their abilities, interests, empathy, skills and experience, so clients need to find the right vet for them and their dog. This book is written to enable you to recognise a caring, knowledgeable, skilled clinician with good communication skills who is also willing and able to listen to your perspectives. If you want to find the right veterinary practice and the right vet to suit you, this book should help.

Information and misinformation about veterinary medicine is all around us; on the internet, on television and in print. Sorting good information from misleading hyperbole is challenging, unless you begin from a secure base. 'Be sceptical and question everything' is a good starting point. Veterinary medicine is a practical science; but in science all knowledge is provisional and incomplete. In the long run it will very probably turn out that some of the guidance in this book is wrong. Some vets may insist they are infallible (none are), others may be unscrupulous charlatans out to make a fast buck from gullible clients, but they are very few indeed. This book is written to help you understand dog health and provide ideal conditions for your dog to thrive. It should also help you recognise good veterinary science, good veterinary medicine and the best practitioners of the veterinary arts.

I am writing this book because when I consult as a vet I often try to pass on a lot of information to my clients, but in the context of a stressful consultation I know that much of this will quickly be forgotten; in the words of my dad, 'it will go in one ear and out the other' (as is the way with much oral communication). When in a social situation I accidentally let slip that I am a vet, I frequently find people later sidle-up to me and say, 'I hope you don't mind me asking but . . . my dog chews his feet a lot / keeps getting ear problems / pants all the time / seems a bit stiff in the morning / pees on the floor when I go out / has suddenly collapsed a couple of times / seems to be quite aggressive when he's on the lead . . .', or ask about any number of other common problems in veterinary medicine. Perhaps their vets have never discussed these problems frankly with the clients, or the clients have not taken in what has been said. Either way, there seems to be a niche for a book covering common veterinary problems targeted at the thoughtful dog owner. I aim to help you and your dog to get the best out of your partnership with your vet. Wherever possible the information and advice herein are based on sound scientific evidence, but often there is little or none. I try to be candid when that is the case. This book is certainly supposed to be a self-help book, but it should never be used in place of a vet.

Here and elsewhere in this text I use the generic names of medicines and medicine classes. I have deliberately avoided using tradenames (even those those might be the ones with which you are most familiar).

A word here on 'alternative medicine'. Some people put a lot of faith in non-conventional medicine, herbs and 'natural' remedies. Many medicines that do work have been discovered by studying natural phenomena: aspirin, antibiotics and the heart drug digitalis are good examples. Science has not turned its back on this path. Recently, for instance, drugs derived from the yew tree, taxoids, have become crucial in treating certain forms of cancer. Some forms of treatment that were regarded as unconventional, say, 40 years ago are now mainstream because they have accrued sound evidence in their favour, this would include acupuncture, hydrotherapy and physiotherapy. That said, a good deal of alternative medicine frankly is snake-oil, peddled by quacks to those who are wary of experts and doubt the whole ethos of science. The vast majority of my profession, myself included, think homeopathy is based on a fatuous idea and utterly without merit. In the words of the Australian comic Tim Minchin, 'Alternative medicine which works is called . . . medicine.'

I believe in evidence. If you are looking for unconventional and alternative medicine then this book may not be for you.

For light-hearted relief look up Tim Minchin 'Storm' and Mitchell and Webb 'Homeopathic ER' on YouTube.

Part I

HEALTHY DOGS

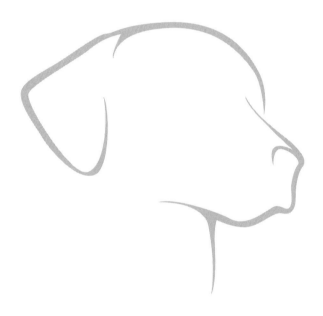

1
INTRODUCTION AND ORIENTATION

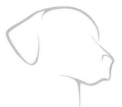

Rudi lay stretched out on the caravan seat breathing noisily. He'd lain like this all morning. He'd hardly moved since Dad had brought him home last night. Around his lips, drool and flecks of foam clung. His eyes were wide, the pupils huge; he was focused on nothing but his own breathing. His gums and tongue were a deep stain of purple, almost beetroot. Suddenly, he let out a long thin painful screeching groan, made a huge gasp, stretched his head backwards and pushed his forelegs forwards. Then he sighed, like a tyre deflating. A stream of frothy fluid dribbled from his mouth, urine splashed to the floor. He was dead. My mother started to cry. I'd never seen Mummy cry.

I was nine. It was July 1968. We were on holiday at the Silversands Caravan Park, near Mallaig on the West coast of Scotland. A few days earlier I had at last learnt to swim, after a fashion, in the chilly waters of the Atlantic. The previous day Rudi and Carlo, our Standard Dachshunds, lifelong insepara-ble companions, had enjoyed a long walk near Loch Morar, leaping through deep heather searching for grouse, rabbits, pipits, everything and anything, but that evening Rudi became withdrawn. He refused his dinner. This was unprecedented. I heard Mummy and Dad talking in low voices. Dad left carrying Rudi, slumped heavy as a sack, to the car. He came back long after my bedtime but I couldn't sleep. More hushed voices. Dad had found a vet who'd given him two white tablets for Rudi. Mummy and Dad tried to get Rudi to swallow them but it was useless. They started to bicker. I fell asleep.

I often recall that day. The day Rudi died was the day I decided I should be a vet.

WHY DO PEOPLE DECIDE TO OWN A DOG AND WHY DO THEY GET SO ATTACHED?

Dogs have lived with people for tens of thousands of years. We have evolved as species together. It's easy to see what dogs get from the arrangement: food, shelter, usually safety and affection too. What do people get? Love, companionship, affection and trust. A short answer; unsatisfactory, too vague, too nebulous, too unscientific for the rationalist, but there are hard-nosed scientific studies that have demonstrated many and various benefits to owning a dog. For instance, when you stroke or pet a dog you have developed a bond with, your own blood pressure and heart rate fall. If you have a heart attack you have a better chance of a full and complete recovery and a longer lifespan afterwards if you already own a pet dog (the evidence is convincing, although the magnitude of the effect is disputed). Folk who own pet dogs make fewer visits to see their doctors. They also do more, and more frequent, exercise than those who don't. They exercise especially in green spaces, which seem to provide the greatest benefit to human health, and do so in all weathers too because they feel an obligation to their dog. They report they feel better for it. People who own a dog are much more likely to talk to other people when they are out with their dog and those conversations tend to be longer and more complex. In other words, dogs seem to act as a social lubricant, they help to reduce loneliness and isolation. Owning a dog carries with it important responsibilities, but these duties are usually shouldered willingly by dog owners and this too seems to be good for the health, wellbeing and happiness of these people. There is evidence that beneficial hormonal changes emerge in both dogs and their owners as their relationship develops. These effects involve oxytocin, sometimes coined 'the cuddle hormone', adrenalin and noradrenalin, key players in the 'Fight, Flight or Freeze' response, and another hormone, cortisol. This illustrates just some of the benefits that can ensue from successful relationships between dogs and their owners.

But there's more.

Children brought up in the presence of dogs have less respiratory, asthmatic and allergic disease. The explanation for this is controversial. Those kids also seem to have a more complex microbiome, which is the teeming bacterial population of the healthy gut. Children who grow up with pet dogs seem to be generally better adjusted socially than those who come from homes devoid of pets. This is especially true of kids with attention deficit and hyperactivity (ADHD) and those with learning difficulties such as autism. People who have grown up with animals often have a much better grasp of the crucial importance of nature and the environment. Those people who are prone to depressive illness have been shown to benefit disproportionately from the presence of a loving dog. Elderly people living on their own report less loneliness if they have a dog. They are also more inclined to look after themselves properly and to live more active lives than those who do not have a canine companion. Some people, especially women and the elderly, say they feel safer when confronted by strangers, if they are accompanied by a companion dog. Research shows this is a two-way thing; dogs themselves feel safer in those situations when their owner is present.

Leaving aside all this science, I believe dogs can cultivate our appetite for being, feeling and empathy. Watching my dogs charge about with wild elation, sprint across a beach or a muddy field, wrestle, romp and play-fight together, brings me joy. When I have been away from home, even for an hour, they throw themselves at me, breathlessly eager to show how deeply I've been missed. At other times, relaxing quietly, torpid and at ease, they exude another sort of happiness; blissful peace.

Dog ownership of course can bring hazards, especially an increased risk of falling for the elderly, and of bite wounds in children. Sometimes owning a dog can be difficult, because not all dogs behave as well as we would like all the time. Keeping a dog costs money. Dogs also deserve a lot of time and effort from their owners. If you are not prepared to invest these in your dog then don't have a dog. Dogs require health care that is frequently expensive, sometimes onerous to deliver, and doesn't always turn out well. Eventually all dogs will die; the sadness which this brings to owners and family members should not be underestimated. We love our dogs; the price of this love can be intense grief.

So, dog ownership needs to be considered carefully.

This book is written to help you navigate both the good and the bad aspects of canine health care and to help you partner with your vet to the benefit of all parties.

ORIENTATION

The book is arranged as follows.

Part I. Healthy dogs

Chapter 1. *Orientation*: this is where you are now.

I hope some readers will choose to read this book right through, but these will probably only be the dedicated few. Others will read chapters, or sections, on their own when that information is most relevant to them, or use this book as a reference; reading parts as they see fit. Most people find dry facts dull and difficult to assimilate. So, the text is peppered with anecdotes and vignettes of cases I have seen (some details have been changed to protect the innocent). I hope this makes it entertaining as well as informative.

Chapter 2. *Choosing your dog*: this tackles the issue of choosing a dog; covering such subjects as the relative lifespans of different breeds of dog, the many advantages of choosing a mixed breed instead of a pedigree, and the important issues you might have to confront if you buy, or re-home, certain breeds and certain types of dog. In this chapter, I will also address how to choose a dog to suit your lifestyle, circumstances and budget. The choosing / purchase process will be discussed with tips to when you should be suspicious about the transaction, because a significant proportion of puppies on sale have come from puppy farms or have been illegally imported. The chapter will discuss preparations for the new family member and how to make the first few days as smooth and stress-free as possible.

Chapter 3. Aims to help you decide ***How to choose your vet***.

Chapter 4. *Your first trips to the vet*: this will deal with your first visits to see a vet with your new puppy or re-homed dog. The chapter will include some basic biology, some information on dog behaviour, and lots of practical advice about parasite control, diet, insurance, toilet training, puppy parties, socialisation, vaccination, neutering, exercise and training.

Chapter 5. *Routine health care*: this is a chapter focused on heathy management of your dog such as choosing diets, how to care for their teeth, skin and coat. Dog behaviour will receive some further attention, which might enhance your enjoyment of your dog and your dog's quality of life. More information will be imparted about neutering, exercise, weight control, dieting to tackle weight problems, vaccination boosters, and important subjects such as holidays, kennelling, taking your dog abroad and the pros and cons of veterinary loyalty schemes.

Part II. Illness

Chapter 6. *Visiting the vet when your dog is ill*: this is devoted to the consultation with your vet when your dog is ill. I start by explaining the diagnostic processes vets employ including the process of interviewing you, the client. I set out exactly what vets do when they examine a dog, and why they are always rather cagey about making a definitive diagnosis, at least until some further investigations are done. This chapter will help you to understand why veterinary medicine always seems so expensive. It will unravel what some different types of diagnostic tests are for, and will give an insight into the costs involved.

Chapter 7. *Common problems*: this is a chapter devoted to the exploration of some of the most common veterinary problems in dogs, such as: recurrent flea infestation, allergic skin diseases, relapsing ear problems, sore eyes, dental disease, recurrent vomiting and/or diarrhoea, urinary incontinence, ruptures of the cruciate ligament in the knee, hip dysplasia, arthritis, bite wounds, grass seed foreign bodies, lumps and rubbing of the bottom on the floor. Other common issues, such as sudden onset lethargy or loss of appetite, excessive thirst, false pregnancy and womb infections in bitches, will be tackled too.

Chapter 8. *Emergencies*: this discusses road accidents, dog-fight wounds, gastrointestinal foreign bodies, poisoning, 'bloat' (gastric-dilatation-volvulus (GDV)), collapse, fainting, seizures, severe breathing difficulties (dyspnoea) and heat-stroke. First-aid for these problems will be discussed. Emergency facilities and treatments will be explained.

Chapter 9. *Chronic diseases*: this will focus on a small number of important persistent medical problems that require very intensive treatments: dry eye (keratoconjunctivitis sicca (KCS)), heart failure, diabetes mellitus, epilepsy, Addison's disease, Cushing's disease and renal failure. These are conditions that can be extremely rewarding to treat and where the outcome is highly dependent on close cooperation between the veterinary team and the dog's owner.

Chapter 10. *Practical nursing of your dog*: this is designed to help you treat your dog when she or he is ill. It will address what you can do to help the vet make a diagnosis and facilitate your dog's recovery. It will explain how to collect urine samples, how to give tablets easily, and how to administer other types of drug, by mouth and other routes. The value of specific diets for gastrointestinal problems, skin conditions, renal disease, pancreatitis, heart problems, liver disease, renal disease and anorexia will be covered.

Chapter 11. *Cancer*: the word 'cancer' brings with it a particular horror for many people but cancer is not a single disease. Dogs have a lifetime risk of developing cancer similar to people. Just as in people, most cancers arise randomly, so it is usually impossible to identify a single cause. The prognosis for the treatment of cancer in dogs is improving. This chapter will explain when cancer might be suspected and how a diagnosis might be reached. It will explain, in broad terms, what might be done to treat the problem; including surgery, drug- and radio-therapy. Monitoring, follow-up, remission and relapses will be discussed.

Chapter 12. *Old age*: this chapter is concerned with geriatrics, age-related disease, cognitive dysfunction, organ failure, euthanasia and death. These issues are best dealt with by frank and honest discussions with your vet. You can help your vet and your dog by being open about your worries and discussing the scenarios before you must face them.

Part III. Frequently asked questions and related issues

Chapter 13. *When things go wrong*: this is a chapter designed to help you when things seem to be going wrong. What should you do if you can't afford the tests and treatments? How to go about changing your vet when the need arises? How to ask for a referral to a specialist? What to expect from a specialist referral. How to make a complaint to, or about, your vet when you feel things are, or have been, badly handled, and how that complaint may be dealt with.

Appendices: this section takes the form of some addenda that address specific issues such as: the law on animal welfare for dogs, the law on veterinary drugs, the

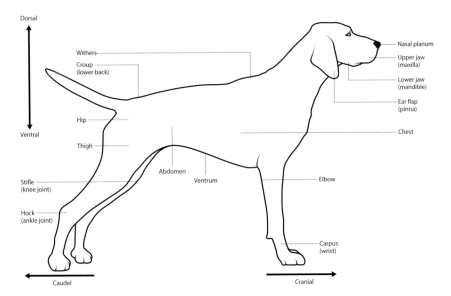

Figure 1.1. Some basic anatomy and veterinary terminology

prescribing cascade, the Royal College of Veterinary Surgeons (RCVS), and other useful contacts, web locations, etc.

Glossary: definitions of some less common veterinary terms.

Selected bibliography: focusing on the key papers, books and online resources that you might find useful.

2

CHOOSING YOUR DOG

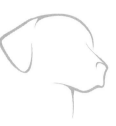

This chapter tackles the issue of choosing a dog; it covers such subjects as the relative lifespans of different breeds of dog, the advantages of choosing a mixed breed, and the important issues you might have to confront if you buy, or re-home, certain breeds and certain types of dogs. In this chapter, I give practical tips to help you choose a dog to suit your lifestyle, circumstances and budget. The choosing / purchase process will be discussed with warnings on when you should be suspicious about circumstances surrounding the purchase of a dog. The chapter will discuss preparations for the new family member and how to make the first few days as smooth and stress-free as possible.

A good vet will be delighted to help you care for your dog irrespective of its type, age or appearance. However, people sometimes make poor choices when they obtain a dog. This can have lasting consequences.

I once knew an elderly pair of sisters who were keen, knowledgeable and dedicated dog owners. They had five big strong female German Shepherd dogs. The dogs were well looked after; walked daily, regularly vaccinated and frequent visitors to our practice. As the dogs aged, they began to exhibit the typical health problems of older dogs: stiffness, dental disease, urinary incontinence. But it was not the dogs alone who aged. The sisters became less vigorous, thinner, frailer; they found the tasks of managing the dogs increasingly onerous, although they always seemed cheerful. One day one of them rang us in a frightful tizzy: her sister had been pulled over by one of the dogs and broken her arm. It was the beginning of the end. Within two years both sisters had passed away and several old infirm dogs were looking for a home.

A family acquired Claude, a large dog, for their elderly father who had recently been widowed. They thought this would help him through his grieving, get him out of doors exercising in the fresh air, and enable him to avoid loneliness. He'd always loved dogs. However, the old man was in declining health; he found Claude was a real handful. He couldn't manage the dog or his own health. Soon, he and the dog joined the family in their home. No-one could give Claude the exercise he needed. The old man had to go to the hospital often, so the dog was frequently left at home for hours at a time. Claude started to vandalise the house when he was left alone. As a temporary solution, the family decided Claude should live outdoors in their large garden. They bought him a luxurious big kennel. However, Claude hated being left outside. He barked and barked almost continuously. The neighbours complained. The police were called. The family decided they couldn't keep Claude and relinquished him to a rehoming centre.

Rosalind's story

My husband's friend bought a Miniature Schnauzer for his parents as a surprise. Shortly after this his father died and our friend found himself sharing the dog care with his mother. He mentioned to my husband that he was considering re-homing the dog as he was often out or away on assignments, as a photographer. He didn't think his mum would want to cope with looking after the dog full time. To my astonishment, my husband volunteered to adopt him. We went to meet the dog, Malcolm, and took him out into the country to visit friends who had three Springer Spaniels. Malcolm came along without a backward glance and had a wonderful day playing with our daughters, then aged 10 and 4, and the other dogs. Malcolm seemed to be the dog for us . . . until our friend mentioned the plan to his mother who was horrified! Malcolm was not going anywhere. So, Malcolm was not for us. But we loved his cheerful personality and within a year we had acquired our own Miniature Schnauzer, Duncan, who was soon confirmed as our perfect dog.

Dogs are a species that diverged from the ancestor of the grey wolf (*Canis lupis*) probably sometime in the last 30,000 years. However, almost all the pedigree breeds of dog we know today are actually a very recent human invention that have emerged from selective breeding and inbreeding over the last 200 years or less. Most dogs certainly appear physically to differ from wolves, but it is surely in their behaviour that the two species have diverged most. In the words of one respected animal behaviourist, Sarah Whitehead: 'Man is not an ape. The dog is not a wolf.'

Choosing a dog is not straightforward. Most people seem to choose their dog based on a few parameters: appearance, familiarity with the breed, availability, perhaps fashion and cost. These may not be the most appropriate criteria. There are more than 200 breeds of dog registered by the Kennel Club and more than twice that number are recognised world-wide; but crossbreeds ('mongrels') are often healthier, just as attractive, affectionate and clever, and make at least as good pets as pedigree dogs. Pedigree dogs are, by their definition, derived from dogs of similar appearance, bred to strict conformational standards, sometimes originating from a quite particular locale. In other words, they invariably derive from a rather small parental stock, a restricted gene pool, which means they are inbred and particularly likely to carry genetic abnormalities. Some breeds come from a foundation stock of only ten or 20 individuals! There is robust evidence throughout biology that the general health and fitness of inbred members of any species is lower than of those that are outbred. This phenomenon is known as inbreeding depression. Crossbreeds (or 'mongrels') are outbred; there is greater genetic diversity between the parents, which tends to be associated with an increase in overall fitness in the offspring. This phenomenon is known as hybrid vigour or heterosis. Genetically determined diseases are much less common in crossbreed than pedigree dogs.

Many people are keen to acquire pedigree dogs. This is, of course, usually because of familiarity with, and affection for, the appearance and character they associate with that breed. However, there is also a widely held misunderstanding that 'well-bred' dogs from reputable breeders who participate in the dog-show circus are likely to be particularly healthy. This is incorrect. Many reputable breeders do take very great care in the selection of the dogs they breed from and try to search thoroughly and carefully for possible genetic or heritable problems. They may also try to avoid close inbreeding, but the plain truth is that genetics is complicated. Sometimes, by avoiding one known genetic trap, breeders may walk straight into another one that was previously unrecognised. Careful testing and careful selection of parent dogs definitely can go some way to mitigate the effects of inbreeding, but pedigree dog breeding is based on the fallacy that dogs that breed 'true' – to produce offspring with a similar phenotype, appearance and behaviour, as the parents – are in some way genetically superior. This is a fundamental biological error. When the genetic pool is restricted, inbreeding depression is inevitable. This does not mean that all pedigree dogs are likely to become sick or develop hereditary diseases, but it does mean that, in general, crossbreed dogs are more robust and live longer. An impressive body of scientific evidence has been published that confirms this.

For those who are particularly interested in this, you might want to look into the science behind a statistic known as the Coefficient of Inbreeding (COI). Briefly, this is a mathematical calculation of the relatedness of dogs based on their pedigree history. Many breeders will use this information when selecting dogs to breed in an attempt to reduce the risk that the offspring puppies will carry inherited diseases. In terms of health, a COI less than 5% is definitely best. Inbreeding levels above 10% will have significant effects. Unfortunately, many breeds of dog currently have high COI values throughout and the problem worsens with every new generation, which is why closed breeding pools, demanded by the Kennel Club, ultimately are very bad for the long-term health of pedigree dogs (see https://www.instituteofcaninebiology.org/blog/coi-faqs-understanding-the-coefficient-of-inbreeding).

For the record, I have a Lurcher, crossed between a saluki and one, or several, other breeds and a cross-bred Terrier.

A dog may live for up to 15 years or more. Small dogs (such as Miniature and Toy Poodles, Yorkshire, Border and Jack Russell terriers) and crossbreeds tend to have significantly longer lives than large purebred ('pedigree') dogs. Indeed, some of the large purebred dogs have average lifespans of only six–nine years (this is true, for instance, of Great Danes, Wolfhounds, Mastiffs and Dogue de Bordeaux). A few of the larger breeds seem to buck this trend; thus, for instance, Border Collies and Bearded Collies often have relatively long lives. Interestingly, differences in the lifespan also occur within breeds; for instance, chocolate coloured Labradors tend to live considerably shorter lives than yellow or black ones do.

NATURE AND NURTURE/GENOTYPE AND PHENOTYPE

The terms 'phenotype' and 'genotype' are useful in understanding genetics and dog breeding. Phenotype is the physical actuality of an animal including its particular appearance, apparent health and behaviour. The phenotype depends on genetics, 'nature', but also upon the total history of the animal: its nutrition, experiences, training, environment, etc. – that is, 'nurture'. The phenotype of an animal (and of people) changes throughout life. The genotype, on the other hand, describes the genetic instructions in the DNA that created that particular dog under those circumstances. Because many genetic instructions have no visible manifestations whatsoever, or have effects only under certain circumstances, it is often completely impossible to recognise a genotype from its phenotype. This is why it is so difficult to recognise inherently healthy or unhealthy stock.

KEY MESSAGE

The anatomy, physiology, behaviour, resilience, health and longevity of a dog depends partly on its genetic makeup: its genome. Purebred dogs tend to have less genetic diversity, poorer genetic health and shorter lives than those who have a more mixed genetic background. This can have negative consequences on the quality of life and overall health of these pedigree dogs. That said, for any individual dog, it is extremely difficult to calculate the impact of their genome on behaviour, life events, their overall health, vigour and longevity.

Dog behaviour, like human behaviour, is partly genetically controlled. There has been an explosion in research into the interactions between genetics and behaviour. It has recently been proved, for example, that dogs are born with some innate abilities to understand human behaviour and body language, such as pointing (see *Current Biology*: doi.org/gkc6wb). Precisely how the proteins coded for by the genome determine specific behaviours is not yet understood, but there is no doubt that they do, which is why a Border Collie is intrinsically better at herding sheep than a Border Terrier. Collies have been honed through many generations to be sheepdogs; they are easily trained to manage livestock, extremely intelligent, have an almost obsessive-compulsive temperament, but very quickly become bored if they do not have enough to occupy them. This is a breed frequently listed for rehoming because of behavioural problems and especially 'separation anxiety' when left alone. They are dogs often best suited to single owners who are willing and able to exercise them vigorously and frequently.

If you are thinking of acquiring a dog, think carefully. Consider your environment, your family, the time, space and financial commitments that a dog brings with it. In a very recent report (PAW PDSA, 2019) the minimum cost of keeping a small dog was estimated at £70 per month. A large dog will be much more expensive to keep. If you live in a small flat in a city then you should probably choose a relatively small dog. There are many examples of breeds and types of dog to choose from weighing less than 10kg when adult; for instance, Toy and Miniature Poodles (Toys are smaller than Miniatures), Maltese Terriers, Yorkshire Terriers, Italian Greyhounds, Shiba Inu, Miniature Pinschers, Pomeranians, Chihuahuas, etc. On the other hand, if you have a large house, live rurally, are willing and able to spend a couple of hours a day exercising the dog, or want them to go running with you, then a big dog might suit you better; for example, a Labrador, Golden Retriever, Standard Poodle, Springer Spaniel, Pointer, Saluki, Setter, Lurcher, etc. Many other dogs from the Working, Sporting and Terrier groups thrive on plenty of exercise.

If you have young family, you must consider the type of dog very carefully. Look for a dog type who is likely to be tolerant and not too demanding. Some dog breeds are intrinsically more likely to bite than others, and obviously if the dog is large with strong jaws, then a dog bite could prove serious. In choosing for a family like this, I would definitely avoid Mastiffs, Chow-Chow, Sharpei, Malamutes, Huskies, American Bulldogs, Akita, Jack Russell Terriers, Chihuahuas and Dachshunds, as well as most of the very powerful dogs such as German Shepherds, Australian Cattle Dogs and Rottweilers (although I have known several very gentle 'Rotties'). Dogs who are more often placid include: Lhasa Apso, Miniature Poodles, Labradors, Golden Retrievers, Irish (Red) Setters, Vizlas and Greyhounds. Many of the 'designer dogs', such as Spaniel, Labrador, Poodle and Golden Retriever crosses, also make excellent family pets; each has a clever epithet, such as the 'Sprocker', 'Labradoodle', 'Cockapoo', etc. I must make particular mention here of the Staffordshire Bull Terrier ('Staffie') because this breed is often mistakenly confounded with the Pit Bull Terrier. In my experience, 'Staffies' can be extremely good with children and make excellent family pets but, on the other hand, they can be rather aggressive with other dogs, which is perhaps why confusion about them is widespread.

In spite of what I have said about the differences between breeds in terms of temperament, the differences in behaviour within breeds can still be enormous. It would be wrong to assume that all Spaniels are gregarious and daft, or that all Labradors are relaxed and friendly. Individual dogs vary enormously. The way that a dog is treated, especially when they are young, will also have profound effects on their temperament and ability to get along in the world. This will be touched upon in much more detail later.

The conformation and anatomy of dogs is extremely diverse. No other mammalian species has such a variable appearance. However, the health and welfare of those dogs that exhibit the most extreme anatomy is often poor. Consider those dogs, for instance, which have very short noses and widely placed prominent forward-facing or bulging eyes, such as Pugs, Boston Terriers, Pekinese, Shih Tsu, French and English Bulldogs. Many of these dogs have serious problems with their breathing (brachycephalic obstructive airway syndrome – BOAS) and with their eyes. This is not simply an occasional health concern; many of these dogs pant continuously and make loud grunting and snoring noises as they breathe. This is not an endearing foible. Those who suggest it is cute are wrong. The noises occur because their airway is obstructed. I often see dogs of this type in which this problem becomes life-threatening, and I have seen some die in agony as a result. These dogs are also unable to regulate their body temperature properly, which means that during even gentle exercise and in hot weather I believe the majority of these dogs suffer because of their conformation.

In 2018, the most popular breed of dog registered with the Kennel Club was the French Bulldog. It is difficult to explain the sudden popularity of this breed except by a desire for a fashionable baby-faced dog. Most French Bulldogs are not born naturally but by Caesarean section because their heads are too big to pass unaided through the mother dog's birth canal. If a bitch of this breed raises several litters her welfare will be seriously compromised. The veterinary profession is horrified by the dramatic increase in popularity of French Bulldogs; they are beset by health problems that can lead to considerable suffering.

No dog breed has ever been improved by the capricious and arbitrary decision that a shorter / longer / flatter / bigger / smaller / curlier 'whatever' is better. Condemning a dog to a lifetime of suffering for the sake of looks is not an improvement; it is torture. (Caen Elegans, 2012)

The dog's nose is quite extraordinary and weird. Technically, the snout, or muzzle, is that part of a dog's face from just in front of the eyes, forward. The region is constructed of three bones on each side. The maxilla forms the roof of the mouth and a large part of the side of the snout. It houses the 20 teeth of the upper jaw, whilst the tip and the roof of the nose is formed from the incisive and nasal bones. The moist patinated black tip of the snout, known as the nasal planum, contains the comma-shaped nostrils. Dogs have the most fantastic sense of smell and their whole world is orientated around this sense, but the canine nasal chamber has other functions too. It is key in temperature regulation. When we humans get too hot, after running for the bus, or when the best days of the summer arrive, we cool ourselves by sweating. Dogs cannot thermoregulate by sweating (although, contrary to popular belief they do have modified sweat glands, especially on their feet, on the nasal planum, in the ear canals and near their bottom). Dogs cool themselves by panting, but the mechanism is complicated and widely misunderstood. Panting dogs breathe in through their noses and expire through the mouth. Each nasal chamber is filled by scrolls of bone known as conchae (or turbinates); these conchae are covered with a fine network of thin blood vessels and are continually moistened with fluid from a gland in the nose. The conchae act like an air-conditioner. Inspired air flows across the conchae where the fluid evaporates rapidly. This evaporation within the nasal chamber cools the body. Evaporation of fluid from the tongue during panting augments temperature regulation. When dogs are hot, they augment this fluid by salivating. However, evaporation from the tongue does not seem to be the primary mechanism to dissipate heat. The normal rate of breathing for a dog at rest is between about 15 and 30 breaths per minute, but during panting that rate can reach 300 per minute or more! Although this is a good way of cooling the body, panting is not very efficient for respiratory function. If you watch a dog in hot weather, you will notice they slobber quite a lot and every few seconds they'll take a proper deep breath. Dogs asleep in the sun don't pant but often breathe much faster than under normal circumstances.

Dogs that have been bred to have very short flat faces, technically known as brachycephalics ('brachy' = short, 'cephalic' = head), have extremely deformed nasal chambers that hardly function at all in thermoregulation. Their upper teeth are also crowded, and their eyes are so prominent that the tear film on the surface of the eye quickly dries out. This means that they are extremely prone to dental disease, conjunctivitis and ulcers of the eyes, which are always painful and frequently cause the eye to rupture completely. They may be very fashionable and look cute, but many of these poor dogs are really profoundly disabled. Their lives are often miserable. The airway obstruction tends to worsen over the years but even young brachycephalic dogs frequently are unable to exercise properly. Recent research shows their sleep patterns are chronically disturbed. Their lives can be an awful struggle, especially in warm weather. Please think very carefully if you really want one of these dogs. If you bought one you would be passively fuelling this suffering. In a later section, I will provide advice about how to manage brachycephalic dogs to try to minimise their problems and what to do in an emergency if they get into serious difficulties with breathing (see page ...).

I wish you could meet Merlin. He's a very wiggly, wriggly, silver grey, French Bulldog, who is extremely pleased to see everyone and loves visits to the vet. My colleague Mike once described a clinical examination he tried to accomplish with Merlin; 'It was like trying to capture a splendid crazy salmon . . .'

I first met Merlin, who is now four, a few months ago, when he was brought in for a persistent cough which had been present for months, day and night. Merlin's breathing was noisy; deep, throaty and bubbling. His family described how he found exercise very tiring and often had to give up when he tried to run about or play. This had gone on for years but it was getting worse. He was in good body condition with normal heart rate and rhythm and a normal body temperature. His lungs and heart seemed heathy. The noises seemed to arise from his throat. These signs and his body shape suggested upper respiratory obstruction. We decided to anaesthetise Merlin, radiograph his head, neck and chest, and explore the possibility of airway surgery. Our fears were confirmed.

Mike, is a particularly accurate, talented and highly qualified surgeon. He performed a series of reconstructive procedures to shorten the soft palate, and reduce the obstructions in the airway. We kept Merlin in for a couple of nights afterwards because after surgery of this sort the tissues in the throat swell, which can exacerbate the problem in the short term. Drugs to reduce the tissue swelling were given for a few days.

Two months on, Merlin is doing splendidly, jumping around, able to run about and barking for the first time in his life.

There are many health problems in dogs that are particularly found in pure-bred dogs; for instance, German Shepherds often have a hip disease known as dysplasia, Dachshunds very often develop back problems, Dalmatians suffer from a condition of the kidneys that predisposes them to bladder stones. Many Dalmatians are also congenitally deaf. Flat-Coat Retrievers are extremely prone to cancer. Greyhounds very commonly are plagued by dental disease. Labradors, Retrievers and 'Westies' often have an allergic skin disease known as atopy, Staffordshire Bull Terriers too frequently develop skin problems, in their case usually due to a parasitic mite, Demodex. But these are just a handful of examples. I could reel off many more. Every known genetic disease can be found in mongrel dogs but occurrences of any one condition are rather rare. On the contrary it has been estimated that one in four purebred dogs are afflicted by genetic disease.

For some breeds of dog, genetic tests and other screening procedures are available to help breeders and purchasers reduce the risks of some of the worst of these diseases. If you decide to buy a pedigree dog you should do some research to find out if that breed has known health problems and to learn if any testing schemes exist (visit www.dogbreedhealth.com). The Kennel Club in the UK runs some Assured Breeders Schemes that can help you to find breeders who are doing their best to avoid inherited disease in their breed.

My own particular specialist interest is veterinary cardiology. There are a few breeds of dog in which death from heart disease is extremely common; particularly Cavalier King Charles Spaniels, Irish Wolfhounds, Boxers, Great Danes and Doberman Pinschers. Most of these dogs appear physically well at least until middle-age, but a very large proportion, perhaps half of them, or more, will die prematurely because of their heart. Unfortunately, there are as yet no genetic tests to identify dogs or bitches from these breeds who are likely to give birth to offspring who will develop heart failure. Some breeders and many vets are trying to find solutions, and there are tests that help to recognise the problems early in their course, but there are no definitive genetic tests presently. I know many people who love these dogs, but every time I meet or hear of another person who has one my heart sinks. Some of these dogs have wonderful characters and I do appreciate that many people develop a deep loyalty to a particular breed of dog despite the problems they have. But why would you deliberately choose a dog who is very probably going to suffer from such a debilitating problem? Think of their welfare. Think of the anxiety you would suffer. Think of the vet bills you might have to pay, or the awful heartache it you cannot afford to treat them.

When choosing a dog some personal criteria will help you to narrow your choice; size, temperament, exercise needs and ability, coat type, grooming requirements, cost of acquisition, feeding costs, known health problems in the breed etc., as well as obvious issues such as appearance and personal familiarity to the breed or circumstances of breeding. If you are undecided about the sort of dog to choose, talk to your vet and to other people who are highly experienced with dogs, such as veterinary nurses, behaviouralists, dog trainers and handlers.

If you decide to acquire a crossbreed (a mongrel) you should still look carefully at their conformation to avoid those who seem most likely to have health problems. Look out for extremely large or extremely small dogs – both are prone to health problems. Avoid dogs who have very short and distorted legs, or very long backs, because these conformations too can lead to problems. Other conformations to be wary of would be those with very flattened faces, bulging eyes, droopy eyelids or very folded skin. If in any doubt, ask a vet to examine the pup or dog before you buy.

SUMMARY

After some research, you should have a clear idea of the breed or type of dog you want, having thought carefully about the practical issues dog ownership entails. Below, I have highlighted a few key questions you ought to consider.

- Are you able to bear the cost of owning a dog?

- Are all members of the household comfortable with dogs?

- Who will be the prime carer for the dog?

- Do you have the necessary time to care for a puppy in the early weeks and in the longer term?

- Might an adult dog be preferable?

- Where will the dog sleep?

- Is there space in a quiet place in the house for a basket or crate for the dog?

- Who will walk the dog?

- Where will the dog go during the day; is there someone who will be at home most of the day, or could the dog go to work with you or another member of the household?

- Will you need to employ a 'dog-walking' service to take the dog out during the day?

- What will you do during holidays; will the dog go with you, or be kennelled, or can you make other arrangements?

- Have you considered all the costs involved in owning a dog above and beyond the purchase price: food, insurance, veterinary care, miscellaneous items such as bedding, leads, collars, toys and possibly kennelling, or the cost of a dog sitting/walking service?

FINDING YOUR DOG

Searching for a puppy to buy, used to begin by looking at adverts in shop windows or in the small ads columns, or by word of mouth, but nowadays people immediately turn to the internet. This is a mixed blessing, because, although there are many, many pups advertised on the net, many from perfectly legitimate businesses or small breeders, puppy farms and crooks who have illegally imported dogs into the country from abroad can be very clever in disguising the seedy and nefarious side of their business from the general public. If you use the internet to search for a puppy, be savvy. Do not buy a puppy online without visiting the breeder; if you do so you are very likely to have bought a pup from a puppy farm. Puppy farms are awful for animal welfare and the puppies often never recover from that experience.

There are two main sources of dogs: direct from a breeder or from a rehoming service, such as the RSPCA, Battersea Dogs and Cats Home, The Dog's Trust or one of many other charities, such as Greyhound Rescue. Puppies are not frequently available from rehoming services, although you might be lucky, so if you are set on getting a puppy, expect to buy it from a breeder. Pedigree dogs registered at the Kennel Club will, in general, cost a good deal more than crossbreeds. Although, having said that, many 'designer' crossbreeds, such as 'Labradoodles' and 'Cockapoos', seem to command very high prices and there are a plethora of neologisms being coined for crossbreeds that seem designed to enable the breeders to charge more than if they were simply called mongrels. I repeat, you should not buy a puppy from a puppy farm where multiple litters of dogs from several breeds are being bred. These puppies tend to be poorly socialised and are often bred in conditions of very poor welfare. They also frequently are heavily parasitised and are unthrifty. Puppy farm owners can be very crafty to hide the fact that they are puppy farmers; for instance, they might suggest they bring a puppy directly to your home, or that you meet in a motorway service station or supermarket car park to get the puppy. If you are made an offer like this, turn it down flat. In Europe, there is a growing form of organised crime involving the breeding of pedigree and 'designer crossbreed' dogs created to fuel the market in the UK for fashionable pups. Puppy farms on the continent exist where the laws on animal welfare are lax and where large numbers of puppies are being bred in very poor conditions. The pups are sometimes weaned very early. They may be given a rabies vaccine, or vaccination certificates might be forged, then shipped legally to the UK, or they could be smuggled into the country under-age with fraudulent papers. These puppies are then sold as if they were UK born and bred. Genuine breeders, be they amateurs breeding crossbreeds, professionals breeding pedigree dogs, or somewhere in between, will expect you to visit their home to see the bitch and the conditions the pups have been bred in. You should expect them to ask you questions so that they can be sure you will provide a good home to their pup, and they will expect you to do so too. It is always a good idea to prepare yourself to interview the breeder by writing down the questions you have before you telephone them. Regular breeders will expect to be phoned about a litter by potential customers even before the puppies are born. It is a good idea at this point to find out if the puppy will be Kennel Club registered. If so, you should ask if the breeder is a member of an Assured Breeders Scheme and also establish if the parents have had any relevant health checks or blood tests before breeding and what the results were. A very good idea is to ask about, and use, the Puppy Contract, which was devised by the RSPCA and The Animal Welfare Foundation as a basis for the safe purchase of puppies from breeders (see http:// bit.ly/PuppyContract).

There are strict and clear laws in the UK concerning dog breeding and welfare, although they do differ slightly between Scotland, England, Wales and Northern Ireland. Breeders who breed more than a small number of litters every year must be licensed by the local authority. Licensed breeders should show you a copy of their licence, or at least give you their licence number. Breeders are only allowed to sell pups they have bred themselves and this must be from the place the pup was born and reared. Pups should be at least 8 weeks old before being sold and should be weaned. Customers must be able to see the pups with their mother (the dam). Ideally, you should see the male dog who sired the puppies too, but this is not always possible. The dam should be an adult dog, no more than six years of age. She should appear well, although she might be a bit gaunt looking having fed a litter of puppies for several weeks. She is likely to have large pendulous mammary glands. If she does not, be suspicious, because she might not be the dam to the litter. A bitch who is, or recently has been, nursing a litter might seem a little wary of you and defensive of her puppies, but she should give the appearance of being happy and very well acquainted with the breeder.

The puppies themselves should be alert and look well without coughing, sneezing or signs of diarrhoea. Eyes and ears should be clean. Their coats should have a good lustre and the skin be clean. Most puppies aged around 6–10 weeks spend their time in one of two states; either asleep, or awake and playing. Pups generally should be bold and curious about you. If they yap or bark excessively, they may not have had much experience of outsiders. If the puppies roll around playing with each other in your presence this suggests they are used to other people and used to family life. Puppies of this age play principally by wrestling and biting / mouthing each other. There might be some growling and yelping. You should not interpret this behaviour as evidence of aggression in the pups; it is normal. Licensed breeders should be able to show you a socialisation plan for the puppies, meaning that they have been gradually introduced to a range of people and experiences. All puppies sold must have been microchipped already and the microchip should have been registered in the name of the breeder. If you purchase a puppy, the chip must be re-registered to you after purchase. This is simply achieved via the internet. Your vet practice can help.

It is a really good idea to see the puppies more than once before buying. If you feel the breeder is pressurising you into buying a pup at the first visit, be very wary. There are a few things you must definitely establish before taking the pup home. What have the puppies been eating since weaning and how many meals have they been getting? Virtually all breeders will provide you with some of this diet for the first few days after going home. Many will also give you detailed long-term diet advice, but that should be taken with a pinch of salt. Your vet has been trained in animal nutrition and will be much better placed to give this advice. Have the puppies been wormed (they should have been), if so what with, and how frequently should this be repeated? Have the puppies had any vaccinations (most pups will have their first vaccines between about 6–9 weeks – see later)? Have the pups been examined by a vet? It is important that the pup is examined by your own vet soon after acquisition, even if this has been done already. A good breeder should offer to take the dog back if there are any problems. Some breeders will provide you with temporary free insurance for the pup for the first four weeks from the Kennel Club, or another source.

Adopting an adult dog from a rehoming centre

Before deciding to get a 'rescue' dog from a rehoming charity, you need to think just as carefully as you would before buying a pup. Rescue dogs are generally housetrained but for many reasons they are still likely to need a good deal of time and attention in the settling-in period. Remember, these dogs may have been surrendered to the rescue centre for behavioural reasons, so you must find this out and establish if your home will suit that dog. The staff in these centres are usually very well appraised of these issues and will be happy to guide you.

When you adopt a dog through a rehoming centre, you will normally follow a protocol designed to match you to a dog that seems appropriate. Most dogs re-homed in this way are adults that have been stray street dogs, or have been relinquished because of a change in circumstances of their owners or because of a bereavement. Sometimes dogs are forfeited because owners in rented accommodation are not permitted to keep a pet (the law on this is changing[1]). Sometimes the original owner's job has changed. Frequently, the owners have been unable to care for them, for some other reason. In many cases the dogs present some behavioural problems. Some of the dogs have difficult phobias or other particular issues associated with their past, but many just need to find a

---

[1] Under the new Model Tenancy Agreement, landlords will no longer be able to issue blanket bans on pets. Instead, consent for pets will be the default position, and landlords will have to object in writing within 28 days of a written pet request from a tenant and provide a good reason. Currently, just 7% of private landlords advertise pet friendly properties, meaning many people struggle to find suitable homes. In some cases, this has meant people have had to give up their pets altogether.

home which is suitable to their temperament and circumstances. The staff at the re-homing facility will have usually carefully assessed each dog to determine their nature and decide what sort of home should suit the dog. When you visit the centre (online or in person) and pick out a dog you'd like to keep, you will not be allowed to take it away at that time. Usually, you will have to fill out a detailed form about your lifestyle and circumstances and then a member of staff will visit your home to check it out. Some centres have very strict criteria about who they feel are appropriate to adopt one of their dogs; for instance, some will not re-home with families who have young children, or to homes where the dog is likely to be left alone for more than an hour or two at a time. Greyhound rescue usually will refuse to re-home to a house with a cat (this is a sensible measure because most greyhounds consider cats to be fair prey and indeed it is not unusual for cats to be killed by greyhounds). These criteria can seem onerous, petty and unnecessary, but the charities who make these stipulations feel they are necessary to avoid a dog serially failing to fit in to one home after another. If you already own a pet, or pets, they might suggest you bring them with you to visit the candidate pooch at the rehoming centre.

Generally, the process to re-home a dog through these charities takes a week or two to complete. On receipt of the dog, they will provide you with up-to-date vaccination records. The dog will usually have been neutered and microchipped too. There will be a fee to adopt the dog, which will go some way to covering the costs of these procedures, around £200–£300. Most dogs are re-homed on the condition that you attend training with the dog. The centre will usually provide post-adoption support and often they will visit you a couple of times in the weeks after the dog has been adopted to make sure things are going well.

(See https://www.rspca.org.uk/findapet/rehomeapet/process/rehomeadog)

Adopting a dog from abroad

Clients sometimes proudly announce to me that their dog has been 'rescued' from overseas (most commonly Spain, Greece, Cyprus or Eastern Europe). They are, I know, quite disappointed when they see my reaction. Some clients have become very aware of the potential risks in the UK of acquiring a dog from a puppy farm, or are put-off by rehoming centres that rarely have puppies available, and sometimes seem to put up barriers that may make it difficult to adopt an adult dog. These are the clients who often decide to import a dog from overseas. I have no fundamental objection to refugee dogs and if, whilst someone is on holiday or working in Europe, they befriend a stray dog, then it is quite understandable that they might wish to bring that dog back to the UK. There are many UK charities that also promote the concept of rescuing dogs from abroad. They will facilitate this for you, for a fee. Unfortunately, however, whilst the law has made it comparatively simple to import a dog, provided that it has been vaccinated against rabies and treated with a drug to prevent a particularly nasty tapeworm that we don't currently have in the UK (*Echinococcus*), that does not mean importation is without considerable risk.

STOP PRESS: *Brucella canis*

Brucella canis is a bacterial disease of the dog that has been absent from the UK until very recently. According to the Animal and Plant Health Agency only three cases of the condition were diagnosed before 2020 but in the 6 months to June 2023 97 cases were diagnosed. All cases identified so far have been in imported dogs, puppies from infected dogs or in dogs mated with those carrying the infection. The disease is important because it is a zoonosis, meaning that can sometimes be transmitted from dogs to humans, especially children, the very elderly and those who are immuno-compromised (such as those being treated for cancer). Laboratory staff are at risk from this disease. Veterinary laboratories have become very wary of handling blood and tissue samples from all imported dogs because of it. The disease is difficult to recognise and to treat, both in people and in dogs. The bacteria itself lives as a parasite within the cells of the host dog (or person) which means it is a very challenging infection to eradicate. The advice from the government is that infected dogs should usually not be treated but should be put to sleep by euthanasia. Anyone who is planning to import a dog from abroad, especially from Eastern Europe, should have it tested for this disease before importation.

Firstly, we know, from experience that many dogs are imported with false documents. Some are brought into the country much younger than the rules allow; customs officials are not trained in the nuances of assessing the age of puppies. In Europe, there are many endemic parasites and vector-borne diseases that are presently absent from the UK; for example, Leishmaniasis, heart-worm, Babesiosis and Ehrlichiosis. It is, of course, possible to test a dog before it is imported to the UK, but no test is perfect, so some cases might slip through. Also, unless you know precisely what to look for, and how, these conditions will be missed. Some of these conditions can remain dormant for long periods; for example, a dog carrying the protozoa *Leishmania infantum* (which is transmitted by biting sand-flies) or *Ehrlichia canis* (an intracellular bacterium) might not become ill at all for years. If and when it does, the cause may be missed by veterinarians in the UK unfamiliar with these problems. For these reasons, these imported 'Rescue' animals have been christened 'Trojan dogs',

Sweet Pea, a cross breed neutered bitch aged about six, was referred to me from another veterinary practice. She had always been a rather quiet dog but in the preceding 10 days she had become dull, listless and lethargic. She was coughing and her breathing was fast. She was not running a fever. My colleagues at the other practice had noticed signs of anaemia, a fast heart and an obvious heart murmur, which was why they chose to send her to me. Some tests they had done showed that although the white blood cell count was a bit depressed there was an elevated proportion of immature inflammatory cells, as well as an unusual protein picture called hyperglobulinaemia. These findings suggested she had a severe inflammatory process which made us all worried she could have endocarditis (an infection in the heart itself, which is extremely difficult to cure).

Sweet Pea was hospitalised and started on supportive treatment including intravenous fluids and antibiotics. An ultrasound study of her heart did show some abnormalities, which explained the heart murmur, but these were not serious. Ultrasound imaging of the abdomen showed up nothing untoward. Chest radiographs were normal.

Over the following week, Sweet Pea improved a bit, but the blood count showed persistent anaemia whilst the protein abnormalities worsened. These proteins were subject to further testing by a process called electrophoresis – they showed a signature typical of a long-standing ('chronic') inflammatory process. The pathologist wondered if she might have Leishmaniasis, a disease that is rare in the UK but found in Southern Europe.

I phoned the owner to talk this over. It was only then that I discovered Sweet Pea had been imported from Romania four years previously. We sent samples to a specialist laboratory who discovered she did not have Leishmaniasis but she did have Ehrlichiosis – a bacterial infection transmitted by a parasite, the Brown Dog Tick, which (until recently) was absent from the UK. Sweet Pea was treated with a prolonged course of the appropriate antibiotic, Doxycycline. She recovered completely.

PREPARING FOR A NEW DOG OR PUPPY

> It's a complete change of lifestyle, like having a new baby, and nothing really prepares you for this. (New dog owner)

If you keep a dog as a pet, you have legal responsibilities governed by The Animal Welfare Act (2006) that states that you must provide a suitable environment and diet for your dog. You should allow your dog to exhibit normal behaviours but should also train it to be a well-adjusted member of the community. Your pet should have reasonable contact with people and other dogs for play and companionship. You must also protect that dog from pain, suffering, injury and disease (see 'Plant and Animal Health' section at www.gov.uk: DEFRA Code of Practice for the Welfare of Dogs, 2017).

In the days before your new dog or puppy comes to live with you, you should prepare yourself and him / her for the move. It can be useful to find an old blanket you are happy to forsake, or perhaps wear an old jumper close to your skin for a few hours, then leave it with the youngster to sleep on. This will help familiarise her / him to your smell. The cloth will also pick up scent from the pup's own bedding and housemates. When you bring the pup home with you bring that now scruffy old rag too for the puppy to cosy up with; it ought to comfort the young dog for the first days in a new home.

You will need some equipment: bowls for food and water, bedding and a basket or perhaps a crate that will become the dog's new safe place. The dog will need a lead and collar, or harness, with a tag labelled with your address and phone number (this is a legal requirement in addition to the microchip that all dogs aged 8 weeks or more must have). Obviously, if you are getting a pup they will grow, so it would be sensible to avoid paying a fortune for a harness or collar that might only fit for a month. Dog toys are essential, especially for puppies and young dogs, but choose these carefully – ideally, they should be rugged and more or less indestructible. Big dogs will be able to destroy items which small puppies cannot. Puppies and young dogs love to chew. They need to do so for dental health as well as amusement. Certainly, you do not want the dog to swallow pieces of rubber, fabric or other material because such foreign bodies in the gut might cause an obstruction or perforate the intestine leading to emergency surgery. A range of toys may be necessary, such as robust cuddly toys, balls, hanks of rope to tug, rubberised gnaw-able items, antler toys, etc. It is very unwise to give the dog shoes or socks to play with because once they have understood these are toys all similar objects in the home will be considered to be fair game.

Think about where in your home you want the dog to sleep at night and rest during the day. It is much easier to establish good habits if bad habits are avoided. Many people are delighted to have puppies on the furniture, in the bedroom, or in the bed, but you need to think very carefully about that because if you allow this when they first arrive it might be impossible to ever revoke that concession. Remember if the dog is going to be big it might take up a lot of room on the furniture that people need to use.

Dog crates are controversial, in my family at least. I know some people consider them to be dog prisons. If you decide to use a crate it must be really comfortable and big enough to allow the dog to turn around easily. Put it in a draught-free place where the dog can be left undisturbed. It is very likely your dog will soon decide this is their own special place and grow to love it, but I can't promise this.

Look around your home and try to put yourself in the mind of a dog. Dogs are naturally curious. Where are the hazards? Is there an open fireplace? Are there steep stairs? Could a puppy fall through the bannisters? Might a stair-guard be an option? Is there a pedal bin in the kitchen where vegetable waste is discarded? Is there a waste-paper bin in the lounge? Are there floor level bookcases or food cupboards that a dog could access? Are chemicals, or drugs, plants, or foods accessible which might be poisonous? If so, store them somewhere safe. Are there loose flexes or electrical cables which a dog could chew? You must find a way to put them out of reach. Could the dog get on the dining table or other furniture? Could she fall off a balcony? Is there a tempting and accessible fish tank or a hamster in a cage? Finally, is there anything really precious that the dog could get hold of, be it a silk scarf or a hand-knotted Indian rug? Remove it. Put it out of reach.

What do we understand of cognition in puppies and dogs? It is difficult to get inside the mind of a dog because they are a different species to us. Their perceptions of the world are bound to differ because their sensory apparatus is so different to ours. Furthermore, the brain of a dog is certainly very different to the human brain. Having said that, there has been a lot of research in the past few decades that has helped us understand some important aspects of how puppies learn and mature. In the first couple of weeks of life a pup is blind and deaf. Their perception of the world around them is principally through touch and smell. Life revolves around feeding, sleeping and growing. Puppies don't even pass urine or faeces except after being stimulated to do so by the dam grooming them. However, by about three weeks of age a puppy will be able to see and hear and will be much more co-ordinated, with rapidly developing motor skills. Play with siblings starts to become important and increasingly boisterous. For the next several weeks, the pup will explore the world with little sense of fear. This is the period when socialisation is critical as they begin to learn about being a dog, interacting with siblings and the people around. This is a great period to introduce puppies to novel experiences. Puppies should be frequently but gently handled for short periods, and introduced to a wide range of people, sights, smells, textures and sounds. The prime time for socialising a puppy actually occurs in the period before they leave their original home because by the time they are 6 or 7 weeks old or more they have begun to become suspicious or even fearful of novelty. This means that the move to a new home and family, at eight weeks or so, can be initially quite distressing for the youngster. In order to minimise distress and smooth the transition to a new life, provide the pup with familiar food, warm surroundings, gentle loving care and, if possible, with something familiar to smell and lie on.

The next few weeks are critical for the puppy in their cognitive and psychological development. Between eight and perhaps 12–16 weeks of age is the critical period during which you can ensure your puppy learns to be a relaxed, amiable, well-behaved citizen. To do this you must be consistent about what behaviours you encourage and discourage. You should also continue to introduce the puppy to new experiences, but in a way that allows them to approach and investigate anything novel at their own pace. Never force the pup to confront something which frightens them. You will only heighten their fear. If, on the other hand, you yourself show the pup that this novelty causes you no anxiety and give them the opportunity to explore each new thing at their own leisure, you will encourage them to become bold and relaxed in the world.

This is not a book about puppy training or canine behaviour. These are not my areas of genuine expertise and there are many excellent texts and websites devoted to such issues, a few of which I have highlighted in the Bibliography and

References later in the book. However, I must now briefly touch on a misunderstanding that has arisen between dog owners and vets for which I believe we vets are responsible. Should puppies be kept in quarantine from all other dogs until a week or more after completing their primary vaccination? The answer I believe is definitely no.

All life engenders risk. There is a genuine risk that a puppy, before being vaccinated and developing immunity to parvovirus, adenovirus, or distemper, might encounter one of these viruses, become infected and die. In the past this risk was much higher than now because these diseases were once much more widespread. As a result, vets have tended to be dogmatic in emphasising the risk. That dogma is no longer appropriate (unless there is a known outbreak of one of these problems in a particular locale). We can minimise that risk by simple strategies. There is another and much greater risk; that a puppy who is wrapped in cotton wool, carried everywhere, isolated from fellow dogs, and who fails to be socialised properly in the first four months of life, grows up to be anxious, fearful and aggressive. Many more dogs fall into this latter category and a high proportion of dogs who are not well socialised go on to have long-standing behaviour problems. Some will be relinquished, or even euthanised, as a result. It is really difficult to manage dogs with behaviour problems caused by lack of socialisation because dogs who have learned to fear interactions with unfamiliar people, novel situations or other dogs find it very hard to 'unlearn' these fears. It follows that we must ensure that all young puppies do get every chance to experience the hustle and bustle of the world, to socialise with people and other dogs throughout that early period in their new home environment, whilst at the same time trying to minimise the risk that they become exposed to contagious disease.

How can we do that?

Most people who acquire a pup have friends, neighbours or family nearby who own a dog (or two). Provided those dogs are already vaccinated and appear healthy they should not pose a significant risk to the pup. Clients should be encouraged to allow their new puppy to meet such dogs in their own home. The encounters often begin nervously and falteringly but usually soon result in mutual fun. Most gardens will not be frequented by roaming dogs or foxes. These too are safe places to exercise the puppy and to allow her to interact with her new friends. Many veterinary practices also hold puppy parties, where they invite pups to meet others of a similar age to interact and play at a time when the practice is otherwise relatively quiet. At first, these events are sometimes a little stressful for a new pup but they can be great fun, especially if they attend regularly over a period of a few weeks. Your principal aim from this process should be that your puppy has fun, becomes confident and delighted to meet other dogs.

Until the pup is 11 or 12 weeks of age it might be unwise for him to walk the streets where other dogs have been because some of those dogs will not have been vaccinated and a few might have been ill. Some vets will advise that puppies have a final vaccination between 12–16 weeks of age because a proportion of puppies (especially of certain breeds) do not show adequate vaccine responses until then. However, whilst this cautious approach is laudable from the immuno-logical perspective, I believe all puppies of 12 weeks and above should be out and about meeting strangers of all species and learning to walk the streets, parks, fields and woods of their home-range. In the same way that we allow our kids to interact with other people and range widely before they are fully vaccinated, I believe we should allow our puppies to do the same (this issue will be touched on again in Chapter 4).

USEFUL INFORMATION WHEN CHOOSING AND BUYING A DOG

Blue Cross: Choosing a dog https://www.bluecross.org.uk/pet-advice/choosing-right-dog

DEFRA Code of Practice for the Welfare of Dogs: https://www.gov.uk/government/publications/code-of-practice-for-the-welfare-of-dogs

Dogs Trust: Buying a dog or puppy https://www.dogstrust.org.uk/help-advice/buyer-advice/

Dogs Trust: Socialisation https://www.dogstrust.org.uk/help-advice/dog-behaviour-health/sound-therapy-for-pets

RSPCA: Buying a puppy https://www.rspca.org.uk/adviceandwelfare/pets/dogs/puppy

RSPCA: Puppy contract https://www.rspca.org.uk/webcontent/staticImages/microsites/PuppyContract/Downloads/PuppyContracctDownload.pdf

3

HOW TO CHOOSE YOUR VET

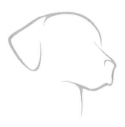

Close proximity to your home should not be the main factor influencing you when you choose your vet.

The usual criteria that people apply to their choice of vet is simple: they choose the practice that is closest to their home, or that is otherwise highly convenient. It's an odd, almost random way to make a decision that might have life or death consequences.

Vets in the UK are closely governed by the Royal College of Veterinary Surgeons (RCVS) and have all reached a high level of clinical competence before they can be registered, but just like doctors, dentists, hairdressers, carpenters and electricians, vets do vary widely in their abilities, skills, knowledge, post-graduate training, experience, empathy, communication skills and prowess. In a recent survey of the profession carried out to look at job satisfaction, many vets said they actually didn't like clients! (see *Veterinary Times* 49(40), 7 October 2019). I wouldn't choose a doctor who didn't like people.

Veterinary surgeons used to be generalists, rather like the Yorkshire vet James Herriot made famous through his novels, TV series and films. They would work with farm animals, horses, dogs, cats, budgies and rabbits. Such general 'mixed' practitioners are now rather rare, especially in towns and cities, where most vets limit themselves to the care of only a few 'companion animal' or 'small animal' species. For the most part, similar to human medicine, routine small animal veterinary practice involves vets who are species specialists, often with particular skills and expertise, who frequently work in collaboration with colleagues in a collegiate atmosphere.

If you are looking for a vet for your dog it is probably best to search for a clutch of dedicated small animal ('companion animal') practices within relatively easy travelling distance of your home. Word of mouth recommendations from friends, colleagues and acquaintances are an excellent starting point to choose a practice; but it is worth drilling down with those sources to understand what it is that they like, or dislike, a practice for, because your needs and preferences may differ from theirs. Most practices will boast websites and social media pages that advertise their services, but you will probably find these are not a particularly useful tool to enable you to discriminate between practices. Often, they may highlight a few well-chosen positive reviews but these reviews may not always be representative. Search engines may uncover other reviews from clients but all these anecdotal reports should probably be taken with a pinch of salt, unless the reviews are very consistent. Most practices will be happy to discuss their fees for routine procedures such as appointments, vaccinations and neutering, which should allow you to make cost comparisons. On the other hand, within a local area these fees are likely to be very similar and many practices run loyalty schemes that can bring down the costs considerably. It would be unwise to choose a practice based on price alone, unless your budget is especially tight. So how else can you proceed?

Importantly, at present, there is no mandatory universal regulation of veterinary practices, (this is likely to change in the foreseeable future) but the RCVS run a very demanding and unbiased practice registration and accreditation scheme, known as the **Practice Standards Scheme (PSS)**. The PSS classifies practices on the basis of their services, expertise, standards of competence and the qualifications of their staff. The most basic level of practice is designated a **Core Standards** practice, the intermediate level is designated as **General Practice**, whereas the highest level of practice is a **Veterinary Hospital**. Over and above this, practices that take part in the scheme can compete for additional awards to demonstrate where they offer excellent standards in six domains:

- team and professional responsibility

- client service

- patient consultation service

- inpatient service

- diagnostic service

- emergency and critical care service.

Under these headings, the best practices are rated as 'Good' or 'Outstanding', in much the same way that schools are rated by Ofsted. The Practice Standards Scheme is voluntary, but well over half of the small animal / companion animal practices in the UK participate. (See https://findavet.rcvs.org.uk)

Once you have a shortlist of practices that you are seriously considering using, it can be useful to ring up to speak to a receptionist or better still to visit the practice(s) to meet staff. This ought to give you a taste of the ethos of the practice. Look for clean, well-presented premises and friendly, helpful, welcoming staff who are willing and able to answer your questions. It is worth knowing that many veterinary surgeons have post-graduate qualifications, such as Certificates of Advanced Veterinary Practice or Diplomas issued by the RCVS, or the European Colleges of Veterinary Internal Medicine or Surgery, which show that they have reached an advanced stage of training and expertise in a particular domain. Similarly, veterinary nurses may have particular skills, qualifications and experience. If a practice has one or several vets and nurses who have reached these advanced standards, it tends to imply that the practice is a good one. Staff turnover is also worth drilling into. Just ask if the vets and nurses have been there for a long time. When a practice has a very stable staffing, that implies it is well managed and the employees are happy, which, in turn, suggests the clinical care should be good. When staff turnover is high, that is generally a bad sign.

Once you've found the practice, you'll want to find the right vets for you in that practice. This must often be a case for trial and error, but it's certainly worth trying to get some steer from the receptionists, nurses and other clients of the practice. Different people will want different things from their vet. Some will want the seasoned old guy who has a wealth of anecdotes to entertain and put clients at ease. Others will want the smart but serious young woman who has a certificate in soft tissue surgery. Be choosy but be open-minded. Ask questions. Also, know that many vets have strengths and weaknesses; for instance, very good with eye cases but not so adept with lameness. It's not always possible to see the same vet every visit (we do get booked up, have time off and occasional holidays). In time you will find one or two who you feel suit you best. Both you and the vet will feel most at ease when a bond of trust has developed. Receptionists are used to clients asking for a particular vet.

A NOTE ON VETERINARY SPECIALISTS

Some vets specialise in a limited field from an early stage in their career, and many of these go on to work in specialist referral hospital practices working at the 'cutting edge' where the facilities are extraordinary (and the costs involved can be 'eye-watering'). These specialists are typically dealing with a limited range of problems in a small number of animals, which invariably are cases referred to them from colleagues in general small animal practices. At present, there is no objective disinterested scheme that classifies these specialised referral veterinary hospitals but there are moves to create a further tier within the RCVS Practice Standards Scheme to address this issue.

4

YOUR FIRST TRIPS TO THE VET

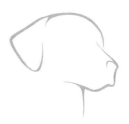

This chapter will deal with your first visits to see a vet with your new puppy or re-homed dog. It will include a bit of basic biology, some insights into canine behaviour, and lots of practical advice about toilet training, socialisation, vaccination, parasite control, puppy diet, insurance, exercise and neutering.

We begin with a short tutorial in some basic biology and some pertinent aspects of canine behaviour. I hope that most people not intimately familiar with biology or medicine will find this section useful, interesting and informative, but I have no wish to patronise you dear reader. If you find the following sections, or parts of this chapter, simplistic and unhelpful please move on.

INFECTIONS AND INFESTATIONS: THE BASICS

In the past, most domestic animals spent most of their lives blighted to a greater or lesser extent by a cocktail of infections and infestations. Thanks to modern medicine many of these ailments are now less common because they can be prevented or treated using a variety of different approaches. So, what are these infections and infestations?

Bacteria

Bacteria are small (usually single celled) living organisms that are ubiquitous on earth. Bacteria have had a bad press. Many people call them 'germs' and believe they are evil. This is a mistake. Most bacteria live in harmony with animals and man and many of these are present as harmless or helpful residents on our skin, in our mouths, in our guts and elsewhere. Millions of different bacteria of many different species are present in and on every person and every pet; different species colonise different animals and different zones of the body and there is a complex web of interactions between these resident bacteria. These bacteria are known as commensals and symbionts. For the most part, these resident microflorae are best left undisturbed, because if the balance within them is disrupted this can led to disease. A small fraction of bacterial species can cause disease. These are known as bacterial pathogens. Bacterial diseases often arise because a species that lives as a commensal in one part of the body has managed to colonise a part of the body from which it is usually excluded; think for instance of a bite wound when bacteria from the mouth of the aggressor enter the victim's soft tissues under the skin, or because a species of bacteria that can live as a commensal in, or on, one mammalian species has managed to colonise another species (e.g. see Leptospirosis later on). A few bacteria cause contagious disease that can be transmitted from dog to dog, or even from dogs to people (these latter bacterial infections are known as zoonoses). Bacterial infections are often treated with antibiotics (see later). Antiseptics differ from antibiotics; they are chemicals used to kill bacteria outside the body, for instance, alcohol hand wipes are antiseptics.

Viruses

Viruses are very different to bacteria. Viruses are much smaller and much simpler than bacteria; most viruses consist only of genetic code, in the form of DNA or RNA, together with a surface coat formed of proteins. Some viruses (like SARS-CoV-2, the cause of Covid-19) also have a lipid envelope. In the words of the Noble Prize winning scientist Sir Peter Medawar: 'Viruses are just bad news wrapped-up in protein. . .'. Viruses are not quite living organisms but are a form of minute parasite. Viruses can enter and subjugate the cells of the living organism, highjacking the cellular machinery to replicate vast numbers of daughter virus particles. Often the highjacked cell is killed in the process. Some viruses, such as the Rabies or Distemper viruses, can cause disease in a wide range of different animal species, whereas other viruses are only pathogenic to one or a few closely related species, such as canine parvovirus or human HIV virus. Viruses cannot be killed by antibiotics, so antibiotics are of no use in treating viral diseases.

However, many antiseptics and soaps used in the environment are effective at neutralising viruses, which is why hand-sanitising or washing has been so central to managing the Covid-19 pandemic.

There are some antiviral drugs but these are relatively few and are appropriate therapy only for a small number of particular problems. New antiviral drugs are becoming available in the wake of Covid. It is likely some of these will be useful in dogs, in time.

Fungi and yeasts

These are another class of living organism that used to be thought of as plants. They are not. Mushrooms and toadstools are the fruiting bodies of certain species of fungi; these are the fungi most familiar to us, but there are many species of fungi of which we are mostly unaware. In nature, the primary job of the fungi is to replenish and enrich the soil by recycling dead plants back into nutrients. As humans, we use some fungi widely in cooking and food preservation. Here, I am talking about yeasts, unicellular fungi that we use to make beer, wine, leavened bread, vinegar, cider and other pickled foodstuffs.

A few fungi and yeasts are found living in niches on healthy dogs, such as Malassezia that live on the skin, especially on the footpads and in the ear canals. Malassezia is generally not a pathogen, but occasionally becomes pathogenic, if the skin environment changes. I will discuss this organism in more detail later when I tackle diseases of the skin and the ear.

Parasites

Few issues in veterinary medicine raise the emotional temperature more than the subject of parasites. Parasites are organisms that live on, or in, other organisms (the host) and that get their food from, or at the expense of, this host. The term is generally reserved for multicellular creatures, 'creepy crawlies' such as roundworms, tapeworms, fleas, ticks and mites. A dog or puppy who is afflicted by parasites is said to be 'infested', a word that packs a very negative punch indeed. Most clients are horrified if they are told that their beloved dog is infested with parasites, but in nature wherever a biological niche exists species have evolved to occupy that niche. The corollary of that is that virtually all animals, and humans, are the home to some parasites unless they are specifically treated to remove these. A small number of parasites probably have little detrimental effects on the dog or puppy who hosts them, and there is indeed a respected argument that these parasite burdens may have a useful modifying effect on the immune system. It might surprise you to hear that the complete elimination of all parasites from your puppy or adult dog may not always be a necessary or helpful goal. On the other hand, many parasites of our pets do cause disease that in certain circumstances can be fatal. Moreover, these parasites are sometimes transferable into our homes and to ourselves as pet owners, where again they can sometimes cause illness, or at least irritation. To compound this further, the parasites themselves sometimes carry other diseases (for example, Lyme disease *Borrelia Burgdorferi* is carried by ticks; *Bartonella* are bacterial pathogens sometimes carried by fleas). In later sections, I will outline in more detail which parasites are likely to occur in our pet dogs and how these should be prevented or treated.

TRAINING AND SOCIALISATION IN PUPPIES AND YOUNG DOGS

I have already warned you this is not a book about puppy care and training, but I know this will be on your mind soon after you get a dog, so what follows is a brief resume of some issues.

Dogs naturally prefer to urinate ('wee') and defecate ('poo') away from their beds but young puppies get very little warning, so, in the first few days after the pup comes home you must be vigilant and give them lots and lots of opportunities. Do not begin toilet training by encouraging the little dog to wee and poo on newspaper. That old-fashioned technique has nothing to recommend it. What you must try to do is quickly establish that wee and poo should be passed out-of-doors. This means that in the first few days, every 20–30 minutes, whilst the pup is awake, you should take her outside to a place where she can toilet. Praise the puppy when she is doing this. There are a few particular times when the pup is almost bound to need to go, namely on waking up, after eating or drinking and after a period of play. So, at these times, make a habit to immediately take him out-doors. If he has a pee or a poo congratulate him whilst he does so. After a short time, you will start to recognise the behaviours and postures which your pup adopts when they are about to go. When you see one of these signals (which can be quite subtle and very brief) scoop the puppy up and take her outside immediately. If she urinates or defecates praise her. If she doesn't, wait. Usually, they will do so within 5 minutes. As the pup learns, so the intervals between journeys outside can be extended. At night, initially you will be lucky to get a three-hour stretch, but soon you will get much longer. You are bound to fail sometimes. Pups are bound to wee and poo indoors sometimes. When it happens, if you catch them in the act, by all means immediately scoop them up to take them outside and praise them if they pass a little out-of-doors. However, know this: there is no value in punishing a dog after it has urinated or defecated inside the house. You will simply make them stressed and confused and might just teach them to wee and poo secretly indoors in the spare room, or under the sofa. One advantage of crate training is that puppies will try to avoid passing wee or poo in their crate, so you might find they learn toilet training more quickly. This is probably especially true at night.

Once your puppy has started toilet training, she should learn to wee and poo in a variety of places. This is important. Some dogs are taught to always urinate on grass and to do so to a command, such as 'Hurry up!', but this can become problematic if they go somewhere where grass is not available, or are supervised by someone who doesn't know the command. It's better if the dog can be flexible, so try to teach that.

Dogs and people can form great partnerships, but no dog innately understands how to behave in a way that exactly suits our needs. They need to be taught. Most dogs will learn quickly if you are consistent but they will learn bad habits as well as good unless you deliberately teach them what you want them to learn. The bare minimum dogs must learn to be good members of the community are: their name, where to urinate and defecate, how to walk on a lead, how to behave around other dogs, people and other species, to come to a call, to sit when asked, and to tolerate veterinary / nursing examinations. Punishment is not helpful in training. Positive reinforcement techniques, using rewards delivered *immediately* a desired behaviour occurs, are effective. There are many excellent classes, videos and books that cover this.

I have already touched on the issue of socialisation. Puppies between the ages of about 4 and 14 weeks are best able to assimilate knowledge about their environment and how to successfully interact with the people and animals they meet.

You should try to introduce your young dog to a wide variety of people, animals, noises, smells, textures and situations in the weeks after acquiring the pup. Much of this will happen quite naturally in the hustle and bustle of daily life, but you do need to try to keep a weather eye on the experiences that you and your puppy have notched up together so that you can plug any glaring gaps before the window of opportunity is closing. Try to avoid situations in which the puppy feels overwhelmed. Never try to push the pup forwards if he is feeling frightened. Give him time and show him that you yourself are not bothered. If the puppy doesn't relax at all, remove them from the situation for a short time, then try again. You ought to get the pup to meet men and women of all ages and a variety of appearances – for example, people wearing hats, sunglasses, bright coats and scarves. Try to expose the puppy to men who are bald and those who have facial hair. It's good if some of these people are carrying things; such as umbrellas, shopping-bags or cases, using walking sticks and rakes, or pushing buggies, lawn-mowers or vacuum cleaners. Also, try to meet people of different sizes, skin colour and ethnicity, and those who are uniformed, doing a variety of different tasks in the community – for example, policewomen, firefighters, lollipop-men and refuse collectors. It's a really good idea to meet children of all ages, but these meetings should be carefully supervised, because young kids especially are prone to lunge and grab at puppies in excitement, which can quickly unnerve a pup. Ideally, the pup should get most of these opportunities when they are on the ground rather than always in your arms. You do not want a dog who only feels safe when you are carrying him.

When you play with your puppy or young dog, sometimes he might become over-excited and hurt you with a vigorous play-bite. This must be discouraged. Use a sharp command like 'Enough!' and cease the game immediately. If the dog stops, give her immediate praise or a tasty treat. The dog will soon learn.

Introductions to other dogs have been mentioned already. These meetings should be supervised, at first, but are essential and often great fun. Growling, biting / mouthing, yapping and chasing are normal; mock battles are not to be completely discouraged but to be watched carefully. When dogs play you will notice that their mouths are almost always partly open in a sort of permanent grin; the puppies are learning to modify their bite so that they communicate without seriously hurting each other. Sometimes the play can seem extremely boisterous, almost brutal, but it rarely is. You will soon learn to recognise many of the postures dogs adopt to communicate. The play-bow is characteristic; in which one dog invites another to play by splaying their forelegs, lowering their head and chest to the floor, whilst keeping their rump elevated and slowly, widely, wagging the tail. This posture is often accompanied by short yaps or brief throaty growls. You will notice that the position of the ears, the cock of the head, the posture of the tail and the corners of the mouth all play a part in this signalling. I will cover the subject of dog body language and behaviour in more detail in Chapter 5.

You should also try to expose the youngster to other species, such as horses, cats, farm animals, etc. Opportunities may come your way easily – for instance, if you live in the country – but if they don't you might have to plan some special visits or days out to tick these boxes.

Travelling by car, bus or train can be quite daunting for puppies. The rapid movements of the vehicle, strange smells, loud noises, etc. might all combine into a frightening mixture. Travel sickness is common in pups, but like children most dogs will quickly learn to handle the experiences. The secret, as with all of these novelties, is to try to lessen the stress by making the initial experience brief, painless, and followed by a reward: praise, a short walk or perhaps a small tasty snack. Most dogs who are travel-sick can be weaned out of it by giving them lots of very short journeys – for example, drive a couple of hundred metres to the park, short walk, drive back. Repeat. Extend the distance a little each time.

One thing you ought to teach your young dog is that they must allow you to handle them all over. As with every lesson we have mentioned, these lessons should be short, followed by praise or a tasty reward. Run your hands all over his body, look in his ears, open her mouth, gently examine her paws, pass a comb through his coat, feel her joints, look under his tail, stare briefly into her eyes. Reward and repeat. Your puppy will soon learn that these intimate examinations are no cause for concern. Soon you can progress to other things, such as brushing the teeth and giving tablets.

Once they have learnt all that, visits to the vet should be a doddle!

There are some excellent short videos on the web you can look at that demonstrate handling techniques for dogs, so that is a resource worth investigating. Later in the book (Chapter 10), there are some also notes and sketches covering this.

FIRST VISIT TO A VET

It is an excellent idea to visit a vet in the first few days after acquiring your new puppy or re-homed dog. I would recommend this to everyone, even if the pet has recently seen a vet. This first visit will introduce the dog to the veterinary environment and staff and enable the vet to examine that puppy or dog in a gentle and thorough manner so that the pet and the vet can become acquainted. This visit also provides an excellent opportunity to discuss health care. Time pressure can be the enemy of good veterinary care so, in our practice at least, we like to provide a double appointment for this first visit. During this visit, depending on the dog's age, vaccination status, and perhaps other factors, further visits to the practice may be planned.

An empathetic vet will try to make this first visit really pleasant for the dog so that they see the veterinary practice as a safe place. I like to begin by stroking and petting the dog whilst talking to them in soft tones so that they feel relaxed. The examination performed will usually be quite detailed in order to disclose any obvious health issues. Thus, for instance, in young puppies the vet will be looking carefully for any congenital disorders, such as abnormal heart sounds, a cleft palate, or an umbilical hernia, and to ascertain if there are any conformational issues, such as dental misalignment, excessive folding of the skin, or disorders of the eyelids (entropion, in which an eyelid rolls inwards so that the lashes rub against the eye, is one of the most frequent conformational disorders seen in dogs). Many practices are able to offer you a short period of free insurance cover after performing this examination. You are not obliged to take it, and if you do there is no obligation to continue to insure the dog through that provider in future. However, most vets will take this opportunity to highlight the benefits of insuring your dog (see later).

The vet will want to understand what (if any) vaccines or other treatments have previously been administered to the puppy / dog before you acquired them. A vaccination certificate and microchip details will have been given to you if these have been done. This should lead into discussions about further vaccinations (if required) and probably also treatment for parasites.

The diet that you wish to feed your dog is an important choice, but in the first few days after acquisition you ought to try to continue to feed the diet the dog is used to. Moving home for a dog is stressful. All too often when a dog or puppy moves to a new home, they will develop diarrhoea as a result of this stress. A change in diet can be stressful too. There is nothing to be gained from combining these stresses.

In the following pages, I will tackle these issues in more detail.

VACCINATION

Vaccination in dogs is the practice of exposing a dog to an agent (usually a modified virus or bacteria) that stimulates the dog's immune system to respond, leading to resistance to an infectious disease. Vaccination is the single most important and effective way to prevent infectious disease. Vaccination against one infectious agent generally provides protection only against that agent and (perhaps) other closely related agents. The immune response consists of the production of antibodies ('immunoglobulins'); specific proteins that neutralise the infectious agent. A second type of immunity, known as cell-mediated immunity, involves the development of a complex series of cell lines within the body that also can neutralise the infectious agent by other means. The immune system is highly complex, so this description is very simplified.

For vaccination to be successful the animal must be in good health with an immune system that is capable of responding to the vaccine. In very young dogs the immune system is unable to mount a response to vaccination. Also, these young puppies will often have acquired some protection against some infectious disease whilst they were growing in the womb, through the placenta, and especially through their mother's milk ('colostrum'); this is known as 'passive immunity' from parental antibodies. This passive immunity can block, or partially block, an immune response to vaccination. For these reasons, there is absolutely no benefit in vaccinating very young puppies. However, as puppies grow and mature, the passive maternal immunity they had gradually wanes. Also, their own immune system matures and soon becomes capable of mounting a good immune response. This means that a window of time opens up during which a puppy can be very vulnerable to infectious disease, because of the loss of maternal passive immunity. This window typically opens at about the age they are weaned and leave home to join a new family. Provided the immune system is sufficiently mature this ought to be the right time to vaccinate the pup to protect them against infections. However, if the puppy's immune system is not yet well enough developed to meet the vaccination challenge, then the vaccination will fail. This is a dilemma. This dilemma means that in any individual pup it is difficult to know when, exactly, is the optimum time to vaccinate them.

The immune system that protects against disease has a memory. This means that once your puppy has been exposed to an infectious agent and mounted an immune response then, if, and when, it meets that agent again the animal will mount a stronger and swifter immune response. Immune memory is the secret to vaccination. Many vaccines are given more than once. The first time a vaccine is given it generally elicits a rather slight response. The second time a vaccine is given the response it elicits is much greater. It is as if the initial vaccination simply alerts the body to the agent but the second vaccination creates a stronger protective reaction that is much more durable and more effective. This is known as the anamnestic response. For some vaccines multiple vaccinations are necessary to develop good protective immunity, but more than a century of vaccine research means that many modern vaccines often provide protective immunity after only a couple of injections.

There are, in theory, many infectious diseases of dogs for which vaccines can be given; in the UK, however, we usually only vaccinate dogs against a limited menu of infections, namely, Distemper, Adenovirus, Parvovirus and Leptospirosis. Some dogs are also vaccinated against Bordetellosis and Parainfluenza (agents that can cause 'kennel cough'). I will explain how these vaccines are generally used and also why your vet might suggest a different vaccine regime for certain circumstances.

Distemper

Distemper, sometimes known as 'hard-pad', is a very serious and often fatal disease of the dog and several other mammals, including the fox and the ferret, which used to be extremely common. It is caused by a virus (canine distemper virus, CDV), which is closely related to human measles. The virus is quite fragile and swiftly dies in the environment, but the disease is highly contagious between dogs, usually through transmission in secretions from coughing and sneezing. Vaccines against this disease have been available for nearly 100 years. Modern vaccines are comprised of a modified live virus that is very safe. The normal schedule of vaccination is to give the first dose, as an injection under the skin, at around

6–9 weeks of age and a second dose 2–4 weeks later. A third dose may be given at 14–16 weeks of age (see below). An additional 'booster' distemper vaccination is usually given at about a year to 15 months of age. This booster is then usually repeated every three years, although such boosters may be unnecessary (see later).

Adenovirus

Two closely related adenoviruses, known as CAV1 and CAV2, can cause fatal liver disease, respiratory infections, kidney disease, an eye condition colloquially known as 'blue eye', or milder signs that are very non-specific, such as brief episodes of fever (high body temperature, technically called 'pyrexia'). If a dog survives the infection these viruses can be shed by that animal for weeks or months, particularly in the urine or via the respiratory tract. Adenoviruses can survive in the environment for long periods of time. Vaccines against this infection have been available for around 60 years. The vaccines have improved over the years and have become very safe. The vaccine given nowadays is a modified live vaccine of CAV2, but there is excellent cross-protection from the vaccine against both strains of the disease. This vaccine is normally given at the same time as vaccination against Distemper and Parvovirus.

Parvovirus

This is a small robust virus that infects rapidly dividing cells, chiefly those of the immune system and those lining the gut. The disease is extremely contagious. It causes vomiting, diarrhoea, dehydration, profound depression and depletion of the cells of the immune system so that the patient becomes immunosuppressed. The disease is rapidly fatal in many cases. Throughout the world, parvovirus infection has become by far the most common fatal infectious disease of the dog. Most animals who get the disease are less than a year of age. The majority who get it either have never been vaccinated or have had an inadequate primary vaccination regime. Certain breeds of dog seem to be more susceptible to the infection than others (especially Rottweilers, Dobermans, Labradors and German Shepherds). Like those against adenovirus and distemper infections, vaccinations to prevent parvovirus are usually first given at the age of 6–9 weeks with a second injection 2–4 weeks later and this is the regime that vaccine manufacturers usually advocate, but there is some evidence that following such a regime means that a substantial fraction (perhaps 10%) of puppies are not adequately protected. Recent research suggests that to develop an effective immune response many dogs should have a third parvovirus vaccine aged at least 12 weeks or older. A booster should be given approximately 9–12 months later when the pup has become about a year old (see WSAVA Vaccine guidance).

Leptospirosis

This is a bacterial infection to which dogs are susceptible. Leptospirosis occurs in many other mammalian species, including cats, cattle, horses and people. Dogs are believed to be the most commonly infected by contact with urine from rats or other rodents, from exposure to water polluted with urine, or directly from wildlife. The disease varies in severity from very mild and transient to severe or fatal. Many mild cases of the condition are probably never recognised, or treated, because spontaneous recovery occurs; however, in severe cases death can be rapid. If a dog with Leptospirosis is treated with antibiotics and supportive fluids etc., recovery is possible, but this depends on how advanced the condition is at the time of diagnosis. If recovery does occur, the infection may nevertheless result in ongoing damage to the kidneys, the eyes or the liver and sometimes to persistent shedding of the bacteria in the urine. In this way, the dog who has apparently been cured may become a source of infection to others. There are multiple strains of Leptospirosis known as serovars, which are grouped into serogroups. Several serogroups of Leptospirosis can affect dogs and it seems that the predominant serogroups to cause disease vary substantially over time and from place to place. In the past, acute infection in dogs the UK was usually due to the serogroups Canicola and Icterohaemorrhagiae, but more recently other serogroups have been implicated. For this reason, vaccines against multiple serogroups of Leptospirosis have been introduced into use in the last few years. Vaccination against Leptospirosis is useful but does not seem to be completely protective – the vaccine only claims to reduce (not prevent) infection and urinary excretion of the pathogen. Initial vaccination is usually given along with the viral vaccines to puppies twice at an interval of about 2–4 weeks (depending on the product). Annual revaccination is recommended because the quality and duration of immunity is shorter than that achieved with the viral vaccines.

TIMING OF VACCINATIONS IN PUPPIES

There has been a lot of controversy and confusion about precisely when puppies should be vaccinated. This, in part, stems from the problem that it is impossible to judge with any real certainty when an individual pup has developed full immune competence and can thus respond most appropriately to the vaccination course. The vaccine manufacturers' recommendations for vaccination are based on the licence they have been granted by the authorities (e.g. Veterinary Medicines Directorate in the UK), which derive from experimental studies of that vaccine submitted to the authorities for review. Many manufacturers suggest that vaccine schedules can be completed by 10 weeks of age with the first vaccine administered at 6–8 weeks of age (which is usually whilst a puppy is still in the care of the breeder). This 'early finish' regime has been popular with vaccine companies and many vets because it facilitates the introduction of these puppies into the wider world at an age where they are particularly programmed for socialisation before the 'adolescent' period when new experiences are potentially more likely to provoke fear. On the other hand, there is evidence that a proportion of dogs (particularly those of certain breeds) do not respond adequately to this approach and that perhaps 10% of puppies fail to respond to vaccination even at 12 weeks of age. For that reason, the vaccination guidelines produced in Europe and the USA now recommend a series of three primary vaccines in the pup starting at 6–9 weeks of age, with a second vaccine 3–4 weeks later, and a final shot given at 14–16 weeks of age (see WSAVA and AAHA Vaccine guidelines; Day et al., 2016). This can create a dilemma for vets and owners because it has become dogma that puppies that are not fully vaccinated should be kept in quarantine, isolated from other dogs, until deemed fully vaccinated, which is likely to be at least a week after the vaccination protocol is complete. However, this problem can be ameliorated by following sensible first principles; puppies who have not yet fully completed their vaccination protocols may still be allowed to meet other dogs provided those dogs themselves are fully vaccinated, appear to be completely healthy, and have had no contact with sick dogs within the preceding 14 days. Until a week after their second vaccination puppies should probably not be exercised in public places because it is conceivable that sick dogs shedding parvovirus (for example) have contaminated those places. In some circumstances, such as evidence of a local outbreak of parvovirus enteritis, vets may advise rigorous isolation of puppies until 16 weeks of age or later. In the end the precise regime and timing of primary vaccination schedules is usually made at the discretion of your vet who will be delighted to discuss this with you.

'KENNEL COUGH' VACCINATION

Contagious respiratory disease is fairly common in dogs. It can be due to various different agents, viral and bacterial. Any infectious respiratory disease of dogs is usually called 'Kennel Cough'. A live vaccine prepared against a bacteria, *Bordetella bronchiseptica,* and a virus, Parainfluenza, exists that claims to reduce the severity and shedding of these agents by infected dogs. However, because the disease often resolves spontaneously and the efficacy of the vaccine is far from perfect, vaccination against 'Kennel Cough' is considered to be optional. However, if your dog is to be kennelled or to visit dog shows, puppy classes or to frequently mix with other dogs then most vets and most kennel owners will recommend vaccination. The bacteria *Bordetella bronchiseptica* is related to *Bordetella pertussis,* the cause of whooping cough in people. Being a live vaccine there is a small risk that the vaccine can infect people, and for this reason people who have underlying serious respiratory disease or are immunocompromised – such as those who have cystic fibrosis, are being treated with chemotherapy, high dose corticosteroids or suffering from HIV infection – should avoid contact with the vaccine and vaccinated dogs for several weeks after vaccination. This vaccine is not administered by injection. Instead, it is delivered into the nose (no needles are required). Immunity to the bacterial component develops quickly after a single dose, within about 3 days, but immunity to the viral component takes around 3 weeks to develop. Mild respiratory signs are sometimes seen in dogs soon after vaccination. Annual revaccination is recommended where risk of infectious respiratory disease remains.

Recently, a new vaccine for kennel cough has become available that is a dead vaccine administered subcutaneously (Nobivac Respira Bb; MSD Animal Health).

WHAT ABOUT VACCINE SIDE-EFFECTS?

Many people reading this will recently have been vaccinated against Covid-19 or Flu. Like all potent and effective medications, vaccines can have side-effects, but these are generally mild and often pass un-noticed. Sometimes, for a day or two after vaccination, puppies are a little less playful and more lethargic or show depressed appetite compared to normal. There might be some slight pain, swelling and inflammation of the tissues close to the injection site. Body temperature may be slightly increased. These signs are transient, for less than three days in nearly all cases. More serious side-effects are very uncommon, but, if a puppy is obviously unwell in the first three days after vaccination, then it must be seen by a vet. If the vet is suspicious that the vaccine might be the cause, then they will inform the manufacturers of the vaccine and treat the puppy. Supportive therapy such as intravenous fluids and anti-inflammatory drugs, or other medications might be required. In cases where the vaccine is held responsible the vaccine manufacturers/suppliers should be expected to pay for this veterinary care. Death following vaccination is very rare indeed.

ARE VACCINATIONS REALLY NECESSARY?

Vaccination has transformed human and veterinary medicine. Conditions that were once common and frequently fatal have become uncommon. The best examples of the success of vaccination are Smallpox and Rinderpest. Smallpox was a highly contagious and deadly disease of humans that was completely eradicated throughout the world by vaccination. By the time the virus was eradicated, in 1979, the disease is estimated to have killed between 300 and 500 million people in the 20th century alone! Rinderpest, a pestilential viral disease of farm animals, was declared to have been completely eradicated throughout the world in May 2011, again by the use of a vaccine.

Hundreds of thousands of dogs' lives have been saved by vaccination. The viruses and bacteria that cause these diseases, however, have not become extinct; they are still around and remain a serious threat to the lives of dogs.

In Finland, around three decades ago, an outbreak of canine Distemper claimed at least 5000 dogs' lives, probably many more. This outbreak has been attributed to use of a poor-quality vaccine and a loss of vigilance against the threat of this infectious disease by the Finnish veterinary profession and dog owners. A similar complacency has developed in much of the world about human infectious disease. Vaccination rates have been falling and in consequence; measles, a disease that had almost become consigned to history, is now once more becoming a major threat to human health. Unvaccinated children are dying from measles.

When you vaccinate a puppy, you protect that puppy against the disease, but you are also doing another thing; you are reducing the proportion of the animals in that population that are susceptible to that infection. Once a certain proportion of a population has become protected then the likelihood of that contagion spreading through that population plummets. Eventually, even though there remain a few susceptible individuals still present in that population, the population as a whole becomes virtually immune to that infection. This phenomenon is called 'herd immunity'. For any particular population, the proportion that must be vaccinated to achieve herd immunity varies with the infection and also the way that the animals in that population interact with each other, but it is expected to be around 80–95%. This is why vets are so keen to vaccinate puppies; because we know that by minimising the numbers of susceptible individuals in a population, we can help to maintain the health of all animals in that population. A report published in the Autumn of 2019 found that whilst in 2016 88% of dogs received a primary course of vaccination, this number had fallen to 72% in 2019. This is a serious trend because it is likely to lead to many more dogs in the future developing these serious and often fatal diseases (PDSA Animal Wellbeing Report [PAW, 2019]).

Regular revaccination of dogs once they have become immune may not always be necessary. Further information on this topic can be found in Chapter 5.

MICROCHIPPING

By law, all dogs over the age of 8 weeks must be microchipped. The microchip implant is technically described as a passive radio-frequency identification device (RFID); quite small, about the size and shape of a grain of rice. It is inert, solid state, non-toxic, has no power source, doesn't break and doesn't wear out. It is enclosed in sterile biocompatible glass. The microchip is inserted using a sterile single-use needle. The procedure is quick. Although not completely painless, microchipping is supported by all the animal welfare charities because missing or homeless dogs are a very serious welfare problem. A microchip has a unique number but stores no other information. Most of the time a microchip is completely inactive. When the chip is read by a scanner the chip 'chirps' that number back to the scanner where it is displayed. The chip must be registered to you. If you move house, change your phone number, or your name, you need to inform the chip register of the change. The weak link in this process means that if a dog with a microchip is picked up by a vet, a dog warden, or the police, for example, we quickly know who the dog is, but sometimes their owner cannot be traced because they've moved or changed their phone number.

ROUNDWORMS

Virtually all puppies have roundworms, typically a species known as *toxocara canis.* Another related species, *toxascaris leonina,* is implicated less frequently. These white worms measure from around 8 cm up to nearly 20 cm in length. They look like cooked spaghetti. Toxocara is a zoonosis; meaning the parasite can affect people. In the UK, this is rarely serious, but in some cases it can have profound consequences. *Toxocara canis* has an elaborate lifecycle. Stay with me on this; what follows may disgust you, but if you understand this parasite's lifecycle you will appreciate both the risks and the treatment.

Adult roundworms live and feed in the intestines of dogs where they are usually tolerated and cause few or no signs of ill-health. The parasite breeds here. Female worms can produce tens of thousands of microscopic eggs ('oocysts') every day. Poo from dogs who have roundworms can contain huge numbers of roundworm eggs. Fortunately, when passed in the poo, these eggs are not immediately infective to other animals, dogs or people. This means that fresh dog faeces is not a potential source of infestation; but, toxocara oocysts can survive in the environment for long periods. Two or three weeks after the faeces have been passed the oocysts have matured. They are now 'embryonated', contain a larva, and they have become infective. If a young dog swallows infective oocysts these larvae break out from the oocyst in the intestine of the new host. The larvae then burrow through the wall of the intestine and begin a migration through the body. As the larvae migrate, they grow and mature. The typical route of migration is following the bloodstream from the intestines to the liver, then from the liver to the lungs. In the lungs, the tiny larvae penetrate into the air-sacs (alveoli) and small airways (bronchi) where they provoke inflammation and coughing. They are coughed up and swallowed by the dog to arrive back in the gut. Here they complete their maturation to adulthood and begin to breed. The adult female worms soon start to produce more eggs; within 3–5 weeks of ingesting the eggs the lifecycle is complete.

The lifecycle I have described indicates events that occur in young dogs who have not been previously heavily parasitised, such dogs are designated 'naive'. However, older dogs, usually over a year of age, who have been previously exposed to infestation, exhibit an immune response to new toxocara. In these cases, the classic migratory cycle is usually not completed. Instead, larvae that emerge from the oocysts and burrow through the wall of the intestine are thwarted in their journey back to the intestine – they migrate more widely; some of them become encysted within the tissues of the body where they survive in a semi-dormant state. It is believed that almost all dogs harbour some encysted toxocara larvae.

When a bitch becomes pregnant a proportion of the encysted larvae become aroused and migrate further around the body. Some of these larvae cross the placenta from the bitch into the liver and lungs of the developing puppies so that the puppies are born with a roundworm burden. What is more, other larvae reach the mammary glands of the pregnant bitch, where they pass into the milk so, in the first few days and weeks of life as the puppies suckle, they acquire additional roundworms through their mother's milk. This elaborate version of the life-cycle ensures that virtually all puppies will have some roundworms and this can sometimes have serious consequences. A heavy roundworm infestation in a pup will cause gastrointestinal disease, diarrhoea and possibly vomiting. The puppy will often appear 'pot-bellied' and may not thrive. Sometimes puppies vomit up a mass of wriggling worms. In very severe cases roundworms can cause complete obstruction of the gut, and even death.

The biology of this parasite has been studied for decades and thoroughly elucidated. It turns out that the lifecycle has yet other branches. Infective oocysts in the soil or on vegetation can be ingested by other species; small mammals, cattle and sheep, birds, and even people. Toxocara are not adapted to breed in these animals. These are so-called 'paratenic hosts', in which the roundworms can begin migration, but in which they are unable to complete the journey from the gut, through the lungs and back to the gut. In these hosts, that larval migration is thwarted but the larvae can survive and encyst, provoking an immune response in the process. If a dog hunts and eats one of these paratenic hosts raw the encysted roundworm larvae can mature in the gut of the new host dog to cause a new infestation in which adult male and female worms breed and further crops of oocysts are shed.

Thankfully, dogs do not eat humans, but humans can easily be exposed to embryonated toxocara oocysts – for example, from garden soil, or perhaps from the hair-coat of a dog. Toxocara larvae do attempt to migrate through the human body but usually die in the process. In some poor countries that have a warm humid climate up to 40% of people have been exposed and developed an immune response to this parasite. Young children, who may play in the earth, and those people who have close contact with dogs, such as vets, veterinary nurses and shepherds, are more frequently exposed. In most cases it seems that no illness follows; however, in a small proportion of individuals this can cause symptoms such as a fever, headaches and stomach pain. Rarely, this parasite can cause seizures ('fits'), or blindness in one eye, if a larva migrates to that site. In the UK, the incidence of human illness from toxocara appears to be very low indeed. For the sake of human health, dog poo should be cleared up promptly. Children should be discouraged from eating soil and should wash their hands thoroughly before meals. Sandpits should be covered when not in use so that they are not used as toilets by dogs (or cats). For their own health, and to reduce contamination of the environment with roundworm eggs, puppies should be treated repeatedly for roundworms in the first months of life. Adult dogs might occasionally have a roundworm burden. This can be checked for by sending a poo sample to a veterinary laboratory to be examined. Alternatively, adult dogs can be treated at intervals, perhaps once or twice a year (controversial – see later).

There are many effective drugs available for treating roundworms in dogs that are safe for those animals and safe for people. Your vet will probably recommend that your young pup or re-homed dog is treated with one of these drugs. Most vets will not carry all these drugs but they will usually consider multiple issues when they recommend a drug; these include animal and human safety, efficacy, ease of use, spectrum and duration of activity and perhaps environmental safety (see later). Some of these products are given by mouth as a paste or a tablet. In other cases, the drug is applied to the skin from where it is absorbed into the body. Some of these drugs are sold in combination with other drugs to widen the spectrum of activity of the product (for instance to include tapeworms, or fleas, etc.), which may, or may not, be appropriate for your pet. When a drug is recommended or dispensed for you, you ought to ask the vet why they have chosen that particular drug. A good vet will be delighted to defend their choice and offer you alternatives if these seem more suited to you, your lifestyle or your dog's circumstances.

FLEAS

Every dog (and cat) will have fleas at some time in their life. This is not an inditement of the cleanliness of your home. Nor is it a tragedy. It is a simple hazard of life.

Fleas are commonly seen on puppies. Fleas feed on blood. A heavy flea infestation can cause serious anaemia and occasionally, though rarely, even death. If your pup or re-homed dog has fleas when you acquire him or her you will soon have a household problem because fleas multiply rapidly and infest their surroundings, so every dog owner will find it useful to understand this parasite.

If a dog has fleas, they are usually cat fleas: *Ctenocephalides felis*. The dog flea, *Ctenocephalides canis,* is less common. Adult fleas live on the dog where they scurry about in the coat. They tend to congregate on the lower back but can be found anywhere on the body. To feed, fleas pierce the skin for a blood meal. These bites are irritating and painful to the dog. Often a dog with fleas will suddenly stop what it is doing to turn around and bite or gnaw at themselves, because they've just been bitten by a flea. A good way to hunt for fleas is to use a fine-toothed flea comb which you can buy cheaply in a pet shop or from your vet (see Figure 4.1). Pass the comb repeatedly through the coat, especially along the back and near the base of the tail. Dander from the skin and shed hair gets caught in the teeth of the comb. If your pup has fleas you will see 'flea dirt', flea droppings, which consist of partially digested blood. This looks black and granular, often in the shape of a tiny comma, if you put some on wet tissue paper it dissolves to leave a red-brown stain. Accompanying the flea dirt will be small pale specks, like salt; these are flea eggs. Sometimes you will come across the fleas themselves, which are

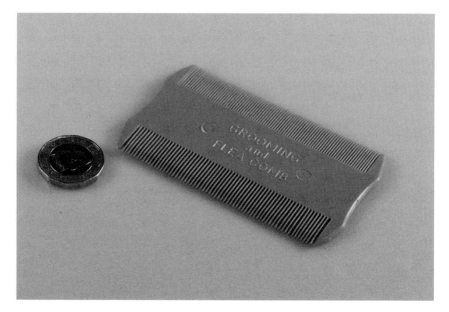

Figure 4.1. Flea comb.

about 2–3 mm in length and reddish-brown to black in colour. They scuttle quickly through the fur and can jump huge distances compared with their body size, certainly 15 cm or more; roughly equivalent to a human jumping over a football stadium!

It is impossible to solve a flea infestation by combing out the fleas. This is because although the adult flea spends their life on the dog, the female flea is a prolific breeder who can lay dozens of eggs every day and will keep doing so throughout her life. Some sources suggest a female flea might produce 300 eggs in her life, whilst others say that number could be 2000, or more. The eggs are white in colour and shiny. They don't stay in the coat for long – they fall off the dog to infest the surroundings, especially when the dog shakes or scratches. In warm houses, flea eggs usually hatch soon after they are laid and a larva emerges. Flea larvae seek darkness and prefer humid environments, often burrowing deep into carpets or into cracks in floorboards; however, in most cases they don't travel very far from where the eggs fell, which means the larval density is highest where dogs spend most of their time. The larvae feed on the partially digested blood of flea-dirt and are cannibals, eating flea eggs that have failed to hatch and even other larvae. It was once believed that flea larvae fed on animal dander, flakes of skin, hair, etc. This is incorrect. They live in the environment for several weeks during which time they moult twice to pass from the first to the third larval instar. In warm, humid conditions the larval phase can be completed in less than three weeks, but in other climatic conditions this phase is more prolonged. The third larval instar weaves a silk cocoon around itself and moults again to become a pupa. This pupa might mature to an adult within 1–2 weeks, but can arrest its development for up to a year. Pupae are virtually impossible to kill with insecticides (see later).

Many, many different drugs are available to kill fleas on your dog without harming either you or your pets. Some can be given by mouth. Others can be applied directly on the skin as sprays, or 'Spot-ons'.

If you have more than one dog, treat them all. If you have cats as well as dogs, you *must* treat all the animals together. Cats are far more often infested with fleas than dogs.

However, if your young dog (or cat) has fleas, treating the animal(s) alone will virtually never solve the problem. You must treat the home too because most of the total flea burden consists of eggs, larvae and pupae in the dog's surroundings.

The single most effective way to reduce this flea burden is to wash all dog bedding in a hot wash (60°C or hotter) and to vacuum thoroughly and repeatedly. Empty the vacuum bag immediately afterwards into an outside bin. Most of the eggs and larvae congregate where dogs lie – so if they sleep on the furniture or on your bed these should be vacuumed too. Thoroughly. Repeatedly. This is hard work. Unfortunately, there is another downside to vacuuming; pupated fleas are awakened by three triggers, carbon dioxide (from our breath), warmth and vibration. When you vacuum a carpet or a sofa, if there are pupae there which are not sucked into the hoover, these pupae will be stimulated to hatch from their cocoon emerging as adults seeking a new host. So, one swift effect of vacuuming can be that you and your dog immediately get flea bites. Do not despair. Keep up the hard work. You are solving the problem.

After you are exhausted from all this washing and vacuuming have a cup of tea, or a glass of wine. Gather your strength. There's more.

Even the most assiduous cleaner will fail to remove every last egg, every final larva, every perishing pupa. So, after all this cleaning, it is almost inevitable that you will have to use an insecticide in your house. Effective insecticides for fleas are sold by vets and pet shops. They're usually composed of at least two different agents. One short-acting chemical kills the majority of the remaining eggs and larvae. The second component is an insect growth regulator (IGR), a persistent chemical that stops the eggs and larvae from hatching and moulting. Larvae that are exposed to an IGR fail to pupate. Most household IGRs persist in the home for months and are very safe for humans and our pets. When using one of these products, follow the labelled directions carefully. You've already vacuumed. Get pets and children out of the way. Close windows and doors. Spray the carpets, floors, skirting boards, and furniture (but not human beds). Be thorough and methodical. Don't spray the air, spray surfaces. Particularly, spray where your dog likes to lie, under heavy furniture that is difficult or impossible to move, and anywhere where dust collects or is tricky to shift. Work your way around the house. If there's a cupboard, a shed, a garage, greenhouse, or a car where dogs (or cats) have been – spray that too. Then go for a walk, some shopping, to the park, or to the pub.

When you get back open the doors and windows. The donkey work is nearly done.

Sadly, even household insecticides containing IGRs will not kill every pupa. But all is not lost. The final stage of this process is easy. Guess what? Vacuum again.

Remember this will stimulate pupae to hatch into adults that should soon be killed by the household insecticide or when they jump on the dog. For the next few weeks, every time you vacuum some pupae will probably hatch but the fleas that emerge will soon die. So, if you see the odd flea after all this work, don't worry, be smug. Know that it's doomed. Continue to treat your dog for at least three months. Different products have different durations of action – some last for only a day or two (for instance, nitenpyram) whereas at least one oral product is effective for a full 12 weeks (fluralaner). If you use a topical spray or 'spot-on' product don't allow your dog to swim for at least a fortnight after you've used the product. At least some of the drug would wash off, which will dilute the efficacy, but, more importantly, these drugs tend to be very toxic to fish and plankton, so you might inadvertently cause an ecological crisis (more of this later).

Some dogs develop an allergic immune reaction to proteins and peptides in flea saliva. This is known a Flea Allergic Dermatitis (FAD). FAD should not occur in puppies. I will tackle this issue elsewhere.

LUNGWORM

The two parasites I've mentioned already are by far the most common ones affecting puppies in the UK but there is another I want to talk about here because it is potentially fatal. This is the lungworm *Angiostrongylus vasorum*, sometimes called the French heartworm. Once considered to be rare and exotic, this parasite has become common in a few parts of the UK over the last 40 years (especially south Wales, the west country and in the south east, around London). *Angiostrongylus* is a roundworm that lives in the blood vessels of the lungs, the pulmonary arterial tree. Despite its other name it does not usually reside in the heart. If you're eating you might like to finish before reading further, because I'm about to describe another parasitic lifecycle.

The adult lungworms live in the pulmonary circulation of dogs; they induce inflammation, breed and lay eggs there, which hatch to the first larval stage (L1). These larvae are coughed up by the dog, swallowed, and eventually passed in the host dog's poo. Slugs and snails in the environment graze on this dog poo. The L1 larvae in the faeces are ingested by these gastropod molluscs where they mature further to the second larval stage, L2, then L3. Later the molluscs themselves may be consumed by dogs, or possibly other animals such as frogs and thrushes, which themselves then become prey to dogs. The L3 larvae eventually reach the intestine of another dog where they penetrate the wall of the gut, migrate around the body, and wind up once more in the pulmonary arterial circulation of a new host where they mature and begin to breed. The life cycle is complete. In the UK, foxes can host lungworms and indeed in parts of the south this infestation is very common in foxes. Much research continues into this parasite because some details of the life cycle are still unclear.

It seems that lungworm infestation is much more common in young dogs than those who are mature or elderly. This is probably due to acquired immunity, but we are uncertain. Some dogs who have lungworm appear to suffer few or no ill effects. Some cough, are breathless, or show other respiratory signs. A few dogs develop catastrophic haemorrhage or neurologic disease (usually due to bleeding into the brain or spinal cord). Deaths are not common but can be sudden and unheralded. Unfortunately, whilst there are faeces and blood tests to confirm if a dog has *Angiostrongylus* the tests are not perfect. Consequently, vets often treat dogs for this parasite on a presumptive basis; for example, if a young dog has unexplained respiratory signs. Several drugs have been used successfully to treat lungworm in dogs. Two commonly used insecticides (moxidectin and milbemycin), which are only available on prescription, have a license that shows they can protect dogs against infestation.

If you live in a part of the country where *Angiostrongylus* is present, your vet will likely recommend that your dog has prophylactic treatment against this parasite at least whilst the dog is young. They might also discuss what you can do to minimise the risk, such as always clearing up your dog's faeces, and never leaving dog-bowls out of doors where slugs and snails might be.

A NOTE ABOUT THE ENVIRONMENT

Although it is often suggested that all dogs should be 'prophylactically' treated for fleas, ticks, worms and other parasites continuously throughout their lives, I believe such an approach is wasteful and neither necessary nor rational. The insecticides that are licensed for use in pets are safe for you, your family and your pets, but they are certainly not completely benign and harmless to the environment. Some are suspected, or proven, to be very dangerous to birds, bees, butterflies, other insects, soil organisms, plankton and fish. This issue may be quite serious but we in the veterinary profession do not yet have a good grasp of it because, until now, the subject has not been seriously confronted by drug companies, researchers or the profession at large. If every dog in the UK were to be on continual 'prophylactic' treatment for all potential parasites the environmental effects might be quite damaging. I will return to this subject later in the book.

DIET FOR THE GROWING/MATURING PUP

Dogs, like wolves, are essentially carnivores, but unlike wolves they are very able to digest carbohydrates (starches and sugars) and this is believed to have been one of the key evolutionary changes that allowed dogs to thrive under domestication. In consequence, dogs are sometimes described as 'omnivores' or 'facultative carnivores'. It is possible, though very challenging, to successfully feed dogs on vegetarian, or even vegan diets, but given the opportunity almost all dogs seem very keen to eat meat. For almost all of our co-evolution together, dogs have fed from human table scraps, food waste, bones, offal and other foodstuffs provided, or scavenged, from our tables and rubbish. There are archaic references to the most appropriate foods for dogs, going back to Roman times, but proprietary dog food is a recent creation dating to the invention of dog biscuits by James Spratt in 1860. This is worth bearing in mind when you read some of the information provided by commercial dog-food companies who often imply that human food is inherently dangerous to dogs. It is certainly true that a few foods that people eat are toxic to dogs (including chocolate, raisins, grapes, onions, garlic, macadamia nuts and nutmeg), but in principle most dogs can survive and thrive on most human food. Like humans, dogs can be rather omnivorous and, historically at least, much of what they eat has been culturally determined by the community they live amongst rather than by science. It is worth bearing this in mind when you meet dog owners who insist that dogs can be made sick by commercial dog food and that all dogs should be fed bones and raw food (BARF) or grain-free diets. There has been a lot of high-quality scientific research into the nutritional requirements of dogs. Much of this has been funded/ sponsored by dog-food companies and should thus be treated with a certain scepticism. However, it would be foolish in the extreme to ignore these data.

Most people will choose to feed their puppy or re-homed dog a proprietary dog food simply because it is convenient and economic. Look for foods that are labelled as appropriate for puppies and 'complete'. Both dry kibbles and canned or semi-moist diets seem quite appropriate; your choice. Commercial pet food companies spend considerable funds researching canine nutrition, often including feed trials to prove their diets are nutritious. They also spend a lot of money trying to persuade you to buy their product. The simple building blocks of a diet are of course proteins, carbohydrates and fats but there are also many micro-nutrients, such as vitamins, minerals, fatty acids, soluble and insoluble fibre, etc. It is interesting that although we know dogs *can* digest carbohydrates, the science does show that dogs (like other carnivores, such as the cat) *can* survive and thrive on diets containing little or no carbohydrate.

It is very important that you feed a puppy food appropriate for puppies, until they are at least 10 months of age. In the first few months of life, puppies have about twice the energy requirements per kilo of body weight compared with adult dogs. Because they are growing and have active but immature immune systems puppies also require a higher protein diet than adult dogs. Nutritional guidelines suggest that adult dog diets should contain a minimum of 18% protein on a dry-matter basis whereas puppies should have at least 22% protein (for the most part complete dog foods will contain more protein than this – usually 24–30%). The mineral content of puppy food too is very important. Adult diets are recommended to contain a minimum of 0.6% calcium whereas puppy food should contain at least 1% calcium. However, too much calcium in the diet can actually cause certain kinds of skeletal abnormalities. Also, the relative proportions of calcium and phosphorus in the diet are crucial (meats are generally very high in phosphorus). This illustrates that the balance between different components of a diet is important and is one reason why correct formulation of home-produced diets (for pups or adult dogs) can be extremely challenging. If you are feeding a good proprietary food, dietary supplements containing additional minerals and vitamins are generally unnecessary and can themselves sometimes be harmful.

Young puppies must be fed frequently, say four times a day at 8 weeks of age, but the number of feeds can be reduced as they grow older and by 6 months of age two meals should be fed. Portion sizes obviously increase. It is quite difficult to judge exactly how much your puppy should be fed at each meal but a good rule of thumb is to feed to body condition so that you should always be able to feel their ribs with ease. In short-haired breeds I would expect to be able to see their ribs too. Underfeeding is much safer than overfeeding. Puppies that are overfed are likely to become obese adults. Those that are very well nourished, or fed ad lib, as they grow are also more prone to joint diseases. I will discuss diet more in Chapter 5.

EXERCISE FOR PUPPIES

Most young dogs seem to have almost boundless energy. When they're not tearing about, they're usually asleep. Learning to wear a collar and to tolerate a lead will take a little while but rarely causes problems. Some types of exercise might not be good for young dogs. Evidence on this is actually rather hard to find. I hate to make pronouncements that are not well supported by evidence. A couple of studies have found that prolonged or jarring activity, such as running up and down stairs, or running after a ball repeatedly, can increase the risks of developing hip dysplasia, elbow arthritis and a joint disorder called osteochondritis dissecans. These conditions are principally seen in large dogs. Each of these are very serious for the dogs involved and can lead to a lifetime of discomfort. There is an aphorism, widely cited, that puppies should have 'No more than five minutes of lead exercise on hard ground, twice a day, for each month of age, until they reach a year of age.' It sounds very sensible. I don't know where the data is to support it. One eminent surgeon has said that, 'Five minutes of bounding around the garden and jumping up and down at the fence to get at the cat next door can be far more damaging than several miles of controlled lead walking' (Hutchinson, 2019: 181).

INSURANCE

I've never insured my dogs. I thought there was no need. I'm a vet after all.

As I write this at my feet lies my elderly lurcher, Tallulah, who has cost me thousands and thousands of pounds, because of all the scrapes she's been in. Five years ago, she was hospitalised at the Queen Mother's Hospital of the Royal Veterinary College in London because of a fracture-dislocation in her neck. The staff there did a superb job (I want to especially thank Brigita, the neurologist). It cost me £7000! Worth every penny. But I wish I'd been insured. Don't do as I did. Do as I say. Insure your dog.

There are four basic types of pet insurance you can buy.

- **Accident only**: This gives no cover at all for illness. It does what it says.
- **Twelve months**: This gives cover for accident and illness but cover only lasts for a maximum of a year after diagnosis.

- **Maximum benefit**: Your dog is covered up to a maximum amount for each condition, which means if they develop a long-standing or incurable problem, such as diabetes, epilepsy, or chronic inflammatory enteropathy ('inflammatory bowel disease'), once you have claimed the full cover all treatment for that problem must be paid for by you.

- **Lifetime cover**: Your dog is covered for life for treatment of each condition. Normally, there is still a maximum amount that you can claim but that amount will be reinstated every year when you renew your insurance.

There are a huge number of insurance companies competing for your business when it comes to pet insurance, which should in theory be good for the buying customer; but it can be quite difficult to compare like-for-like when you are trying to make comparisons. This is partly because the headline figures that are quoted as maximum cover vary between suppliers and almost all suppliers will deduct a fixed excess from every claim (say £100 or £150) and will additionally also often deduct a variable excess (usually around 10%). So, you need to be very savvy when you look into this. In the words of the songwriter Tom Waits, '... The large print giveth, and the small print taketh away ...'.

When we were insuring my daughter's puppy, Lyra, we found an easy way to compare different insurers was to begin by deciding how much we were willing to spend every month on insurance. That done, we decided that Lifetime Insurance would give us the most security and peace of mind. We then sought out half-a-dozen reputable insurers and plugged Lyra's particulars into their websites to get a quote. By tweaking the fixed and variable excesses we were willing to pay, we were able to select an insurer we felt would give us good value for the money we were willing to spend. This approach might not suit you, but it suited us. A few months after taking out the insurance we had to make a claim. The cover did what it said on the tin.

> Dear Chris,
>
> Thanks for seeing this puppy so promptly. Mr N has just lost his wife to cancer. He lives with his mother and daughter. He bought this puppy a few days ago for £500 (he's not well off, so I think this was quite a stretch). The pup is not insured. He's about 11 weeks old now. When I saw the pup for the first time I heard a heart murmur. I do hope it's not too serious.

Best wishes, thanks again,

Z. S.

Veterinary Surgeon

The normal heart makes two distinct sounds every time it beats: 'lub-dup, lub-dup, lub-dup'. Murmurs are unusual sounds caused by irregular blood flow through the chambers of the heart. A puppy with a heart murmur could have one of several different congenital anatomic abnormalities, but sometimes the murmur is not caused by a serious condition at all. Blood is thicker than water – which means it is also less prone to turbulence. Young puppies are often slightly anaemic between the aged of about 8 and 16 weeks. This is a normal 'physiologic' anaemia that requires no treatment and will resolve completely, but, whilst they are anaemic the blood is less viscous, more likely to flow irregularly, which can lead to a 'physiologic' heart murmur. If a vet hears a heart murmur in a puppy, they will often refer the pup to a cardiologist like me because diagnosing of the cause of the murmur is difficult. It is essential to know the cause so that an accurate prognosis can be given and treatment provided if necessary.

I am introduced to Baldrick, a German Shepherd Puppy who is lively, alert, full of mischief. He's a bit nervous of me. His heart rate, 160 beats per minute, is a little fast but that could be quite normal in an excited pup. His pulses feel fine. He's a good colour, well grown. I listen with my stetho-scope. There is a very obvious murmur. I have a long frank talk with Mr N.

Ultrasonography of the heart, often called echocardiography, is painless, the best way to examine a heart to determine the cause of a heart murmur. Technically this is a form of echolocation, like sonar, which submarines use to find their way around underwater, and which bats navigate by. My equip-ment is expensive and delicate, an electronic masterpiece without which I couldn't function as a cardiologist. I scan Baldrick's heart whilst he's gently held by Morag my veterinary nurse.

The problem is clear. The murmur is arising from the pulmonary artery, the tube that carries the blood from the right heart to the lungs. There is a constriction in this vessel at the level of the pulmonic valve. This means that the blood must accelerate through this region, which is what causes the turbulence and the heart murmur. The right heart wall is hypertrophied, becoming thickened, in response to this obstruction to blood flow. The pressure within the right ventricle, the pumping chamber that drives this blood flow is much higher than normal, and the other valve in the right heart, which usually ensures that blood flows one way only, has started to leak too so that a proportion of the blood ejected from the ventricle is regurgitating backwards into the right atrium. The prognosis is difficult to judge with certainty. I have seen many worse cases than this but the pressure and flow measurements I have made suggest Baldrick would benefit from heart surgery.

I have another talk with Mr N. Although surgical treatment would offer the best outlook it's not going to be possible. Finances won't stretch. We decide to regularly check Baldrick's progress. We do so for a nominal fee.

NEUTERING

The decision whether or not to neuter your dog is a personal one. It's basically a management decision, but it will have health implications either way. If you want to breed, then the decision is clear. If you don't want to breed, then the decision is complex. No-one but you should make the decision. If a vet tries to bully you about it, resist. Whilst it is possible to neuter quite young dogs, and some people are evangelical about doing so, the decision usually does not have to be made soon after you acquire a dog. However, you might like to start thinking about this quite soon. More on this in Chapter 5.

5

ROUTINE HEALTH CARE

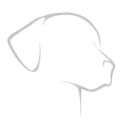

This chapter focuses on healthy management of your dog. Dog behaviour will receive some attention, which ought to enhance your understanding of your dog. Issues such as nutrition, how to care for their teeth, skin and coat will be tackled. More information will be imparted about neutering, exercise, weight control, dieting to tackle weight problems, regular check-ups and vaccination boosters. Also, holidays, kennelling, taking your dog abroad and the advantages/disadvantages of veterinary loyalty schemes.

The principles of good preventative canine care are easily stated.

- An appropriate diet should be fed in appropriate amounts in one or two meals a day to maintain body weight but avoid obesity.

- Every dog should have exercise, ideally both on and off the lead, every day.

- Most dogs will appreciate regular opportunities to meet other dogs and other people, provided they have been well socialised as puppies.

- All dogs should be given opportunities to exhibit normal behaviour and to rest in comfort.

- Dental care by brushing the teeth and regular opportunities to chew or gnaw are good for your dog.

- Regular veterinary check-ups are advisable when preventative medicines such as vaccinations may be provided in agreement with your vet.

- If you are not intending to breed your dog then you ought to consider neutering them. This is by no means essential. For bitches at least, the benefit can be considerable but in every case this should be carefully weighed up.

There are two things almost every dog loves: exercise and food.

If you socialise your puppy early under careful supervision by maximising opportunities for the pup to freely and safely interact with other dogs of various breeds and ages, and to meet people from all walks of life, your dog should swiftly become a well-adjusted member of canine society.

Meetings between dogs often first occur whilst they are on leads but this is often not ideal because dogs who are on a leash are not fully able to express themselves and can't run away when frightened. Also, the pace and proximity of these meetings is determined by the action of the dogs' owners not the dogs themselves. Despite their owner's best intentions, meetings between dogs on leash can sometimes be highly stressful for both dogs, often involve tangled leads, and may degenerate into hackle-raised barking matches, or worse. So, let's look at the way these meetings usually unfold when the dogs are free, off lead.

When a well-socialised dog meets another relaxed, well-adjusted dog they don't know, or have not recently met, there are some typical behaviours that follow. If you've never been aware of these, try to get the opportunity to watch. Firstly, as they approach each other, still several metres apart, the dogs will usually slow down, falter or briefly stop. They will also usually deliberately, but briefly, look away from each other. Both of these are signals of non-aggressive intent. The dogs' ears may be moved forward and the tails lifted and fluffed out. These are certainly signs of arousal, though not necessarily aggression. When the tails are wagged widely back and forth in a soft relaxed manner this tends to signify benign intent. Dogs seem to prefer to avoid direct 'head-on' meetings (which is one reason why meetings on leads can be fraught); instead, they usually approach each other obliquely. Provided aggressive signals are absent, as the dogs get close they will sniff and snuffle each other's muzzles and ears, often quite vigorously. Then, in turn, they will usually each sniff around the other dog's backside. As they do so they tend to circle each other. During these first moments of interaction, frequently one or the other dog will turn away to do something else. These interruptions seem to lower the emotional temperature between the dogs and are part and parcel of the normal behaviour.

After this greeting ceremony, sometimes a pair of dogs decide by mutual consent that they are disinterested in each other, or would rather carry on with their own plans, so they disengage. On the contrary, after the initial contact a pair of dogs may decide to play. This might be signalled by one or other dog performing a play-bow, in which they lower their chest towards the ground whilst remaining more upright on their hind legs and swishing their tail widely, or by one dog bumping against the other with their haunches as if to say: 'right, come-on, let's run around' (see Figure 5.1). During play, some dogs make rumbling breathy sounds that might be 'dog laughter'. Much play between dogs involves high speed chases and mock battle in which the dogs rear up on their hind legs whilst growling deeply and 'mouthing' each other. Well socialised dogs learn as puppies to inhibit their bite so that they don't hurt one another during play. Sometimes after a few

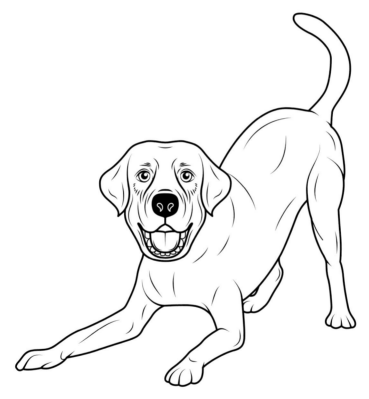

Figure 5.1. Play-bow. This behaviour is often used between dogs to invite play. The dog lowers their fore quarters and raises their hind quarters. They tend to raise the tail and wag it. Often they cock their head slightly. Their facial features are relaxed and sometimes the mouth will be slightly open. These postures might be accompanied by throaty light growls and energetic rocking or twisting of the body.

minutes of play the dogs stop, perhaps to get their breath back, but in doing so they often turn away from each other and sniff the ground, or stand still panting. Such breaks in the games, like turning the head aside to avoid a stare, seem to prevent vigorous play-fighting games escalating into real violence.

Frequently, a pair of dogs will adopt dominant and submissive roles. The dog who wishes to assert themselves will get their head above the other dog and might try to mount or bowl the more submissive dog over. The more submissive of the pair might stand still whilst the dominant dog actively sniffs at it and might raise one forepaw, or roll-over completely, to allow the dominant dog to stand over it. Although you might be tempted to intervene, it is usually best to let the dogs sort out the pecking order between them. Dogs have complex and subtle body language and usually understand each other well. It is interesting that during play, dogs often seem to take turns to display dominance and submission as they chase around together and mouth each other.

Once you know the normal greeting behaviours of dogs, it becomes easier to recognise when one or both parties are not so happy with the meeting. Stiff postures or very rapid movements can indicate that one or both dogs are anxious or fearful. When dogs are uncertain but assertive, they tend to lean forward, and their hackles often go up along their back so they look larger and more powerful. Tails tend to be elevated. By contrast, a dog who is definitely fearful or frightened will slink close to the ground with their ears flattened back and their tail tucked under. A dog who is anxious will often lick their own lips or yawn. If an anxious dog wishes to appease another dog it might lick at their face and will avoid looking directly at it.

The dog who is frankly aggressive will not pause as it approaches another; instead, it will lunge forward, staring at the other dog. Aggressors hold their ears very forward with their eyebrows close together and show bristling hackles. Sometimes the lips of the aggressor seem pursed. The aggressor's tail may be stiffly erect with the tip of the tail twitching rapidly.

There is a well-established set of appeasement signals that dogs display when they are feeling anxious and stressed. This starts with yawning, blinking, lip-licking and turning the head and body away from the perceived threat. If these signals are ignored, or the dog still feels threatened, they will try to distance themselves from the threat by walking or running away. If this is prevented – for instance, by a leash, or by being forced to confront the threat in a tight corner – then they may crouch with the ears flattened and the tail tucked under or might raise one fore-leg or roll over to expose their abdomen. If these signals too are ignored, or the threat persists, the dog will stiffen up, and growl or snarl with the teeth together and the upper lip curled back and trembling. This is a final warning sign that they intend to bite. This stereotyped series of signals is normally understood and results in de-escalation and the prevention of violence between dogs. If you recognise these signals and take note, confrontations and bloodshed can usually be avoided. If you have children, teach them about these signals. They are warnings children should not ignore.

Ideally, all dogs should frequently be given opportunities to meet other dogs off the lead in safe circumstances, away from roads and other major hazards. This is actually a legal duty for owners of pet dogs enshrined in the Animal Welfare Act (2006) (see www.gov.uk: Code of Practice for the Welfare of Dogs). Understandably, many owners find this difficult to organise and challenging too. However, left to themselves, aggression between dogs is actually not very common because most dogs understand other dogs' signals. Just like humans, dogs are naturally social creatures who thrive in groups. Their normal behaviour promotes cooperation within the group. It is dogs who are isolated and who miss the opportunities to bond with other dogs who most often become fearful and stressed in social situations. Those who are most likely to get into difficulties are those who have had little opportunity to meet and interact with other dogs, are permanently on a lead when not at home, and / or are picked up by their owners whenever they meet another dog. It is ironic that the owners of these dogs often feel their dogs are at awful risk because the other dogs are being deliberately aggressive, whereas the truth is rather the opposite.

However, if you and your dog on a walk meet another dog who is on a leash it is important to realise that the dog who is on a lead might feel uncomfortable and threatened (even if they are usually relaxed and gregarious with other dogs) because they are unable to display a full range of signals and behaviours to keep themselves safe. If you have excellent control of your own dog then you might be able to persuade your pooch to ignore the one who's on a lead, but many dogs unfortunately seem to revel in the opportunity to tease a dog that is on a lead by barking and taunting the leashed dog. I have a terrier who loves to meet new dogs for vigorous play-fighting sessions. However, she also tends to enjoy 'winding-up' dogs who are on a lead. Such situations can quickly degenerate into conflict if I am unable to get my own dog leashed to prevent a debacle.

Walking dogs with other people can be enormous fun and a really good communal experience but, as most seasoned dog owners will allow, there can be personal politics tangled up in this activity. When all the owners and all the dogs are familiar with each other the atmosphere might be very relaxed, but inevitably the relationships between dogs and owners tend to be in constant flux. A bitch might be on heat – that will change the dynamics of the group. Another dog might have been injured or be unwell for some reason. There might be a newcomer dog who is very anxious, or rather too bold. In my experience, dogs are better able, or perhaps simply more willing, to cope with this flux than many owners. However, there are multiple stakeholders in these interactions and sometimes leashing some or all the dogs is the most practical and least stressful approach to preventing problems. It is also important to be aware that dogs are pack animals; sometimes when a few dogs are together, if the emotional temperature rises, one dog might be picked on by all the others. Those who exercise their dog with others must be alert to this possible scenario.

Occassionally a pair of dogs will become sworn enemies. The cause is often opaque. It is tempting to blame the other dog, the other owner, or both. This is not helpful.

As a vet, I often meet dogs who are anxious, frightened, or in pain. My experience is that most dogs would prefer to avoid violence, but some feel they need to be aggressive when their signals are ignored. In the clinical setting we do our best to prevent fear, anxiety and violence, but there are situations where I find we have to use a muzzle on a dog to prevent my staff or myself being hurt. When we disarm a dog in this way, they obviously feel vulnerable. It is incumbent upon us to respect their feelings, to avoid inflicting unnecessary pain, and to try to swiftly relieve their distress so that in future they are less likely to feel the same way. This can be a difficult circle to square.

EXERCISE

Dogs are exceptionally athletic animals. For instance, greyhounds are said to be the second fastest land animal after the cheetah. They can reach speeds of more than 40 miles per hour during a 250-metre sprint. Dogs can also exhibit feats of extraordinary stamina; the sled dogs who take part in the Alaskan Iditarod race each winter pull a sled for over 100 miles a day over a course stretching for around 1000 miles! Working sheepdogs may run 40 or 50 miles in a day. These are elite athletes; but pet dogs are also capable of remarkable effort. Jemima, my terrier cross, can easily clock-up four hours or more of vigorous exercise when out for the day in the woods or the beaches of Kent. Their athletic prowess depends on their anatomy, physiology and attitude to the world. Clearly, some types are capable of more strenuous or sustained exercise than others; some are better equipped to swim and some more adjusted to sprint. But all dogs derive from the same basic stock; an animal evolved for rapid and sustained activity. A dog who is denied exercise is an animal whose welfare is at risk. How much exercise should I give my dog? Is there good evidence-based data available?

Most people who get a dog expect to walk it at least once a day and almost all healthy adult dogs enjoy this. Some small dogs, such as Chihuahuas, Pomeranians, Yorkshire Terriers and miniature Dachshunds, will be quite satisfied with 20 or 30 minutes daily but most other breeds will benefit from one or two hours each day. Of necessity, some of this walking must be done on the lead, especially if there are livestock in the vicinity, but most dogs do love off-lead exercise, especially in the company of other dogs or where they have the opportunity to explore or hunt. We know from studies in humans that for our physical wellbeing the more walking exercise we get the better, and that brisk walking seems to give greater benefits than ambling. Whether these observations are true for dogs has not been proven, but I think it's highly likely.

DIET

Dogs are essentially carnivores; their dentition is adapted to a carnivorous diet and they have a short gut that is unsuitable for the digestion of many plants. Nevertheless, in the long history of co-existence between dogs and humans, dogs dietary requirements have changed so that many authorities now consider them as 'omnivores' – who thrive on a diet more akin to that chosen by pigs, rats and humans. Obligate carnivores (cats for instance) must obtain certain nutrients from their diet; particularly taurine, arachidonic acid and Vitamin A. In contrast, dogs can synthesise these substances from dietary precursors. Twenty-two amino acids, the building blocks of protein, are required by dogs. Ten are essential – that is, they are absolutely required in the diet – the others can be synthesised by the dog (in their liver, by modifying other dietary amino acids, provided the overall protein content of the food is high enough).

Because dogs have evolved from the ancestor of the Grey Wolf, it is often sug-gested that the diets we feed our dogs should be modelled around the diet that wolves eat in the wild. Modern Grey Wolves hunt in packs. Their preferred prey are large hoofed mammals such as deer, elk, caribou and bison. When a pack successfully kills one of these large ungulates, they feast initially on the organ meat in the carcass, such as the liver, heart and spleen, followed by the large skeletal muscles. Over the next 48 hours, they will consume bone, tendon, cartilage and hide, leaving the rumen and unbreakable bones behind. In summer months their diet becomes more varied and includes small mammals, occasional birds, invertebrates and plant material. Fish form a tiny proportion of the diet of wild Grey Wolves.

When offered the opportunities, wolves and dogs favour fat and protein over carbohydrate in the diet. Both species appear to be well adapted to a feast and famine mode of eating, in which they are capable of gorging on food when it is available but can also go for days, even a week or more, with little or nothing to eat. Wolves will eat carrion when alternative foodstuffs are in short supply. Dietary fibre does not appear to be of much importance to either species. Contrary to popular belief, increasing fibre in a dog's diet does not appear to affect satiety to any marked degree.

Although they derive from a common ancestor, the DNA of the dog and the Grey Wolf differ in several respects. Many of the genetic differences appear particularly related to behaviour. Dogs have also acquired multiple copies of three key genes (AMY2B, MGAM & SGLT1), which code for digestive enzymes for dietary starches, and these genes appear to have originated in the dog population as agricultural techniques spread through human civilisations.

An awful lot of myth and misinformation circulates about canine nutrition. I do not wish to add to it. In my experience, much of the information provided by dog food manufacturers to their customers is confusing or trite and should be treated with scepticism. On the other hand, some of the material provided by those who disparage the dog food industry should also not be swallowed whole. It seems that many people chose how to feed their dog based on ideology rather than evidence. Vets are not alone in this.

Here, I will try to set down some key facts that clients should know about dogs and their diet.

1. Dogs are not strict or obligate carnivores. They are described by some biologists as 'facultative carnivores', meaning carnivores who are able to eat a

wide variety of other foods. The dog food industry and many vets describe dogs as 'omnivores' but personally I don't think that description is wholly accurate. Dogs can and do thrive on diets containing plant materials and carbohydrates but struggle on diets entirely free from meats and fish. Vegan diets for dogs exist but it is a challenge to make these completely balanced and highly palatable.

2. Dogs are metabolically programmed for a feast-and-famine dietary strategy in which the time intervals between meals are variable and can be very long (days). This strategy is found in their ancestry. A corollary of this is that dogs are willing and able to gorge at any one time, eating very large meals; their appetite is not well designed to regulate food intake. Consequently, any dog which is fed 'to appetite' will almost inevitably, and quickly, become fat. The amount of food fed to your pet must be regulated by you. This can be helped by regularly weighing your dog and measuring the amount of food you feed. Regular body condition scoring (by you, your vet or vet nurse) should guide you in this (Figure 5.2).

3. Dogs tend to prefer high protein and high fat foods. Given the option they do not tend to choose to eat carbohydrates. Their taste buds are tuned to recognise four basic flavours: sweet, sour, bitter and umami ('savoury'). There is disagreement in the scientific literature whether dogs can taste salt.

4. Dogs can live and thrive on both raw and cooked foods. Commercial pet diets make up over 90% of all food fed to companion dogs. This food is highly processed and cooked; usually bought as dry kibble or wet tinned. Many dogs are happy with both. Wet food tends to be somewhat more palatable, are obviously high in moisture (70–80% or more), usually are principally meat-based but often contain some carbohydrates. Dry foods keep better for longer and may be better for oral health (see later). Weight for weight, dry 'kibble' dog food is usually around four times as nutrient dense as wet tinned dog food. Kibble is almost always very high in carbohydrates.

5. Many dogs are delighted to be fed raw meaty diets. There are some potential hazards in feeding raw food, especially to the people preparing the food and to their families. This is because raw meats tend to have a high microbial content and some of these microbes, such as salmonella and some strains of *E. coli*, can be dangerous to people (especially children, the elderly, and those who are immunocompromised from disease or, for example, during

therapy for cancer). Raw foods also increase the risk of parasite transfer to dogs and family members. Raw bones when eaten by dogs can sometimes obstruct the gullet (oesophagus), small intestine (usually causing a vomiting syndrome) or the large intestine – leading to constipation. These obstructions can be fatal (see Chapter 7). However, the risks associated with cooked bones appear to be far greater than those due to raw bones.

6. There are downsides to cooking food for dogs because it can degrade some nutrients (especially vitamins). On the other hand, cooking increases the digestibility of many foods, both plants and meats. Archeologists are uncertain when cooking was first invented, or for how long people have been habitually cooking their food, but it seems this practice was widespread long before the Dog diverged from the ancestors of the Grey Wolf. In other words, dogs have been eating some cooked foods probably for as long as they have associated with people.

7. Most dog food sold in the UK is labelled 'Complete', which has a legal definition, meaning that it reaches a minimum standard and provides *all* the nutrients that dogs are believed to require in a healthy diet. However, this means that the dietary composition of these foods is constrained. Contrast this with human diets. You and I do not eat a complete and balanced diet at every meal. It is very possible for dogs to thrive on diets that are 'complete and balanced' over a given time period but in which individual meals vary widely in their nutritional content (just like people do).

8. If you want to understand what is in a dog food we are told to read the label: Ingredients are listed in order from highest to lowest, so if the top ingredient is 'cereals' and the second ingredient is meat and animal derivatives (minimum 4% chicken) then obviously the food is principally made from cereals. Try as I might, I find it is practically impossible to fully understand the constituents of any dog food from these labels (try this out yourself). For instance, one very popular brand of canned food, loudly proclaims on its packaging that it is made with 'Natural Ingredients*'. Further down the label is the opaque message '*Meat and Animal Derivatives, 36% Natural.' Helpful? Not.

9. All is not as it seems when you properly look at dog food. So, for example, the tinned food you have just bought might describe itself as 'Meaty chunks in jelly.' When you give the contents a cursory look it might appear to be largely

composed of chunks of cooked meat. But those chunks themselves are probably not 100% meat at all; they are more likely a processed composite, often primarily made from cereals with added meat meal that have been made to appear like chunks of meat. As another example, the can might be labelled 'With Lamb and Kidney' but when you examine the small print the composition is 'Chicken 42%, Lamb 4%, Kidney 4% . . .' When you add up the ingredients listed on cans of dog food you often find the numbers fall well short of 100%. I quizzed a few companies about this. Those that candidly replied to my emails admitted that the missing fraction in a can of dog food is usually added water (apparently, they are not obliged to state this on the label). These tricks are all legal but I would argue they are at best unclear, bordering on dishonest.

10. Dogs seem very capable of surviving and thriving on foodstuffs made from ingredients that are completely or largely absent from the diets of the Grey Wolf – such as the protein sources poultry, fish, soy and even insects, and other ingredients rich in carbohydrates that have a less than ideal protein composition (e.g. rice, potatoes, oats, wheat, tapioca, sugar beet, etc.). Many scientists argue that dogs have no need for carbohydrates at all. It is very conceivable that obesity in pet dogs is largely due to high carbohydrate intake. The role of carbohydrates in the development of human obesity is still disputed and contentious so it is no wonder we are even less sure about dogs.

11. Dogs can eat most foods which humans eat, with notable exceptions (see below). They can eat 'Dairy' foods, such as eggs, cheese, milk and yoghurt, although this does vary; some dogs are lactose intolerant. Most dogs are also perfectly able to digest gluten, which is present in many grains/cereals.

12. In a world where food resources are being stretched, where ever more land is being used for food production and where it is estimated that at least 30% of all the food grown / produced is wasted, it would seem wanton, even immoral, to throw away edible food that was purchased to feed people, whilst refusing to feed some or all of this surplus to dogs, based on a misunderstanding that human foods and 'table scraps' should not be fed to dogs. Obviously, if you do feed table scraps to your dog, you should reduce the amount of conventional dog food fed.

13. The costs of prepared dog food is quite variable. It is quite possible to feed dogs cheap and nutritious foods of relatively poor 'quality' and for the dogs

to nevertheless thrive. On the other hand, some 'boutique' dog foods can be four or five times the price of basic dog foods. It has been said that up to 20% of owners feed their dogs meals that are more costly than their own food!

14. Some dog food manufacturers produce diets that are supposed to be particularly suited to certain breeds of dogs, to dogs of certain type, or for particular market niches such as 'neutered bitches'. These vary in nutritional profiles. In most cases, genuinely robust scientific evidence does not support the concept that dogs fed such bespoke diets or 'high quality' foods live healthier or longer lives. On the other hand, it would be expected that diet will have a significant contribution to the development of disease in the dog just as in humans. Research into this issue is continuing.

15. Most dogs do not savour their foods. Interestingly, although dogs have very highly developed sense of smell, they have far fewer taste-buds than people do (on average a dog has about 1700 taste buds in the mouth whereas people have around 9000). In a large proportion of dogs, the food is gobbled down quickly. This behaviour too is likely a remnant behaviour from their ancestry – in a wolf-pack if a member fails to eat quickly the best of any prize kill will be devoured by another wolf before they know it. Only a few studies have been done to examine what dogs choose to eat when offered alternatives but these have consistently shown that dogs do not volunteer to eat carbohydrate-rich foods when protein and fat are available. Palatability of foods for dogs tends to be greater for wet foods fed warm rather than cold.

16. A small number of very good quality scientific studies have been published that have made serious and radical contributions to understanding the effects canine nutrition on health and longevity in pet dogs. One landmark study of a colony of Labrador retrievers, conducted by a dog food company and published about 20 years ago, showed that life-long and quite radical dietary restriction can significantly increase canine longevity. In this well-designed study, dogs who were fed only 75% of the food given to their matched controls lived on average nearly two years longer (13 years cf. 11.2 years). The dogs fed a restricted diet also developed fewer chronic diseases.

17. There are several common chronic diseases of dogs that appear to be ameliorated by feeding specific diets. Indeed, individualised nutritional therapy can be central in the treatment of certain conditions (see later).

However, you should beware that these veterinary prescription diets for problems such as bladder stones, kidney disease, diabetes mellitus, and gut problems are often very expensive indeed.

18. The food eaten by your pet dog will make a sizeable contribution to the environmental impact of that dog. Some journalists have suggested the environmental impact of an average dog is equivalent to, or more than, that of a Sports Utility Vehicle (SUV) driven 10,000 miles per annum, based on the fact that most that dog foods are rich in farmed animal protein. However, little robust data has been published and this estimate might be wildly inaccurate because it is actually very difficult to establish the exact meat content of most commercial dog foods. Although dogs fed commercial diets do tend to eat a higher proportion of meat than humans do, the meat in that diet is often principally that which is of low value to human consumers – 'offal' – organ meat such as liver, heart, lungs, meat and bone meal and mechanically recovered meat-scraps removed from the carcass as the final phase after conventional butchering. Generally, dry dog foods – in which the kibble has been created by a cooking process of extrusion – contain a much lower proportion of meat/poultry/fish than wet dog foods do.

19. Dogs fed 'Boutique' dog foods, sometimes designated as 'Gourmet', which contain a very proportion high of 'human-grade meat' might be expected to be healthier than dogs fed less expensive diets. However, as far as I can ascertain, there are no good scientific data to support this concept.

20. Developments in dog food nutrition continue. Recent work, for example, has shown that certain carbohydrates and soluble fibres can act as prebiotics, which can enhance the microbiome of the large bowel by promoting growth of 'good' bacteria in preference to those which are harmful. This aids digestion and gut health. Naturally occurring polysaccharides found in chicory, bananas, Jerusalem artichokes, and many other plants, contain inulin, or related dietary fibres known as fructooligosaccharides (FOS). These plants, or their extracts, are now being added to some dog foods.

SCAVENGING

When free, off lead, dogs love to explore the world around them. If they find something smelly, they might try to eat it. Dogs and their ancestors have always eaten some carrion. Decomposing material seems especially attractive to dogs. Most of the time this behaviour is not dangerous but occasionally can be; for instance, rotting compost can contain mycotoxins, which, if ingested in sufficient amounts, can cause tremors, convulsions and sometimes death. Scavenging and eating of unsuitable material, often described as 'dietary indiscretion', is probably the most common reason for a dog to develop vomiting and diarrhoea (signs of gastroenteritis) that may necessitate that you visit your vet (see later). Also, if a dog comes across a picnic-site or abandoned barbecue they will frequently find something hazardous they want to eat, such as part of a chicken carcass, corn-on-the-cob, or perhaps a peach-stone, all of which if swallowed might cause an acute obstruction in the gut (see later). There is no foolproof way to avoid this happening, but for repeat offenders we sometimes recommend they are fitted with a basket muzzle when off lead – this should prevent them eating such delicacies.

Wallace

One evening the police brought a dog in who had been hit by a car; an unusual mixed breed, probably part sight-hound, part terrier. Rough sandy brown coat, pale face, one black ear. He had been badly knocked about – a crushed tail, lacerations on the legs, a ripped dew-claw, and several missing or broken teeth. Judging by those teeth that remained, he was a young adult. He had not been castrated, very skinny, nervous, but seemed quite affectionate. No collar, no microchip.

Over the next few days, we gave the dog pain relief, tended the wounds, amputated the crushed tail and fixed him up. Despite sending word around to other vets, the RSPCA and via social media, nobody claimed this waif. He was adopted by Sinnead, our practice manager, who christened him Wallace.

Wallace is wonderful but wayward. He has a lovely goofy temperament but is utterly obsessed about food. Perhaps he had been living rough on the streets for some time? Sinnead used to regale us with stories of his food obsession. If toast popped out from the toaster Wallace would seize it and scarper. If butter, bread, apples, bananas, tomatoes or a cake were left unattended, even for a moment, Wallace was in there, quick as a cat, running off with his spoils.

Unfortunately, this proclivity to larceny did not stop at food.

One day, within a few months of being adopted, Wallace started to be sick. Some food was brought up, then pieces of wood, coal, a food wrapper. No foreign body was obvious on palpation of Wallace's abdomen, but vomiting continued the next day. Wallace was anaesthetised. My colleague passed an endoscope into Wallace's stomach where she found a tangle of rope and string. This had to be surgically removed. Wallace recovered.

A month or two later, Wallace presented with vomiting again. This time we found a partly digested dishcloth in his upper intestine. Surgery was necessary again. So it continued: bits of plastic, a piece of corn on the cob, a squash-ball. Each episode meant further surgery.

As I write this it occurs to me it has been more than a year since we have had to remove a foreign body from Wallace. I hope he's learned his lesson.

FOODS TO AVOID

- **Chocolate**: contains theobromine, can cause heart failure.

- **Garlic, onions, leeks, chives** (all members of the Allium family): are toxic, with garlic being the most potent – contain organosulphoxides, which are rapidly metabolised to compounds causing damage to the red blood cells.

- **'Vine fruits' – Grapes, raisins, currants and sultanas**: toxic substance not definitively identified, **possibly tartaric acid**. Can cause acute renal failure, variable / idiosyncratic toxicity.

- **Macadamia nuts**: non-fatal syndrome causing vomiting, diarrhoea, hind-limb weakness, staggering, 'drunken' gait, etc. (toxin unknown).

- **Nutmeg**: contains myristicin a neurotoxin that is a hallucinogen (in humans), causes tremors and seizures.

- **Xylitol**: artificial sweetener used in chewing-gum and other confectionary. Ingestion can be rapidly fatal in dogs due to a sudden drop in blood glucose, also liver failure.

- **Star fruit and rhubarb**: these contain oxalate, which, when absorbed from the gut, cause a sudden drop in circulating calcium. Actual poisoning from rhubarb stalks is almost unheard of, but if a dog were to eat the leaves where the oxalate concentration is much higher this would be dangerous. Signs of this type of poisoning include a depressed appetite, vomiting, lethargy, weakness, tremors, bloody urine, changes in thirst and urination.

Incidentally, contrary to some reports, avocado flesh is not toxic to dogs, although it does contain a substance, persin, which is toxic to some species.

Contrary to folklore, glutens from grains are not a source of digestive upsets to many dogs. Indeed, there are very few conditions in dogs which have been shown to be exacerbated by glutens (gluten enteropathy of Irish Setters, Border Terrier Gluten Dyskinesia).

Finally: it is not always immediately obvious that a foodstuff in your kitchen or on your plate might be toxic to your dog, but chocolate biscuits or cake, muesli, fruit cakes (containing vine fruits) and hot-cross buns (vine fruits, nutmeg) are common examples.

CARE OF THE TEETH

Dental disease is extremely common in dogs. It is much more common in small breed dogs though certain other breeds, particularly greyhounds, are also blighted. Severe disease is limited to only a small proportion of the dog population. There is a widespread belief in the veterinary profession that those dogs with bad teeth might be more prone to diseases of the heart and possibly other organs. This idea has been taught to veterinary undergraduates for years and might be true, but the concept is not very well supported by evidence. The cause of dental disease in dogs is not completely understood. However, there are similarities to, and differences from, human dental disease that are proving to be of a rich area for research.

Human dental disease is dominated by dental caries, holes in the teeth, which arise from the accumulation of food materials, especially sugars, on and between the teeth combined with the action of saliva, salivary enzymes and oral microbes. Human saliva is acidic. The oral environment is a complex ecosystem in which a slimy material, plaque, coats the mouth and covers the teeth. Plaque is a biofilm composed of vast numbers of bacteria and other organisms, including yeasts, comprising hundreds (!) of different species, embedded in a matrix of fluid and polymers. Microbes in biofilms are much more difficult to kill than free-living microbes. The microbes in plaque are believed to be central to the development of dental caries in people. Certain microbes are more commonly present on the surface of the teeth whereas others are more common below the gum-line, in the so-called gingival sulcus. Brushing the teeth can remove food debris and plaque and reduce the number of bacteria in the mouth. Regular brushing reduces dental disease.

Caries are not a common problem in dogs. Dental tartar or calculus, a yellowish-brown crusty material, is one of the most obvious signs of dental disease in dogs. Tartar is hardened dental plaque. It is formed from precipitation of minerals, principally calcium carbonate and calcium phosphate, from the breath, saliva, and plaque coating the teeth. In dogs, tartar most commonly develops on the outer surface of the upper cheek teeth and the inner surface of the lower cheek teeth. These areas are bathed in saliva from the salivary glands. The rough hard surface of tartar provides an ideal surface for further plaque formation. This leads to further calculus build-up, in layers, which compromises the health of the gingiva, the gums. Calculus can form both above the gum-line, and within the narrow crevice between the teeth and the gingiva, where it is referred to as sub-gingival. Deposits of tartar above the gum-line might be unsightly, but they seem to play no important role in the development of serious dental disease. Sub-gingival calculus, on the other hand, and separation of the gingival margins from the teeth creates pockets between the teeth and the support structures. As these pockets deepen, the periodontal membrane, which anchors the tooth root into the jaw, becomes damaged. Eventually, this causes loosening and loss of the teeth.

The anatomy of dogs' teeth, designed for tearing flesh, means that food particles do not regularly lodge in the mouth. Also, the saliva of dogs is alkaline (unlike humans) and the microbial community of canine plaque is very different to that of the human mouth, so obviously the processes by which dental diseases progress differ between these species. Nevertheless, regular brushing of dogs' teeth has been shown to reduce tartar, gingivitis – inflammation of the gums – and damage to the periodontal membranes. In this way, bad breath, dental pain and loss of the teeth can be prevented, or at least reduced.

So, the best way to look after your dog's teeth is to brush them every day. This is ideally done using a soft toothbrush or a finger-brush and tasty flavoured toothpaste formulated for the purpose. Unfortunately, although this strategy definitely works, in my experience most people do not persist in brushing their dog's teeth for more than a few weeks. This is because, unless you train your dog to accept this when she / he is a puppy, you might find it onerous, tiresome and difficult to do.

Various passive approaches to improving canine dental health have been studied. These tend to centre around the use of specially formulated dry kibbles or physical chews (usually made from cereals) that are particularly abrasive so that they scrub the surfaces of the teeth, sometimes combined with various polyphosphates, chemicals that bind oral calcium and reduce the substrate available to form dental tartar. Other approaches use antiseptics, such as chlorhexidine, which may favourably diminish the microbial load in dental plaque.

Another approach to dental health favoured by some is the provision of raw-hide chews, raw bones, pig-ears, cow-hooves, duck-necks or antlers – things that dogs naturally enjoy gnawing. In my experience, most adult dogs continue to enjoy chewing after they have grown up, so to me this approach sounds promising. Darwin has taught us that behaviours which are normal and widespread within a species are unlikely to cause them serious ill-health. Some veterinary dentists deride this approach because they allege these products can cause damage to the teeth including slab-fractures and gingival bruising; also, there is no doubt that some dogs can destroy almost anything they chew. Occasionally, they can break chunks off these chew-toys that might lodge in the gullet or the intestine. However, several good scientific studies have shown that the abrasion from gnawing does indeed effectively clean dental tartar from dogs' teeth. Moreover, the greater the frequency and duration of gnawing the better the oral health. I know many dogs who chew this kind of thing frequently, but I cannot vouch that they are always safe for all dogs. Veterinary dentists often say that dogs should not chew anything that you cannot dent easily with a thumbnail. I don't know if this rule of thumb (sorry) has the backing of rigorous science, but have found no well-designed studies that provide proof. My personal view is that the commercial dental treats made by the big dog food companies are frankly pretty useless because most dogs chomp them down with very little effort and in short order. If you find brushing your dog's teeth impossible or impractical, find a variety of robust things that they enjoy gnawing and give them the opportunity frequently.

Recently, a fascinating and well-designed randomised double-blinded trial performed in pet dogs was published that examined the effect of giving edible treats containing the brown algae, *Ascophyllum nodosum*, on plaque and dental calculus accumulation on the teeth, over a three-month period (*Frontiers in Veterinary Science*, 27 July 2018). Sixty pet dogs from five small-breeds of dog were involved. Beneficial effects were seen on all parameters studied in the treated dogs compared with those on placebo. The mechanism of action is not fully understood. *A. nodosum* is rich in compounds that seem to interfere with bacterial growth. These, and other compounds indigenous to the alga, are absorbed in the intestine and seemingly are excreted into the oral cavity via the saliva. In contrast to dental chews, these algal treats do not appear to act locally in the mouth.

As will be obvious, preventative measures to reduce dental disease in dogs are an active area of veterinary research.

CARE OF COAT, EARS AND CLAWS

Dogs groom themselves naturally, but excessive licking, nibbling and scratching of the skin is abnormal. Often these are the first signs of skin parasites or other skin diseases, so if you notice these behaviours see your vet. Most dogs enjoy being brushed. It aids the shedding of dead hair and can help to remove dirt, especially from long-haired dogs such as Spaniels and Retrievers. Brambles, burrs and pieces of twig can become entangled in the coat especially in breeds with long fine hair; when left the hair can become matted, which prevents the dog grooming itself properly. Nevertheless, few dogs require any more specialist or regular care of the coat than simple brushing. Hound breeds with smooth coats do not require brushing at all, although a wet hand stroked over the coat can help shed dead hair. Shampooing and clipping are performed more often for appearance's sake than for health reasons, although no doubt some dogs are delighted to be clipped (or stripped) in the warm months of Summer. It is worth noting that the pH of a dog's skin (around 6.8) is different from humans who have an 'acid mantle' pH nearer 5. For this reason, human shampoo, even baby shampoo, may not be ideal in this regard. For dogs that seem to need regular baths, such as those who habitually roll in smelly things on walks, it is probably best to use plain water or choose a proprietary dog shampoo. Medicated shampoos can also be very useful in the treatment of some canine skin diseases.

Many owners are very keen to keep their dog's ears clean, but in fact the dark slightly crumbly waxy material seen in the ear canal, cerumen, is a normal secretion.

It plays a healthy role in the physiology of the ear transporting cell debris from the outer surface of the ear drum, and the deep portion of the ear canal, to the outside. More than 70 years ago, in a classical experiment, which would probably no longer be permissible, it was shown that repeated wetting of the ear canal of dogs with water, or soap solutions, will actually swiftly cause inflammation of the ear (Witter, 1949). For this reason, I have always taken the view that if the ears are not inflamed, show no excessive discharge, give off no obvious odour, and are not causing the dog to scratch, shake the head, or exhibit pain, then they should not be cleaned. The causes of external ear disease, sometimes known as 'canker', are complex. This will be discussed further later in the text. Suffice to say, for now, routine ear care should consist mainly of benign neglect, unless your vet tells you otherwise.

Similarly, few dogs require routine care of the claws. Most dogs, who are frequently exercised on hard surfaces such as pavements and roads, will wear their claws. Some dogs, particularly those with very soft pads, such as dachshunds, those who are elderly suffering from joint disease, and those who are exercised solely on soft ground, may need their claws to be clipped from time to time. Your vet or veterinary nurse can do this at a routine visit.

NEUTERING

Some vets believe all dogs should be neutered. Many vets will open up a conversation with you about neutering at the first opportunity, because in some clinics they are keen on early neutering, so that bitches never experience a season at all. I hope to give you evidence, as we currently understand it, so that you yourself can decide what to do about the sex of your dog. Before that it is worth explaining the sexual cycles of dogs.

Dogs achieve sexual maturity from about 7 months of age in small breeds, whereas some large breed dogs are not sexually mature until well after a year of age. Once they have passed puberty, intact males (those that have not been neutered / castrated) will be willing, indeed keen, to mate with any female dog who is on heat. A healthy male who has the opportunity will often break out of a garden, or run off during a walk, then travel several miles to suitor a bitch. Obviously, this can cause trouble. Road accidents for instance.

Bitches after puberty, on the other hand, are only sexually receptive to males for a period of about 7–10 days whilst they are 'on heat' or 'in season'. Technically, this period is called oestrus. It is the period of time when eggs have been freshly delivered into the uterus awaiting fertilisation by sperm. In the week or so preceding oestrus the bitch is in a stage known as pro-oestrus. Owners who have an un-neutered bitch come to recognise this phase because she shows changes in behaviour and appearance. Male dogs will start to find her very attractive; indeed, she will become of more interest to dogs of both sexes, but bitches in pro-oestrus will not allow mating. During pro-oestrus the vulva tends to become swollen and a bloody discharge is seen. This stage of the sexual cycle is driven by increasing concentrations of hormones, known as FSH and LH originating from the pituitary gland at the base of the brain and oestrogen, which is secreted from the ovaries. Nests of cells within the ovaries, called follicles, are stimulated by these pituitary hormones. Each follicle will produce an egg. The vagina and uterus are prepared for mating and pregnancy by these hormones. Just prior to oestrus there is a dramatic change in the hormone signature of the body. At the onset of oestrus, the ovarian follicles rupture to deliver the unfertilised eggs (ova) into the uterus. This is ovulation. Oestrogen levels plummet. Progesterone concentration rise and this hormone begins to dominate. Soon after ovulation most bitches will become receptive to males and willing to mate. In the ovaries, the follicles that supplied the ova change to become tissues called corpora lutea. These are the source of progesterone.

If a bitch is mated and conceives, she will usually be pregnant for two months; the average is 63 days. This is a period during which progesterone levels are high.

If a bitch is not mated, or fails to conceive, this period is called dioestrus. During late dioestrus some bitches show moody or 'mothering' behaviour – as if they feel pregnant. This is known as 'pseudo' – or 'false-pregnancy'. In some cases, the bitch might produce milk in her mammary glands. Bitches displaying pseudopregnancy may make nests and become very attentive to their toys. Their appetite may become wayward. Certain drug treatments can be used to suppress these signs but for some dogs pseudopregnancy does seem to make them miserable (see p. 187).

After two months in dioestrus the progesterone concentrations fall. The bitch enters a stage called anoestrus. During anoestrus there is no sexual activity.

This phase lasts for a variable period – generally about 3–4 months. So, most bitches come into season twice a year, although this is by no means fixed. Large-breed dogs tend to come into season less frequently, often only once a year.

Recently, a dog owner described her dog's pro-oestrus and oestrus period to me as 'three or four weeks of purgatory'. It was quite clear to her that she wanted the dog to be neutered before this occurred again.

SO, WHAT ARE THE PROS AND CONS OF NEUTERING BITCHES?

Some owners believe it is unethical to neuter a bitch or a dog. I do not agree, but this is a practical text. If you have an ethical objection to neutering, I do not expect to persuade you otherwise.

Any bitch who is neutered obviously cannot conceive and raise puppies. One primary argument for neutering is to prevent unwanted pregnancies. This is certainly a good reason to neuter stray or free-roaming dogs. Interestingly, most canine pregnancies in the UK, and in many developed countries, appear to be intentional, although this issue has not been very thoroughly studied.

An important and consistent finding from multiple studies, in the UK and USA, is that neutered female dogs live longer lives that those that are intact. This effect is substantial. Neutered bitches, on average, live about six to 18 months longer than un-neutered ('intact') bitches. The reasons for this are complex and are not yet completely understood, but there are several conditions to which entire bitches are prone, which are less common or completely absent from neutered bitches. Intact bitches often develop womb infections later in life – known as endometritis and pyometra. These conditions are very common and extremely serious, often fatal (see p. 187). Thirty or forty years ago this was the most common surgical emergency in small animal practice in the UK. In one very large and fairly recent study, reported from Sweden, where very few bitches are neutered because it is considered to be unethical, 19% of intact female dogs had developed pyometra by 10 years of age (Jitpean et al., 2012). Mammary tumours also appear to be more common in bitches that are not neutered. The same Swedish study showed that 13% of 260,000 entire female dogs developed mammary tumours by the age of 10 years. It is important to say, however, that about half of these mammary tumours are benign (not cancerous). Also, a recent in-depth analysis in the UK concluded that the evidence to show a protective effect of neutering against mammary tumours is rather weak (Beauvais et al., 2012). Against this, it is worth reminding ourselves that lack of strong evidence itself does not mean that there is no effect. In veterinary medicine, unlike western human medicine, detailed evidence is absent, or weak, in many domains. There is a role for anecdote here. Neutering of bitches has become very common practice in the UK over the last few decades, whereas in the past it was performed much less frequently. My experience from 40 years of practice is that both malignant and benign mammary tumours are now rather infrequently seen in bitches; on the other hand, I saw many cases in the 1980s.

Tumours of certain other types appear to be somewhat more common in bitches who have been neutered compared with those that have not. The list includes osteosarcoma – a bone cancer; haemangiosarcoma – a cancer of the blood vessels; and lymphoma – a cancer of the immune system. These are all relatively common tumours, but the increased risk of a bitch developing these tumours is difficult to judge based on current data because the published studies have derived from only a few breeds of dog.

There is good evidence that a common joint problem, rupture of the cranial cruciate ligament, which affects the stifle (knee) joint, is substantially more common

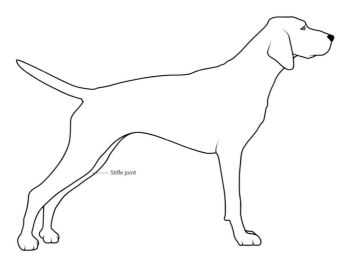

Stifle joint

Figure 5.2. The cruciate ligaments lie within the stifle (knee) joints. The kneecap or patella slides across the front of this joint.

in the veterinary profession changed to recommend earlier neutering, from about 6 months of age. More recently, the pendulum has swung back again, because robust and rather consistent data has been published that suggest that, especially in large breeds of dog, orthopaedic problems such as hip dysplasia and cruciate disease are much more common after early neutering, so many vets now recommend that dogs should not be neutered until their long-bones have stopped growing. This will vary with breed; so, for instance, a Cocker Spaniel will reach adult body size by 9 months of age but a Great Dane may not do so until 18 months or later.

CONVENTIONAL OR 'KEYHOLE' SURGERY?

Laparoscopic or 'keyhole' ovariectomy is a technique becoming more widespread throughout the veterinary profession. Those who offer this approach claim there are numerous advantages:

- smaller wounds

- reduced pain

- less risk of wound breakdown

- a faster recovery time

- reduced stress.

However, there are critics who warn that a keyhole approach can lead to big problems hidden behind small holes. I believe laparoscopic spaying is a preferable technique, but few studies have been published to resolve this issue once and for all (I've listed a couple in the references). Keyhole surgery is considerably more expensive than conventional open surgery because it requires costly equipment and a highly skilled surgeon. I have no doubt that this price differential will decrease and laparoscopic neutering will become a much more common approach in future.

WHAT DO VETS DO WHEN THEY NEUTER A BITCH?

Prior to the operation your vet will examine your dog carefully to ascertain that they appear healthy. Particular attention will be paid to listening to their heart and lungs with a stethoscope, palpating the pulse rate and quality, examining the breathing and assessing body condition.

The dogs must be fasted for at least 8–12 hours before surgery. Drinks are permitted except in the hour or two before the operation.

Many vets will recommend that blood samples are taken before surgery to evaluate the dog's biochemical health and look for evidence of anaemia. They will need your permission for this. However, this blood sampling can add considerable expense to the procedure and the value of this sort of 'screening test' is often quite low (controversial – see later), so if you are working to a tight budget it is worth asking your vet if they can justify the need for pre-surgical blood tests. Listen carefully to their answer before making a decision.

Neutering of a female dog is usually performed when the bitch is midway between seasons. Neutering involves abdominal surgery, which is called a laparotomy. The most common technique used in the UK to neuter a bitch is ovario-hysterectomy in which both ovaries and the uterus are removed. This is done under general anaesthesia, which may come in the form of intravenous or gaseous agents, usually both. During the anaesthetic your dog will be completely unaware of what is going on. A tube will be inserted into their windpipe to allow the administration of oxygen and other gases. Various monitors to assess heart rate, blood pressure, breathing, oxygen saturation, depth of anaesthesia, etc., will be used. The surgical incision is usually made in the midline of the abdomen, just behind the 'belly button' (umbilicus), although a 'flank' approach – through the side of the abdomen can be employed. This surgery requires a high degree of skill and is certainly not without risk, which is why vets take it very seriously. Many vets, in candid moments, will tell you that their single greatest professional fears involve serious complications after neutering a female dog. The chief risks involve haemorrhage from the blood vessels supplying the reproductive tract. In rare cases this can be fatal. Other complications include swelling of the abdominal wound, localised wound infections, wound breakdowns and in some cases a failure to completely remove the reproductive tissue. Complications are more common in large bitches, especially if they are overweight. Some minor complications occur in about 10% of cases. Surgical complication rates are much lower for highly experienced surgeons.

It is technically quite possible to neuter a female dog simply by surgically removing the ovaries. Ovariectomy is a less radial procedure than ovario-hysterectomy.

In such cases, the uterus will gradually shrink away to become vestigial. This approach is commonly employed on the continent of Europe and is what is done during laparoscopic neutering too, but is not fashionable with UK vets, for reasons I cannot fathom. We offer all these different techniques in our practice.

A few vets recommend that bitches be neutered by surgically removing the womb (uterus) leaving the ovaries intact. This is not a popular technique in the UK. I have not discovered any recent peer-reviewed scientific articles about the technique. In theory, the bitch will continue to show reproductive cycles but will be unable to conceive.

NEUTERING MALE DOGS

Castration of the male dog is a much simpler, quicker, cheaper and less risky procedure than neutering a bitch. As for the bitch, the vet will perform a pre-surgical clinical examination to make sure they feel the dog is a good surgical risk. Again, the procedure itself is done under general anaesthesia with similar monitoring. A surgical incision is usually made in the skin in front of the scrotum. Some surgeons remove the scrotal sac completely. Post-operative complications; including bleeding, wound swelling, etc., do occur, but are less frequent than in the case of the bitch.

For both of these procedures pain relief is central to good technique. Drugs to reduce discomfort are given, usually about half-an-hour before the surgery, in a 'pre-med'. The drugs that anaesthetise your dog also act as pain-relievers. Additional analgesics are given during and after the surgery to speed recovery with a minimum of discomfort. Some dogs require much more analgesia than others, so an essential part of the nursing of these animals after neutering is assessment of their pain level so that appropriate pain-relief can be given in a timely fashion. For this reason, after a bitch or dog is neutered they will not be permitted to go home until thorough post-surgical assessments have been performed. When the dog goes home, he/she may have to wear an 'Elizabethan collar' (famously christened 'the cone of shame' in the film *Up*), which is a sleeve fitted over the head to prevent the dog licking the surgical wound. Some surgeons use intra-dermal sutures that are buried out of sight, but many surgeons close the wound with conventional sutures or sterile metal staples.

After your dog has been neutered, they need time to recover. Complete recovery takes a few days for males, two or three weeks for females. Your vet or veterinary nurse will explain the recovery process to you. Within 24 hrs of surgery most young patients will be eating and fairly bright but they may be disorientated and feel pretty miserable at first. They will have some mild discomfort. The skin wound might be tender. They should not be exercised in the first day or two except to go to the toilet. Most vets like a post-operative check to be done on the patient within 2–5 days. At that point, provided healing is proceeding well, the vet or nurse will advise you further about exercise. Skin sutures, or staples, if present, are usually removed 10–14 days after surgery.

After neutering a dog's metabolism slows down. This is particularly true in bitches. All neutered dogs should be fed less than they were before being neutered – on average a 10% reduction in calories is required.

PREVENTING WEIGHT GAIN AND OBESITY

Obesity is an excess of body fat so that it compromises health. **The single most important thing you can do to prolong your dog's life is to prevent them getting fat**. Obese dogs have markedly reduced lifespans to the extent of 2–3 years. Moreover, dogs who are obese, or overweight, are likely to develop other diseases which shorten and often dramatically reduce the quality of their lives; there is strong evidence that osteoarthritis, diabetes mellitus, cancer and heart diseases, amongst others, are much more common in dogs who are overweight. Some authorities consider obesity itself to be a chronic and ultimately incurable disease.

There is disagreement about how common obesity is in dogs but estimates suggest between 25–60% of adult dogs in the UK are overweight or truly obese. A well validated body condition scoring system (BCS) exists for dogs in which animals are graded on a scale from 1–9, with points 4 or 5 being considered ideal. Each point above the ideal represents a 10–15% increase in body weight, so a dog scored as 6 or 7 is definitely overweight, those scored higher than this are obese. This system, which is almost universally used by companion animal vets, is illustrated in Figure 5.3.

When asked about their dog, more than half of the owners of obese dogs do not consider them to be overweight. This misperception is important because to

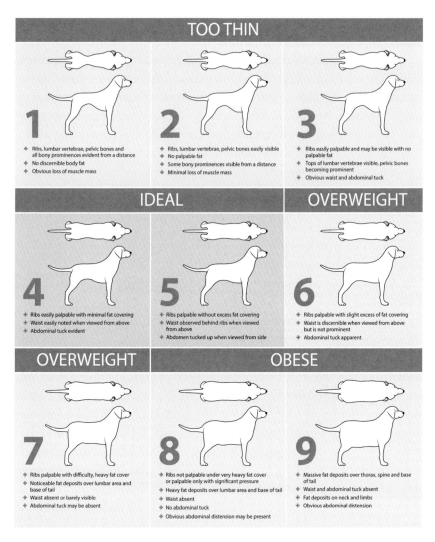

Figure 5.3. Body condition scoring.

maintain optimum health owners must have a correct appreciation of the normal body shape for their dog. If obesity becomes considered to be normal then the welfare of the whole dog population is at risk.

The cause of obesity is almost always an intake of food and calories in excess of the needs of the body. It follows that obesity can be avoided if a dog is never fed to excess, but this blunt statement is very much complicated by the individual circumstances of the dog and its environment. Firstly, the calorific needs of dogs of the same weight and age can differ by a factor of two or more. Secondly, there are some very strong predispositions to obesity. For example, certain breeds, including the Labrador Retriever, Pug, English Bulldog, Shetland Sheepdog, Yorkshire Terrier, Cocker Spaniel, Cavalier King Charles Spaniel and Rottweiler are prone to obesity, whereas Greyhounds, Salukis and other sighthounds are much less likely to become overweight. Other factors that have been documented to predispose to obesity include feeding the dog to appetite (or ad lib), feeding 'leftovers' or table scraps, feeding dogs from the table, giving in to 'begging', and regularly giving treats, including 'dental chews'. Older and heavier owners are more likely to have dogs who carry too much weight. Dogs who have restricted exercise are more likely to be overweight probably because they have a lower metabolic rate. Neutered dogs, particularly bitches, are liable to gain weight rapidly in the months after neutering, so it is incumbent upon every owner to reduce the food they give to their dogs following neutering. A good vet should warn you about this when you have your dog neutered.

A few dogs that are obese have other medical problems, such as hypothyroidism, and in a small proportion of cases obesity stems from the long-standing use of drugs (especially corticosteroids or drugs to treat epilepsy – see later).

In order to prevent obesity every puppy should be weighed regularly as it grows up. Healthy normal growth curves for dogs have been published. These are freely available on the web. The most comprehensive scientific work looked at the growth of more than 6 million dogs in five general size categories with an adult weight of less than 40 kg (Salt et al., 2017). Body condition scoring and weighing should be done at every veterinary examination, and owners should be taught how to do this themselves (see page 95, Figure 5.2). All owners of new puppies should appreciate that dogs should never be fed ad lib and that they should not be fed 'to appetite'. Once past puppyhood, a dog should only be fed once or twice a day. For those people who are training their dogs using positive rewards the weight/volume of food required for each day should be measured out and all rewards/treats should be taken from this.

If a dog has become overweight, the sooner this is recognised and acted upon the better. Initial assessment is best done by a vet or a veterinary nurse. Usually, this will centre around a detailed dietary history, evaluation of exercise; frequency, duration, and intensity, as well as objective measurements of the body weight and BCS. Laboratory investigations are rarely required. The dog food companies are keen to promote 'weight-loss' diets that have been specially designed to be fed to overweight dogs. These tend to be relatively high in protein and may have enhanced levels of some essential nutrients such as L-Carnitine and conjugated linoleic acid. Some of these diets are rich in fibre (in the hope that bulking the food will increase satiety) although the value of this is doubtful. However, in many cases it is quite acceptable simply to begin a weight loss programme by giving the usual diet but reducing the food volume / weight offered to the dog by 20% for a month. The aim would be for body weight to fall by 1–2% a week. If the calorific value of the food being given to the dog is known, a good starting point is to feed 80% of resting energy requirements (RER), which is calculated by the following formula:

Daily RER (calories) = 70 × ideal weight in kg

e.g. Daily RER for a 10 kg dog is 700 calories

80% of Daily RER for 10 kg dog is 560 calories

Useful tips

For owners and carers, it is psychologically much easier to feed smaller meals if the food is given in a smaller bowl. This is proven. A trick used in restaurants. I recommend to all my owners that if their dog is overweight that they should begin that day by buying a smaller bowl. Buying a smaller food scoop also helps. Dogs themselves have some ability to count, but are not adept at measuring volume. Some good science confirms this.

Increasing exercise is unlikely on its own to contribute much to a weight reduction programme, but if this increase is maintained over time, it should go some way to increasing your dog's metabolic rate. As a dog loses weight, they tend to become more active, thus completing a virtuous circle.

Dogs can get enormous pleasure, and more exercise, if they have to work for their food. Providing a large part, or all, of the daily ration in a puzzle-toy or crammed into a 'Kong' can keep dogs amused for hours. Ian Dunbar, the vet, behaviourist and dog-trainer, recommends using wet kibble pressed into the hollow centre of a marrowbone then frozen in your freezer.

Almost all owners feed their dog some treats. Both parties gain pleasure from this. It seems mean to ban treats entirely. If these treats are replaced with kibble (or other food) taken from (*not* in addition to) the daily ration, that change in itself can make a major contribution to a diet. 'Dental chews' based on cereals and sold as dental health products can be very calorie-rich, equivalent to 10% or more of the daily RER (resting energy requirement). They are usually principally carbohydrate and, in my experience, consumed very rapidly.

The success of weight control regimes depends on careful monitoring (weight and BCS) and readjustment repeatedly over months. Unfortunately, for most dogs that do become overweight, restrictions and monitoring must usually be lifelong thereafter.

REGULAR VETERINARY CHECK-UPS AND BOOSTER VACCINATIONS

I believe every dog who appears to be in good health should nevertheless have a veterinary examination at least every 6–12 months. Remembering that dog's lives are much shorter than ours, it is only sensible that routine check-ups should be done as least as frequently as you see a dentist.

Vets often sell routine check-ups as 'Vaccination Booster Visits' because most owners are aware of the value of vaccination protection against parvovirus, and other contagions, but in fact vaccination might be the least useful part of this visit. The principal aim of these check-ups is to monitor dogs' health as they age so that any illnesses can be identified early on in their development.

Each clinician will have their own routine for a visit of this sort. For myself, I use this opportunity first to check body weight and to confirm whether their BCS is in the normal range (i.e. 4–5 on a nine-point scale – see page 96, Figure 5.3 for a refresher). You will recall that many dogs are overweight or obese and that this problem has important ramifications for their health and wellbeing (see p. 95). It is not unusual for body weight to increase over time stealthily so that owners are only dimly aware; regular objective measurement of body weight and BCS allows this to be identified. Contrariwise, if an animal loses weight gradually over several months this too can go unnoticed by clients. Unexpected weight loss is often a sign of serious unrecognised disease so, once we know it is occurring, we can take steps to investigate the cause. Once a dog's weight and BCS are known, discussions around nutrition and diet may be called for.

At these routine visits, clinicians will enquire about appetite, thirst, urination and defecation habits, because any abnormalities in these might indicate a loss of health. Similarly, they will ask about exercise/activity and whether the dog has a cough, exhibits breathing difficulties or shows evidence of stiffness/lameness.

A clinical examination will be performed, particularly to evaluate vital signs (colour, pulse rate and rhythm, heart sounds, breathing effort and rate, etc.). Heart sounds are listened to carefully because heart disease becomes common in middle-aged and older dogs. One of the earliest signs of heart disease in dogs is a murmur, an abnormal sound heard with a stethoscope. The normal heart makes two sounds in quick succession each time it beats: lub-dup, lub-dup. A heart murmur is a new sound superimposed on this rhythm, usually between these two sounds. Quiet murmurs are common but often of little or no significance, whereas louder sounds tend to imply more serious disease. Certainly, loud heart murmurs should never be ignored. The body temperature might be taken (although in the absence of other signs of illness many vets choose not to do this to minimise the dog's distress). Your clinician will also examine the mouth, teeth, eyes, ears, coat and skin and may make brief neurologic and behavioural assessments. I find this is a great opportunity to check for fleas using a flea comb.

Routine visits of this kind are an ideal opportunity for you, the client, to ask about anything that concerns you, be it in the realms of health or behaviour. I usually also like to discuss parasite control. Whilst it has become fashionable in the veterinary profession to advise that broad-spectrum anti-parasitic agents be given to all dogs frequently throughout their lives, I personally do not believe this is justified or good clinical practice. Most dogs most of the time have no serious parasite infestations. When such infestations are present, they ought to be identified and treated, but the blanket and continuous use of anti-parasitic agents seems to me both wanton and illogical. Blanket use of similar agents in agriculture has caused serious environmental damage and also led to drug-resistance in the parasites. All these agents can potentially have deleterious effects on the species around us, which may include bees, butterflies, fish-stocks and birds. Why contaminate the world with these potent chemicals if there is no clinical need?

WHAT ABOUT BOOSTER VACCINATIONS?

In Chapter 3, I discussed primary (puppy) vaccinations that, in the UK, are normally directed against Distemper, Adenovirus, Parvovirus, Leptospirosis and often Kennel Cough. An additional 'booster' vaccine against these agents is usually given at around 12–15 months of age. Thereafter, the vaccine manufacturers now recommend that further 'boosters' against Distemper, Adenovirus and Parvovirus (DAP) are given at three yearly intervals. This is controversial. There is good evidence that many dogs, probably a large majority, remain protected against these viruses for many years, probably often for life, even if they are never given 'boosters'. There are ways of testing this using blood samples to measure the concentration of protective antibodies a dog has, and indeed if you wish it, vets will usually be delighted to do this. However, the cost of performing these 'serological titre tests' tends to be higher than the cost of the vaccine itself.

In contrast to the DAP viral vaccines, the duration of protective immunity to the bacterial infection Leptospirosis after vaccination is rather short-lived. Annual revaccination is advised. Similarly, the duration of immunity to *Bordetella bronchiseptica* and parainfluenza (the agents in the 'Kennel Cough' vaccine) is also such that annual revaccination is generally recommended.

Rabies vaccination is not routinely done in the UK because the disease has been absent for a century. However, dogs who travel elsewhere in the world will need to be vaccinated (see later).

HOLIDAYS

Some dogs love to go on holiday, others get stressed by the change in circumstances and routine. If you're planning a holiday away from home, here are a few things to think about. Is your dog used to travelling? Do they get travel sickness?

Most dogs can be trained to cope with travelling by car (see Chapter 4, p. 43). For those who do suffer from travel sickness, there are drugs that can help to mitigate this but long journeys and road trips should be avoided. I would hate to subject my dog to this day after day.

Where are you going and what will you be doing when you get there?

If you have a vigorous dog an active holiday in the UK could be ideal, but a hillwalking holiday during the lambing season might be a foolish choice. Many beaches are closed to dogs in high season, but in most areas there will still be somewhere dogs are allowed to exercise off lead. Some hotels and guesthouses are 'dog friendly' but these are not as widespread as you might wish. Certainly, don't assume you can take a dog with you into catered accommodation. Self-catering cottages, flats, etc., on the other hand, are very often quite willing to allow 'well-behaved' dogs. If you want to lounge by a pool on the Algarve, or to visit museums in Liverpool then neither you nor the dog would enjoy the experience together. Whatever your choice, if the dog would be bored, stressed, or a nuisance then think about kennelling or perhaps a house-sitter to look after your hairy friend whilst you enjoy the break.

Are there likely to be particular health hazards that you should plan for?

In the UK, there are few particular health hazards not mentioned elsewhere in this book, but it might be wise to consider whether your dog might be exposed to ticks, which are most prevalent in rough terrain such as the New Forest, the Lake District and the Scottish Highlands. If you exercise your dog anywhere where ticks are common it is prudent to examine them regularly for ticks that attach very firmly to the skin and feed on blood. At the time of attachment, the tick is only 2–3mm across, dark and hard. Removal is easy using a tick hook, a very nifty and cheap device (see Figure 5.4). Other methods of removal are not recommended because they can leave the mouthparts of the tick behind that can transmit disease. As it feeds, the tick body enlarges to become a bloated grey/blue sack up to the size of a small olive. If you find engorged ticks of this description on your dog they will have been feeding for some days. Various products are excellent to repel and / or kill ticks – get advice from your vet.

HOLIDAYS ABROAD

If you want to take your dog abroad, you should do some research about your destination(s) to find out if there are any parasitic infestations that you might need to plan for.

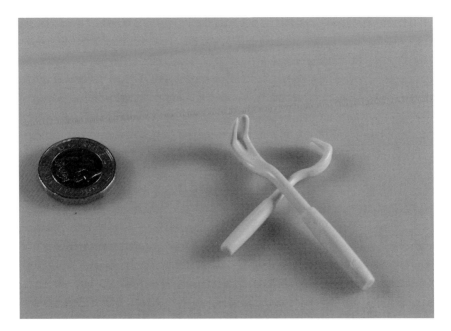

Figure 5.4. Tick hooks. These come with full instructions.

Heartworm (*Dirofilaria immitis*), which is transmitted from dog to dog by mosquito bites, is found in much of southern Europe, including Portugal, Spain, France, Italy, Croatia, Serbia, Greece and Turkey. The parasite is not present in every region of these countries. Prevention of heartworm can be simply achieved by the use of various drugs (usually those containing Selamectin or Moxidectin) applied to the skin once a month for three months, starting *before* you travel out of the UK. When in these countries, avoiding contact with mosquitoes is advisable but not always easily achieved.

Red-water (Babesiosis) is a group of inter-related conditions in which the red blood cells of the dog are parasitised. The disease is called red-water because, when severe, it causes the urine to appear bloody. It is transmitted by various tick species that are found on the European mainland (particularly *Dermacentor reticulatus*). The disease is most common in central and southern Europe (although has recently occurred in the UK in Essex). Tick repellents and drugs that kill ticks (see above) are effective at preventing the disease but if ticks are found attached to a dog they should be removed (see p. 102). The dog should be monitored for signs of illness in the following weeks.

Leishmaniasis is a nasty and basically incurable disease caused by a protozoa (*Leishmania infantum*), not found in the UK, which is carried by sandflies, typically found in southern Europe. Sandflies are biting insects that, despite their name, are particularly common in woodland. They are most usually active in the evening. If you travel to an area where the disease is found, you should keep your dog indoors from early evening and overnight. There are vaccines available against Leishmaniasis that are not perfect but might be an option to consider, particularly if you travel to an affected region frequently or for a long period.

Also, when going abroad you need to research carefully the legal requirements for bringing your dog into that country.

Travel from the UK to Europe with your dog used to be relatively simple as a result of the PETS passport system. However, since 1 January 2021 this has become some-what more complicated and certainly a good deal more expensive than it was.

Firstly, all dogs must be microchipped and the microchip registered to you the owner. This is now a legal requirement for all UK dogs anyway (see p. 52).

Secondly, the dog must have been vaccinated against Rabies (which must have been done when the dog was 12 weeks of age or older), and this vaccination must have been done at least 21 days before travelling.

Thirdly, you will need an Animal Health Certificate (AHC) from your vet, which must be issued no sooner than ten days before you travel.

The first two requirements are relatively easily accomplished but the Animal Health Certificate is causing headaches for vets and owners alike. This is a com-plicated ten-page document that is quite onerous to fill out. Only vets qualified as local veterinary inspectors can issue an AHC. Your vet will do this at an appoint-ment but often they will need a long appointment to complete this. Warn your vet in advance that this is what you are attending for. The vet will want you to bring some documentation. I have seen prices from £99–£250. An AHC will last for up to four months.

Incidentally, for travel to Northern Ireland (or the Republic) with a dog you will need to follow the same rules because under the Brexit Agreement, Northern Ireland, in this regard, is considered to be part of the EU.

Take the AHC with you wherever you travel in Europe with your dog.

Before returning to the UK from Europe with your dog it must be treated with a drug effective against the tapeworm Echinococcus. This is usually given as a tablet and must be administered between 5 days and 24 hrs before returning to the UK. You have to attend a vet for the drug to be given and certification obtained.

For travel to countries outside of Europe with a dog there are a huge range of different rules which can apply. Do not expect your vet to know what they are. Look at the relevant website or contact the embassy or consulate of the country well before you intend to travel, or leave your dog behind.

KENNELLING OR HOUSE-SITTERS

If you decide to put your dog in a boarding kennel whilst you are away from home for a while, finding convenient and sound kennels can be a challenge. Your first instinct might be to use the web for advice. Be wary of using internet recommendations exclusively. Ask friends, colleagues and family for recommendations. Ask your vet or the other staff at the practice too. Vets sometimes have to be a bit cagey about giving recommendations because they have to be seen to be even-handed and won't want to upset kennel businesses who might be clients. All kennels must be registered with the local authority and inspected. They must properly provide for your dog's welfare, as follows.

- Each dog must have access to their own sleeping area at all times.

- Sufficient space to allow them to sit, stand at full height, lie down fully, stretch out, wag their tail, walk and turn around.

- At least one daily walk outside of their kennel.

- Their own separate kennel, unless you specifically ask for your own dogs to be allowed to share.

- Access to toys.

- Kennels who aspire to higher standards will offer two (or more) walks per day each lasting for at least 20 minutes.

A visit to the kennels to take stock of their facilities, their service and staff is definitely a good idea. Ask the staff questions, such as why they work there and how they deal with sick animals, etc. Many kennels are run by people with a veterinary background and / or a thorough grounding in animal handling. When you think you've found a good place, book your dog(s) in for a couple of nights as a trial run. I've used several different boarding kennels in my time. Feedback from the staff afterwards has given me quite an insight into how the visit has gone. When the staff forgot my dogs' names that did not go down well. One kennels I used was definitely a big hit with the dogs because they were always absolutely delighted to go back and the staff got to know them well.

I've often used house-sitters instead of a kennels. Obviously, you must find someone trustworthy who likes dogs and knows about them. I have found this can work well but I'm lucky because when I was an academic it was easy to find a vet student willing to do the job for a handy sum. I always said they were free to use the house and its contents as their own. On a couple of occasions this meant I came home to an empty fridge and freezer with only a tin of pilchards left in the larder (!), but the dogs always seemed to have been well cared for. As a clinician in practice, again, it's been a piece of cake because my nurses are often delighted to be paid to live for a week or two in a decent gaff close to the practice.

I always advise my friends to ask at their vets if they are in two minds about how their dogs should be looked after whilst they are away. In my experience, many veterinary nurses like to house-sit. Obviously, they will expect remuneration.

VET LOYALTY SCHEMES

Loyalty schemes are run by many veterinary practices and on the face of it often seem to be a very good deal indeed. For a regular monthly fee, the schemes usually cover you for 'routine health care', such as annual vaccination visits, regular prophylaxis against parasites, a 'health check' at six monthly intervals, and often some discount on drugs, non-routine visits, surgical procedures and diets. What's not to like?

These schemes are designed to bind you to the practice and encourage you to use the practice frequently, but might not always represent ideal veterinary care. Let me give you an example to think about.

It is definitely good practice to treat all young dogs for roundworms (because virtually all young dogs will have a worm burden (see page ...). It is also good practice, in areas where lungworm are prevalent (some locations in south-west England, south Wales and parts of the south east), to treat young dogs for that parasite, because it can sometimes be deadly. On the other hand, most adult dogs do not have a worm burden, or skin parasites, most of the time and the drugs used to treat dogs for parasites, whilst very safe for people and dogs, are deliberately designed to be very toxic to insect life. It is likely that routine use of these drugs offers very little if any benefit to most dogs and may inadvertently be killing beneficial insects such as bees, butterflies, ladybirds, etc. Even if you don't personally like insects, these drugs might be having serious knock-on effects on the environment. It would be much better if such drugs were used strategically. In other words, anti-parasitics should really only be used where your vet has good evidence that your dog needs treatment, ideally from lab tests, or at least a careful individualised risk assessment. **Dogs that swim regularly must not be treated with sprays or 'spot-on' anti-parasitic agents because the drugs wash off into the water.** The environmental effects of these drugs can be horrendous; for instance, the drug imidacloprid, is widely used as a 'Spot-on'. The routine 250mg dose applied to a large dog such as a Labrador is the same as the LD50 for around 50 million honeybees (based on an LD50 of 5ng/bee)! That is not a misprint. Other insects are probably just as susceptible (LD50 is the dose found to kill 50% of the test animals). Loss of pollinators and other insects threatens agriculture and the whole biosphere (Goulson, 2013). Insectivorous birds, like swifts, starlings, swallows and thrushes are in steep decline. These drugs should not be treated as trivial.

Don't blithely treat your dog every month with these drugs. At your routine appointments ask your vet to examine your dog for parasites and to make a careful risk assessment before prescribing anti-parasitic agents. Flea treatment should be used only in animals with fleas, or flea allergic dermatitis, or where they are at high risk of becoming infested, such as a dog going to kennels. Similarly, ideally dogs should be treated for roundworms and lungworms only where lab tests indicate they have a worm burden, or where a proper risk-assessment has been done. In most of the UK, tapeworm infestations in dogs are uncommon and do not cause ill-health, so routine use of drugs against these parasites is generally pointless. Similarly, ticks are not a serious pest in most part of the country, so there is no need to treat most dogs against these unless you live in or are visiting a tick hot-spot.

Recently, several of the veterinary bodies in the UK came together to produce an easy-to-follow document on this issue: **Responsible use of parasiticides for cats and dogs**. You can download this plan at www.bva.co.uk. All companion animal vets in the UK should now be following this plan, designed to minimise the environmental impact and unnecessary use of these agents.

The European Scientific Counsel for Companion Animal Parasites (ESCCAP) sounds like a respectable body from which to get disinterested information about this subject. Unfortunately, the body is entirely funded by the veterinary drugs companies and tends to recommend monthly treatment of virtually all dogs for parasites despite the fact there is very little scientific evidence for these recommendations and contrary to the advice of the BSAVA, BVA and BVZS.

Some vets will be taken aback if you ask them to justify their routine use of anti-parasitic agents but, as a rule, vets are thoughtful. A decent vet will try to manage parasites without damaging the environment. They should be happy to talk this through with you.

At the risk of repeating myself, **be sceptical, question everything**. You owe it to your dog. A good vet will be delighted to have a grown-up conversation about your dog's health.

Part II

ILLNESS

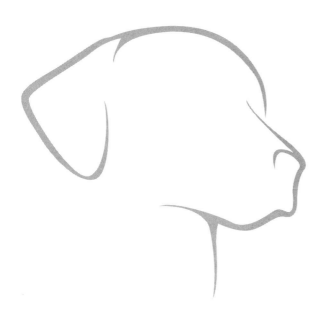

will be seen by a vet you and your dog already know and feel you can trust. Before you visit, you might want to take a few minutes to collect your thoughts about your dog's problem. Sometimes it is helpful to write down bullet points you want to remember.

Here are a few simple ways to help the appointment go smoothly.

Try to arrive on time for your appointment. I know we vets often run late. Usually, this is because another patient has a complicated or difficult problem, but sometimes it is because other clients have arrived late.

If your dog can be defensive or snappy, please let the staff know, especially anyone who will handle the dog. If you have a muzzle for your dog, please bring that and perhaps fit it to your dog before going in to the consulting room.

If your dog tends to bark or can be aggressive to other dogs then for everyone's benefit you are often best to wait outside for your appointment.

If you have brought your dog because they seem unwell, try to avoid complicating the appointment with additional issues such as asking about vaccinations, parasite control, neutering or an odd patch of hair loss.

Don't bring along another pet for an unrelated issue 'while you're here'.

For the sake of this illustration, let's assume you have a 4-year-old male neutered Cockapoo called Harry.

The vet will start the consultation by greeting you and your dog then asking rather general 'open' questions such as: 'What can I do for you today?' or 'What seems to be the trouble?' This type of question is asked so that you can provide a really clear steer to the consultation. So, for example, if Harry has suddenly developed a limp, or a cough, a swelling, or diarrhoea, then the vet can immediately focus their attention on the clinical signs that you have highlighted. There will be times when you might find it hard to be specific about what is going on, but you shouldn't worry about this; non-specific clinical signs, which are vague or nebulous, are rather common. Your vet will not be phased by this. The clinician will probably ask further questions whilst, or before, examining Harry in detail. The questioning tends to be of a rather general nature early on in the course of the consultation, which should allow you to give an overview of the problem(s) you have noticed. This will also enable the vet to gauge how worried you are about your dog. Later questioning tends to become more specific and focused as the consultation proceeds, often consisting of 'closed' questions that usually require quite specific short answers such as: 'When did you first notice that Harry was ill?', or 'Has he been sick today?', or 'Is he drinking normally?' Try to give direct and truthful answers to these questions.

Initially, when Harry is first approached, your vet will try to calm and befriend Harry with gentle handling and quiet words so that the dog does not become too fearful or excited. During the examination itself, the vet will tend to follow a rather personalised and particular routine which suits them. Some might start from the head working back towards the tail. Other vets might focus on different body systems in turn, such as the skin, then the respiratory system, then the nervous system, and so forth. This approach will vary between individuals. In spite of what some people expect, it is highly unlikely that in a period of only a few minutes, the vet will be able to perform a complete and exhaustive examination of your dog, but they will rather tend to examine Harry depending on the main clinical sign(s) that you have mentioned. So, it is crucial that you try to help the vet by giving answers that are accurate. It is a mistake to try to please the vet by giving answers that you think the vet would like to hear. So, again, by example, if Harry has had a swelling on his paw for two weeks, please don't say it has been present for only two or three days, because if you give misleading information the vet will not be able to properly evaluate his problem.

There are a few very crucial measurements that vets usually want to take almost every time they examine a dog. These are known as 'vital signs' and usually include: body weight, some assessment of body condition, heart and pulse rate, respiratory effort and rate, body temperature (a rectal thermometer will be used; the ear thermometers used in people do not work well in dogs) and general state of arousal. The vet will also be looking carefully for any signs of pain. These general findings can often be used to get a good handle on the severity of the problem and the need, or not, for urgent investigation / treatment.

Again, it is important to understand that the clinical examination that is performed will depend particularly on the original presenting signs, their duration, intensity and if/how they are changing over time. So, if Harry were to have a lump on the paw, then the vet will probably examine that lump very carefully (looking for size, shape, colour, heat, pain, fluid, etc.) and also watch him to see if he walks normally or if he is lame. If he has a normal body temperature, that will impact the vet's assessment of Harry compared, for instance, with a similar situation in the presence of a high body temperature. If the lump is changing in size, shape or appearance, this is another important part of the puzzle.

During the examination, it is likely that your vet will ask you to help by steadying or petting Harry whilst he is on the examination table, or holding Harry on a short leash on the floor, so the vet can examine each part of him they feel is relevant. If the vet uses a stethoscope to listen to the heart, lungs, or the gut; don't talk whilst they doing this, they will not be able to hear you properly and might miss a crucial finding, such as the presence of abnormal lung sounds.

This process, the taking of a history and clinical examination, has been shown to be very efficient in terms of time, money and resources.

After your vet has examined Harry, in the light of your history – that is, the clinical signs which you have described – it is possible they will have come to a diagnosis. However, it is much more likely that they have not reached a firm diagnosis. More probably, they will have several possible diagnoses in mind and this 'differential diagnosis list' will in effect be a list of hypotheses – educated guesses – to explain their illness.

In many cases, the vet will continue to ask supplementary questions to clarify Harry's history. Most of these questions will seem logical, for instance: 'Harry is lame, has that worsened recently?' and 'Has Harry been licking this lump?' – but don't be surprised if some of these questions might seem irrelevant such as: 'Has Harry ever had surgery to this leg?', 'Can you tell me about Harry's diet?' or 'Has Harry ever travelled abroad?' or 'Harry's breathing seems a little laboured – is this normal for him?' These types of supplementary questions sometimes can clarify the case because they bring other issues into focus. For instance, in a dog with a lump on the foot, a history of previous surgery, even years ago, might be relevant, or the presence of respiratory signs may redirect attention to the chest, the 'thorax', even though you have been aware of the lump on the paw only.

During the consultation, most vets will focus their attention on two particular issues, namely: diagnosis and prognosis. The diagnosis is a specific classification of the illness that enables the clinician to understand the cause of that condition and how it might be most effectively treated. The prognosis is different; it is a definition of the disease in terms of the likelihood of a cure being reached (depending on the treatment given). In some respects, as far as an owner is concerned, prognosis is far more important than diagnosis, but from a mature veterinary perspective it is impossible to speculate rationally about prognosis unless or until a diagnosis has been reached.

At this stage, decisions will have to be reached about how to proceed. If the vet is fairly certain about the diagnosis, or has a menu of only a few possible diagnoses for your dog's problem, they will explain the findings they have made and what the implications might be. But, in many cases the vet will remain uncertain as to the precise diagnosis because the physical findings and history associated with the problem are often not specific enough to allow the clinician to be certain. So, for a lump on the foot, for example, there are a range of possibilities, including: a bacterial or fungal infection of the claw, a bite abscess or other form of local infection, an interdigital foreign body (such as a grass seed), interdigital cyst, traumatic damage (such as a fracture or dislocation involving the bones of the foot), and a range of tumours (such as melanoma, histiocytoma, mast cell tumour, squamous cell carcinoma, plasmacytoma, soft-tissue sarcoma etc.). In these instances, where the diagnosis remains uncertain, the vet might recommend various tests to narrow the diagnosis. They ought to explain what they are thinking and why they want to do these tests.

It is at this point in the consultation when many clients become anxious because they feel they have little control and that they might be facing large bills without any guarantee of success. This is the stage where a good clinician should be able to provide support and guidance by setting out for you, the client, a simple 'road-map' for the future care of your dog. So, again, thinking of the lump on Harry's foot, the clinician may have noticed it is painful and feel that the most likely diagnosis is trauma; for such a case the most useful diagnostic tool would probably be to take X-ray image(s) of the foot. In a few (rather rare) cases, chest radiography might be advised in addition because occasionally limb tumours spread to the lungs early in the course of disease and also certain diseases of the chest can cause bony lumps on the limbs – a condition known as 'Hypertrophic Pulmonary Osteo-Arthropathy' (HPOA). In other cases, your vet might recommend a procedure called 'aspiration cytology' in which a sterile needle is introduced into the lump to harvest some cells from the mass which are then examined under a microscope – either by the vet, or more often, by a specialist pathologist; one who is specially trained, to make diagnoses from microscopic samples. In yet other cases, the vet might recommend either 'symptomatic treatment', using a 'best guess' approach to the diagnosis, or a 'wait and see' approach. Some clients might consider this last option to be rather cavalier, but an experienced clinician might, for example, be very suspicious that the lump they are interested in is, in fact, an histiocytoma. Histiocytoma is a form of skin tumour. It is not an especially common lump, but it does have a rather stereotypical appearance and behaviour. Importantly, in almost all cases, histiocytomas flare up over a few weeks, initially appearing quite angry and aggressive, but the disease almost always spontaneously resolves without (or in spite of) treatment.

I hope this illustration gives you some understanding of the way that vets are thinking and working during a consultation. The vet's aim is, above all, to treat your pet appropriately, in a way which you agree to, and can afford. To do so, the clinician will pay very close attention to the history you volunteer, the answers you give to their questions, and how this information seems to fit alongside the objective findings they make during the examination of your dog. The vet will seek to reach a firm diagnosis and prognosis, wherever possible, but this in turn often means that the clinician may want to do some particular tests, to try to reach that diagnosis. Generally, they will aim to choose the cheapest, quickest, least invasive and most appropriate tests to try to reach the diagnosis and to 'rule-out' alternative diagnoses. The tests chosen will depend on the whole constellation of clinical signs and historical findings that are present, because individual signs are rarely diagnostic on their own, but a cluster of signs is much more likely to be caused by only one, or a few, conditions.

This approach will probably fall short of the 'no stones unturned' schemes that many students learn in academia. The vet's aim is often to be practical and economic rather than exhaustive. Young vets entering practice from university sometimes are uncomfortable with this approach but soon learn that few clients are willing or able to fund a more academic investigation, unless they are well-heeled and the dog is thoroughly insured. In some cases, this must be a sequential or iterative process, in which a series of tests are selected in turn to reach that goal. In the present example, if a painful swelling is radiographed to reveal more information, a fine needle aspirate might then be deemed useful.

There are unfortunately many cases where the diagnostic route is highly complex, or very expensive, or sometimes where the magnitude of the problem does not seem to justify this process. It is always a good idea to try to tease this out with your vet before, and during, this process, so that you can be confident that the plan that is being followed seems appropriate for you and your dog.

A useful motto for every client at the vets is: **be sceptical, question everything.** Good clinicians will, on the whole, be delighted to share their thinking with you and know this is the easiest way to maintain their client's trust. Also, if you have your own theory of what might be wrong, please share that with your vet. Good rapport between clients and their vet is generally helpful.

Another thing: **never leave the practice without a clear plan of how things are expected to proceed.** Usually, a plan can be articulated by the vet in one sentence, such as:

'Everything seems fine now, only come back if the problem comes back or a new one arises.'

or

'Use these ear drops for two weeks then come back to see me for a recheck.'

or

'We expect the lab results by Thursday afternoon. If you've heard nothing by Friday give me a ring.'

For every clinical scenario, the option to do nothing should always be considered. We know well from experiences in both veterinary and human medicine that many conditions resolve spontaneously, or do not benefit from treatment. It is always sensible to ask your vet what they think would be likely to happen if no investigations and no treatments are performed. Some vets will be taken aback by this sort of question, but they shouldn't be.

You might like to ask your vet another question, which is the flip side of the same coin: 'What do you think could be the worst possible diagnosis or outcome from this case?' The answer you get might be shocking, or comforting, but either way it should help you and your vet come to a mutual understanding of the issues you are facing.

I'm trying to come clean with you about the consultation process because, like most vets, I am conflicted over it. As I have grown older and more experienced, there is no doubt that I frequently approach each new diagnostic challenge as a simple pattern recognition problem. Pattern recognition is quick and dirty, driven by hunch, backed by experience, and often steered using simple aphorisms:

Common things are common.

Don't go looking for unicorns.

The answer is usually in the history and physical examination findings.

A strong intuition is much more powerful than a weak test.[1]

Pattern recognition is fast and lazy, frequently correct, but also very prone to error. A much more methodical, analytical and scientific approach would be to weigh up all the evidence through detailed hypothesis testing and calculation by 'leaving no stone unturned'. This latter technique is the way students are often taught and one that feels more authentic, scientific and rational. The central problem though is that such an analytic approach requires greater resources – more time, more mental energy, more cash and far more testing. In voicing this conflict, I want to acknowledge that clinicians honestly grapple with this conundrum every single day. For much of the time, pattern recognition is fine, elegant, accurate and relatively cheap. On the other hand, every clinician must be humble in the face of biology; willing and able to change tack if circumstances demand it; for instance, when some of the history or clinical findings are unusual or seem out of place, and especially if an illness evolves in an unexpected direction. It is the mark of an able clinician that they pay especial attention to these dissonant signals. When the going is tough the more analytic approach has much to recommend it.

Another issue I'd like to raise here is that the meaning of diagnostic tests results from blood samples, radiographs, electrocardiograms, ultrasound scans, etc. can

---

[1] This one's from *The Laws of Medicine; Field Notes from an Uncertain Science* by Siddhartha Mukherjee. It's shorthand for some important ideas from probability theory and some elegant maths.

be ambiguous. When a disease is common, or when there is a lot of supporting evidence that a disease is likely to be present, then tests can be very useful to confirm or refute a diagnosis. However, this is the crux; no test is perfect at identifying either all diseased animals, or all healthy animals. In other words, there are always some false-positive and some false-negative results. Furthermore, many tests do not give simple yes / no binary answers. Instead, they provide numerical or visual results that require careful evaluation in the light of all the other data collected from a case. The magnitude of these effects also often depends on the skill and previous experience of the vet with each particular diagnostic test, the quality of the equipment, and the frequency of normal or abnormal patients amongst the dogs being tested. So, for instance, when a disease is rare, or the clinical suspicion of a disease is low, then there is often little point in performing diagnostic tests because even if the result is positive, it is very likely that will be a false positive.

These are issues of practical importance because if several different tests are done the chances are that one or other will deliver misleading results, or be mis-interpreted, which, in spite of everyone's best efforts, could lead to diagnostic error. This is one reason why all blanket testing and screening profiles must be employed wisely. It is another reason we are often cautious about making definitive diagnoses. It also helps explain why many vets choose to specialise; so that they can become masters of a limited domain.

There is a lot to be said for sticking with the same vet when treating a problem that your dog has because this should mean that you don't have to repeat yourself endlessly and, if the condition does not immediately resolve, the unravelling of your dog's problem can be progressed forwards rather than stuttering and stumbling through reiteration and repetition.

On the other hand, if you feel your own vet is not sufficiently skilled in dealing with your dog's present problem it is never wrong to ask for a second opinion from one of their colleagues, from a vet at another practice, or to be referred to a specialist (see later, Chapter 13). Good clinicians will not be offended by this sort of request. Indeed, sometimes they will be extremely relieved to pass the responsibility on.

SUMMARY

Try to be very clear why you have brought your dog. Be honest when asked about the history. When you don't understand your vet's thinking, or what they plan to do, ask them to explain. Be sceptical, question everything. If finances are an issue tell the vet. Always go home with a plan.

WHY IS VETERINARY MEDICINE SO COSTLY?

I think this is an appropriate point in my narrative to tackle the question of the cost of veterinary care because it is a sore subject with many clients and is probably one reason why you bought this book.

In the scenario I have just described, I indicated that by the end of a short consultation a vet may have reached a diagnosis, or more probably will have reached a series of possible hypotheses to explain the clinical signs that your dog is exhibiting. The cost of reaching this stage is usually the fixed cost of a routine appointment and relatively low, say £40–£60. The next stage of the process is usually the creation of a plan by which a more definitive diagnosis can be made and treatment chosen. Vets are in the business of trying to reach definitive diagnoses in order to treat each problem most effectively with the expectation of deriving the best outcome for the patient in terms of pain control and ongoing health, but they have to do this with full the consent and support of the owner. This is where the costs of veterinary care often become contentious because sadly sometimes vets do not take the time, or make the effort, to fully explain what they want to do and what this will cost. The best way for an owner to prevent bills skyrocketing is to question their vets closely, asking them to explain the rationale for each and every procedure. A good vet will be easily able to justify what they are recommending. Most vets are also willing to compromise in the diagnostic plan but will want you to understand that this compromise might not represent their ideal approach.

To return to the scenario I have just sketched out, what sort of costs are we talking about? Well, imagine that between you and your vet it is decided that the most appropriate next step might be to simply take a sample of cells from the lump; this is known as an aspiration biopsy, which is frequently quickly performed without anaesthetic (sometimes some form of sedation or local anaesthesia is required). The sample is usually acquired with a needle, transferred to a microscope slide, fixed to preserve the cells, stained with special dyes, then examined under a microscope. Sometimes this examination is performed in-house by a vet, but often such samples are sent away to specialist veterinary pathologists who are much more experienced and knowledgeable in this field. The cost of this might range from, say, £100 to £160. Importantly, the results of aspiration cytology are usually not available for at least 24 hours, and are not always diagnostically helpful; indeed, in only about two-thirds of cases is a diagnosis reached. In the case of 'Harry's Lump', this procedure might then have increased the total cost for you to around £200. Was this cost justified? In some ways that depends on the results. Say the pathologist reports that the sample is definitely a histiocytoma. Well, this is a clear diagnosis and excellent news for your dog because a complete and spontaneous recovery is very likely. On the other hand, the pathologist might say that this is definitely a mast cell tumour. This diagnosis too is important because mast cell tumours can be very serious indeed. In some cases, with mast cell tumours of the lower limb or foot, treatment can be given with a new drug (tigilanol tiglate) that is injected directly into the lump. In other cases, radical surgery may need to be performed quickly, followed by treatment with expensive drugs (but this will depend on how aggressive this tumour appears to be). In the case of 'high grade' mast cell tumours, the costs involved in treatment can sometimes run into many hundreds or even thousands of pounds. Even then the long-term outcomes are far from perfect in every case. Then again, the pathologist's report might be ambiguous and conclude that they are unable to make a diagnosis at all. Was the aspiration cytology a complete waste of time and money? These are issues that a good clinician should be sharing and discussing with his/her clients along the way. When vets and clients partner together, then the outcome tends to be better for the patient and there is much less likelihood that clients will feel they have been ripped-off or misled.

Turning back to the virtual case we have just been discussing; imagine that it was decided that the most useful investigation was thought to be radiography – X-ray pictures – of the foot. Radiography is potentially dangerous since it uses high energy ionising radiation. This procedure is commonly performed, but the health and safety of veterinary staff, and UK law, mean that staff exposure to radiation must be minimised. For that reason, staff are not allowed to hold animals for radiography, and because dogs will not routinely adopt the perfect position

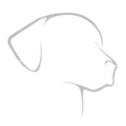

7

COMMON PROBLEMS

This chapter is devoted to the exploration of some common veterinary problems in dogs. I will start by discussing skin irritation; persistent itching / scratching, which can often be caused by external parasites such as a flea infestation. Another extremely common cause of an itch is an 'allergic' skin disease known as atopic dermatitis. This condition, in turn, must be differentiated from food sensitivities and allergies that are much less common but are best treated by dietary manipulation. 'Scooting', rubbing of the bottom on the floor (usually caused by irritation of the anal sacs), is sometimes the first or principle sign of generalised itching. Ear problems, sore eyes, vomiting and / or diarrhoea will be addressed as well as urinary problems, the lame dog, sudden onset dullness and loss of appetite, dental disease, wounds, grass seed foreign bodies, coughing, lumps in the skin, false pregnancy and womb infections.

THE ITCHY DOG

Tis better than riches to scratch where it itches.

Common things are common.

Itching (technically called pruritus) is one of the most common problems that dogs present with to the vet. There are many causes of itching but most often these can be identified through the vet taking a thorough history and performing a clinical examination. The most common cause of canine pruritus is a flea infestation. If there are several dogs in the household and only one dog exhibits the itch then parasitic disease is not likely to be the explanation, whereas if all dogs (and possibly cats or people) in the household are itching then a parasitic problem is highly likely. All itchy skin conditions cause dogs to scratch or bite at themselves, which in turn leads to skin trauma, which then begets further itching: the so-called 'itch-scratch cycle'. This self-reinforcing syndrome makes diagnosis and treatment of the primary problem more challenging.

Although the whole skin is on display for the vet to look at, it is not always easy to make a diagnosis simply from an examination. On the other hand, most common skin conditions present with a particular distribution of skin 'lesions'. A lesion is a part of the body that has suffered damage through injury or disease, such as a wound, an ulcer, abscess or tumour. So, for instance, if a dog has fleas, then typically the irritation will be localised to the dog's back, especially the lower back near the tail (the rump or 'croup'), and at this site there may be skin thickening and scurf. Very often 'flea dirt' can be seen – small comma-shaped black crusts (which are flea faeces – partially digested dog-blood) and white specks (which are flea eggs). In a proportion of cases, when a fine-toothed 'flea comb' is passed through the coat, fleas will be found. In such a case the diagnosis is secure. However, there are often cases where no fleas are immediately obvious and the characteristic scurf and flea dirt is absent. In such cases, if the distribution of the lesions is suggestive, and the dog(s) is (are) not being regularly and appropriately treated with anti-parasitic drugs, then a flea problem might still be the cause. Such hidden ('occult') flea problems can be due to the dog having a low parasite burden but exhibiting an allergic reaction to fleas. In other cases, the dog might have recently been bathed (or swum) so that the characteristic scurf / dander is absent.

In any case, if a vet is suspicious that fleas might be at least part of the explanation for the pruritus, many clinicians will start by using trial therapy with anti-flea medication. Please don't be offended. Dermatologists say it is never wrong in a case like this to begin with trial anti-parasitic treatment. People are often a bit embarrassed to be told that their dog might have fleas. You shouldn't be because it is absolutely no reflection on the cleanliness of your home. Many, many different anti-flea products are on the market. When treating fleas, or a presumed flea problem, it is essential to treat the dog in question, the household, and any other dogs or cats who live with them. A detailed description of a flea treatment regime for the environment is given in Chapter 4 (p. 55). If a dog has an allergy to fleas, then treatment will probably require religious anti-flea treatment for life.

There are several other skin parasites that can cause pruritus. For instance, in the part of Kent where I live, another parasite – a mite called *Sarcoptes scabiei* – is quite common. Locally, the condition is known as 'Fox Mange' because a large proportion of the fox population in this part of England is infested with this parasite. Sarcoptic mange is due to these mites burrowing into the dog's skin. The condition is highly contagious (often owners can catch it from their dogs) and intensely itchy, but again the distribution of lesions can be helpful in making a diagnosis. Thickening and crusting of the skin on the edge of the ear flap, on the elbows, hocks ('ankles'), and sometimes on the lower part of the abdomen are characteristic. Skin scrapings can be taken to find this parasite, and if they are found the diagnosis is certain, but it has been shown repeatedly that even in the absence of parasites in scrapings, the parasite is often the cause; in other words, this test has a very high proportion of false-negative results. A simpler test, known as the 'pinnal-scratch-reflex', in which a clinician watches the dog's reaction to rubbing the edge of their ear, may in fact be a better diagnostic test if the condition is advanced. Sarcoptic mange can also be confirmed via a blood test. As with a suspected flea infestation, if your vet suspects that your dog might have sarcoptic mange they will usually perform trial therapy with an appropriate anti-parasitic drug.

Other parasites can cause itching. One, known as *Cheyletiella yasguri,* causes particularly marked scaling of the skin on the back. The parasite can be found by examining this scurf under a microscope. It is not common except perhaps in puppies. Owners of affected animals may develop skin lesions themselves.

*Trombicula autumnalis (*sometimes called *Chiggers)* is a bright orange mite that can also cause pruritus. The larvae of the mite are responsible for the trouble which usually occurs in late summer or early autumn in the UK, hence the other name for this parasite: 'the harvest mite'. These mites make shallow burrows in the skin, release various tissue fluids that provoke intense itching and often a rash in the patient. There are a few areas of the body where the mites are most often seen, sometimes in small clumps; namely, in the webs between the digits of the feet, and around the face / ears (especially in a little fold towards the back of the ear flap called 'Henri's pocket'). Most anti-parasitic agents will kill both of these mites successfully.

I am looking through our microscope at a daub of crumbly, sticky brown gunk from a dog's ear, which I've smeared onto a glass slide. The material has been fixed and stained with a chemical cocktail that might enable me to make some sense of the grot. What I see is actually rather enlightening and brings a small smile to my lips; clumps and small islands of purple cells shaped like footprints together with dead skin cells (called 'squames'), smaller numbers of (much smaller) bacteria, debris, and a swirling blue haze caused by proteinaceous exudate. Eureka! I have the rudiments of a diagnosis. This is what I was trained for.

There are many pleasures, and some pains, attached to being a vet in small animal practice. I find the pleasure of reaching a diagnosis to be one of the most exquisite. Once you have a firm diagnosis to explain the features of a case, you can relax a little because you can be confident that the most unsettling speculative part of the clinician's job is over. Of course, in practice some diagnoses we make will be wrong and quite frequently we do make presumptive diagnoses in the face of incomplete data; it can be sometimes quite difficult to know for certain that you have reached a firm and accurate diagnosis. This is a zone where academic rigour and practical veterinary medicine collide. When I reach the stage of making a diagnosis, I often hear a small voice in my head crying to me:

'Can you REALLY be sure? Shouldn't you do further tests? Have you ruled out ALL the alternatives . . . ?'

Indeed, it is particularly difficult for most of us to be honest with ourselves and to retrace our steps to give up on a diagnosis that we have made when the natural history of a disease unfolds to show we were mistaken. On the other hand, it is not my money I am spending when I do these tests. It is not my skin that is pricked when a blood sample is taken. I need to reach a diagnosis at a reasonable cost with minimal discomfort and distress to the dog. This is an issue I wrestle with.

The purple footprint-shaped cells I was looking at are a yeast, *Malassezia canis*, which is frequently found in the inflamed ears of dogs. When the yeast is found in large numbers we can be rather sure that this yeast is what I might call the 'proximate cause' of the inflammation. Treatment with an anti-fungal agent is justified and will almost certainly provide rapid relief to the dog. But that is not enough.

Otitis externa, inflammation of the external ear canal, is common in dogs, and usually amenable to treatment, but is very commonly recurrent, returning again and again to irritate and hurt the dog and to disappoint or enrage the client. Recognition of the 'proximate cause' is not enough. What is also needed is an effort to discover the 'ultimate cause', the underlying problem(s) that have led to this yeast proliferation.

I spent three years of my life, whilst I was young and fit, researching the causes and consequences of long-standing and recurrent ear disease in dogs. It earned me a PhD and gave me the opportunity to meet Denise, who is now my partner, mother to our children. I published several papers and helped to develop some radical surgical techniques during those years, but it was probably a decade or more later before I fully grasped the importance of Malassezia to the development of otitis externa in dogs.

Rosie, a bright, cheerful, middle-aged, West Highland White Terrier ('Westie') came to me today. Her right ear was painful. Dark crumbly discharge was clogging the canal. The skin of the canal was reddened, fragile, ulcerated and sore. The other ear looked almost normal, just slightly reddened at the opening and on the hairless surface of the 'pinna' (the flap of the ear). Rosie is a regular patient with a fairly typical history; regular vaccinations, a few episodes of enteritis thought to have been diet related, and several episodes of ear problems in the past. Also, Rosie has had episodic skin irritation for years which seemed to be seasonal. At home she was given the nickname 'blackfoot', a slightly cruel slur, because her feet were stained a deep brown. This discolouration is common in pale dogs if they lick their feet frequently; saliva staining, associated with itchy and inflamed skin between the toes, very typically due to allergic skin disease. This tell-tale sign should not be ignored. The underlying cause of Rosie's recurrent ear problems is the chronic inflammatory/allergic skin disease known as atopic dermatitis (or atopy) in which there are immunological abnormalities and the skin appears to form an incompetent barrier. Dogs with atopy often develop secondary otitis externa associated with overgrowth of yeasts (e.g. *Malassezia canis*) and/or bacteria in the ears.

Atopy

Atopy (also called canine atopic disease or CAD) is the second most common cause of skin irritation in dogs after fleas. This is an incurable condition. It may affect more than 10% of the dog population. This disease presents as scratching, licking and rubbing of the skin. Some dogs with the condition also rub their backside on the ground; 'scooting'. The pruritus usually develops first in dogs who are young, less than three years of age, often as a seasonal problem (most commonly in the spring and summer). Initially, the skin can seem quite normal in appearance but as the condition progresses changes start to develop in the skin, especially reddening, hair-loss and thickening. Sometimes there are little papules on the skin that can become infected. If the condition is long-standing the skin becomes very thickened ('lichenified') and darkly pigmented. Atopy most frequently affects the folds of skin between the digits of the feet, the skin over the carpus ('wrist') and hock ('ankle'), the axillae ('armpits'), the face, ears and the less hairy parts of the lower abdomen. It is likely that atopy is a genetic disorder because most dogs with this problem come from a few breeds: Labradors, Golden Retrievers, Terriers (especially West Highland, Staffordshire-Bull, and Cairn Terriers), Boxers, Bulldogs, German Shepherds, English and Irish (Red) Setters, Lhasa Apso, Shi Tzu, and a few others.

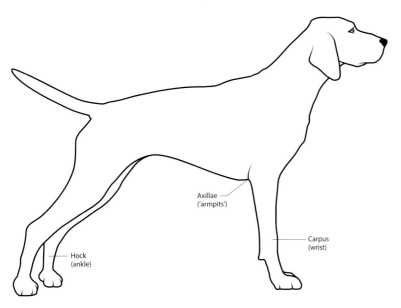

Figure 7.1. Typical sites for skin lesions associated with atopy: the carpus (wrist), hock (ankle) and the axillae ('armpits').

Diagnosis of atopy was challenging and contentious in the past, but following some large-scale trials published about a decade ago the diagnosis can now usually be made from the history and clinical signs, perhaps after employing trial therapy to rule out fleas (and flea allergic dermatitis) and finding that there is good responsiveness to trial treatment with the anti-inflammatory drugs known as corticosteroids. There are skin tests that can be used to confirm the diagnosis by identifying allergens that cause an inflammatory reaction in the skin. Blood tests to identify antibodies to certain allergens can also be done. Sadly, neither test is entirely reliable, showing both false-positive and false-negative results; so, for diagnosis, it is preferable to use the criteria listed below.

Diagnostic criteria for canine atopic dermatitis (Favrot, 2010):

1. Onset of signs under 3 years of age.

2. Dog living mostly indoors.

3. Glucocorticoid ('steroid')-responsive pruritus.

4. Pruritus without skin lesions at onset.

5. Front feet affected.

6. Ear pinnae affected.

7. Ear margins not affected.

8. Lower back ('dorso-lumbar area') not affected.

At least five of these criteria should normally be met to make a diagnosis of atopy. When more are met the diagnosis is more secure. Ideally, food allergic dermatitis should be ruled out before finally making this diagnosis (see later), but unfortunately, in my experience, often owners are very keen to get a quick fix for this problem because pruritus is clearly distressing to their pet. It can be very frustrating to live with a dog who licks and scratches themselves constantly and/or has recurrent ear disease.

When I see a dog who appears to have atopy, I explain my fears. Owners need to know that the condition is incurable and be warned there is no quick fix. This can be difficult for owners to accept. Treatment of atopy is challenging and will be expensive; often several different therapies must be used in combination and invariably some forms of therapy must be life long. The disease tends to flare up at intervals (as in Rosie's case), consequently strategies must be developed for each dog to try to manage these. Close cooperation between vet and owner can definitely enhance the management of atopy. Fortunately, there has been really fantastic progress in the management of this disease in the last 20 years or so. This gives me a great deal of hope. I now find most dogs with atopy can be managed very successfully. Below, I will discuss the pros and cons of the main different treatment options for canine atopic disease as I see them.

Hyposensitisation (allergen specific immunotherapy)

The skin and/or blood tests performed on some dogs with atopy are done to pin-point which allergens provoke an inflammatory reaction in that dog's skin. A variety of mites, pollens, moulds, and perhaps other environmental proteins to which the dog may have been exposed, are tested. Once the allergens are identified, a vaccine – individualised to that patient – is prepared that contains small, measured, amounts of each allergen. Hyposensitisation involves giving this vaccine repeatedly, by sub-cutaneous injections, delivering increasing doses of the allergens regularly to 'teach' the immune system to recognise these proteins and become desensitised to their effects. This process is not completely understood. It works well in around two-thirds of cases, but must be continued indefinitely. There is a lag of several months, possibly up to a year, before the therapy works. This can prove very frustrating and may necessitate additional treatment. Even after hyposensitisation is successful, some additional drug therapy is usually required at intervals when the problem flares up. Hyposensitisation can be very effective. It is not cheap.

Corticosteroids

Corticosteroids are broad-spectrum anti-inflammatory agents that have dramatic effects on the body, especially the immune system. The drugs have been available for decades and are remarkably effective in the short-term at reducing pruritus caused by this disease. They can be given by injection, by mouth and topically (as sprays, creams, ear drops, etc.). Corticosteroids are quite cheap. Some of the injectable forms have a long duration of action. Unfortunately, although they are very effective, corticosteroids have numerous side-effects that limit their long-term usefulness. These side-effects include excessive thirst and appetite, suppression of inflammatory and immune reactions, impaired wound healing, thinning of the skin and hair coat, weakening of the muscles and bones, and changes in behaviour / personality. Side effects tend to be more severe with high doses given over long periods. Some dogs are much more prone to side-effects than others. Oral or topical corticosteroids given every other, or every third day, cause fewer side-effects.

Ciclosporin

Ciclosporin is another immunosuppressant drug that is used in human medicine to treat transplant patients, people with rheumatoid arthritis and the human version of atopic skin disease. It has been in use to treat dogs with atopy for about 20 years and is licensed for this purpose. Ciclosporin has been shown to be very effective. Unfortunately, it is quite expensive and there are side-effects in some patients, especially vomiting or diarrhoea. The drug is usually given daily, but as the condition responds it may be possible to use the drug less frequently.

Oclacitinib

Oclacitinib, technically known as a Janus Kinase (JAK) inhibitor, has a modifying effect on the immune system. It inhibits the reception of messenger chemicals, called cytokines, which are proteins released by some cells to regulate the function of other cells in the immune system. In particular, Oclacitinib inhibits a messenger called IL-31, among others. In so doing it can very effectively stop itching. The drug has a fairly rapid onset of effect. It is initially given twice daily, reduced to once daily after a fortnight. Side effects are uncommon although benign (non-cancerous) skin tumours may be more common in dogs receiving this drug. Oclacitinib has now been licensed for the treatment of atopy in dogs for about eight years. It is quite costly.

Lokivetmab

Lokivetmab is a newly introduced drug, an antibody, which acts specifically against the cytokine IL-31. The drug is given once monthly by injection. Initial results with this drug are very impressive but at present the drug is very costly.

As you can see, there are quite a range of options available to treat atopic skin disease in dogs. Several of these options have become available only recently so they are still being fully evaluated. Other therapies can also help in managing this condition, including essential (omega 3 and omega 6) fatty acids added to the diet, which can improve skin barrier function. In the past, antihistamine ther-apy was fairly commonly used, and some vets continue to find them useful. A drug preparation derived from Chinese medical herbs has shown some success in treating a minority of dogs. Moisturising shampoos and antibacterial and/or anti-fungal shampoos also have a role to play because secondary skin infections often cause the condition to flare up. Some of these products must be used at intervals in many atopic dogs to manage flares in the disease.

Dogs with atopic dermatitis often develop various forms of flare-up; such flares may present with classical signs (as described above); however, these flares can also occur as localised problems; inflammation of the ear 'otitis externa' (see later), acute moist dermatitis (often called 'hot spots'), bacterial skin infections, or localised infections with *Malassezia canis* (particularly in the interdigital webs of the feet). All of these conditions can also develop in dogs who are not atopic but who have other predisposing conditions.

Adverse food reactions (sometimes described as 'food allergy' although this condition does not appear to be a true allergy)

This is an itchy inflammatory skin disease associated with diet. It is a reaction of the body to large protein or starch molecules in the food. There is some doubt about how frequent this condition is; certainly, much less common that atopy, but some atopic dogs are also 'food allergic'. The condition presents with itching usu-ally affecting the same parts of the body as atopy. A few dogs have signs of itchy ears ('otitis externa') alone. A proportion of dogs also have signs of a food related enteritis (i.e. diarrhoea). Most studies suggest that dogs with 'food allergy' usually present with signs at less than one year old. On the other hand, the condition is also reported in mature dogs up to old age and sometimes they have been eating the offending food for years before developing clinical signs. It is said that in most cases the itch does not respond to corticosteroid therapy, which could be a very useful observation in suggesting the diagnosis because the pruritus of atopy is usually quickly interrupted by giving the dog these drugs. My personal experience does not chime with this observation.

There is sadly only one way to definitively make a diagnosis of 'food allergy'. The dog in question must be fed a novel diet, EXCLUSIVELY (no treats, no table scraps, no scavenging), ideally one to which it has never previously been exposed. This diet is fed until the pruritus decreases dramatically or vanishes completely. Once that has occurred the condition can be more securely confirmed by re-exposing the dog to different foods, one a time. As you will know from Chapter 5, commercial diets often contain quite a variety of different ingredients but are rarely clearly labelled to show all constituents, so it is very difficult to know precisely all foods that a dog has previously been exposed to. Consequently, choosing a completely novel diet for this food trial can be difficult. The diet should be composed of protein(s) and starch(es) to which the dog has never been exposed. There are proprietary veterinary diets available for this purpose that your vet will offer you (e.g. venison and potato, tilapia and tapioca, duck and rice, etc.). Another approach (possibly preferable), is to feed a specially prepared proprietary 'hydrolysed' diet in which the proteins have been chemically treated, so that they are comprised only of short chains of amino acids rather than much larger complex proteins. These polypeptides are highly unlikely to provoke an immunologic reaction. Hydrolysed diets are really expensive because of all the science and technology behind their preparation. On the other hand, some specialist dermatologists recommend a novel home-cooked diet as most effective for the food trial. This diet does not need to be perfectly balanced. It is not to be fed long-term, just for the duration of the trial. Unfortunately, it will take 4–6 weeks in most cases, sometimes up to 12 weeks (!), before the pruritus reduces on a novel diet. This can be very frustrating indeed because it means it is difficult to exclude or confirm food allergy as a possible cause of the skin signs for that length of time. Recently, a protocol for shorter food trials to diagnose this problem has been published, which would obviously be preferable. The protocol also permits the use of drugs during the initiation of the trial. Results from recent papers on the subject are encouraging. The efficacy of this approach is still controversial, so further work is necessary before it becomes accepted.

The most common foods that seem to provoke allergies are beef, chicken, lamb, eggs, maize ('corn'), wheat, soy and milk. Contrary to popular belief, glutens – from grains – do not appear to be a common cause of adverse food reactions. If a food trial is successful, it should be followed-up by introducing one food at a time, whilst continuing to feed the trial diet as the main food. The offending 'allergens' will usually provoke new pruritus within a few days (sometimes within hours). Bear in mind that the dog may show this reaction to several foodstuffs. If a dog's pruritus is solely due to a food sensitivity / allergy, it can be extremely rewarding to identify the problem and manage the skin disease via the dog's diet.

Pyoderma

Pus is a collection of inflammatory cells, fluids and proteins which is (usually but not invariably) rich in bacteria. Pyoderma literally means 'pus in the skin'. Superficial pyoderma is common. A second form of the disease, deep pyoderma, is relatively uncommon but can be very serious.

In general, pyoderma can result from any disruption of the skin's normal defence mechanisms, or of the immune system's ability to keep bacteria from growing on the skin in large numbers. In most cases, it is the commensal bacteria, *Staphylococcus pseudointermedius,* which are normally present in small numbers on the healthy body, which are responsible for superficial pyodermas. These bacteria colonise the hair follicles and skin glands where they multiply. Initially, small red bumps like goosepimples – papules – or 'micoabscesses' – pustules – form a rash across the body. Often the hairless skin of the lower abdomen and groin is where this is seen. These lesions spread out to form inflamed rings of hair-loss surrounded by a rim of dry crust that have a characteristic 'cigarette-burn' appearance, technically known as epidermal collarettes.

All pyodermas have an underlying ('ultimate') cause, such as: local trauma, scratching, parasitic infestation, local irritants or allergies (atopy and food allergy).

Treatment with antibiotics can be given but in superficial pyoderma, because the peripheral skin (which has a poor blood supply) is affected, high doses of these drugs are usually required for a period of several weeks. Fortunately, most simple 'superficial' pyodermas respond as well, or better, to direct treatment with antibacterial shampoos or washes. If an underlying ('ultimate') cause is suspected and identified that also needs to be treated. Some cases of superficial pyoderma are recurrent and difficult to manage. In all such cases, a thorough search for underlying disease is mandatory and bacterial skin culture may also be required.

Deep pyodermas are generally much more serious skin infections that involve all layers of the skin and the associated glands. Often, they occur in association with other chronic inflammatory skin conditions (e.g. Demodex mite infestations) or in certain breeds and specific sites (for example, a form of deep pyoderma, called anal furunculosis, is seen around the bottom almost exclusively in German Shepherd Dogs). Investigation and treatment of deep pyodermas usually necessitates further investigation including bacterial culture and sensitivity testing to identify the causal agents and the drugs that can be used in treatment. These cases often require specialist care by a veterinary dermatologist.

Impaction of the anal sacs and anal sacculitis

The anal sacs, or 'glands', are two scent organs, similar to those owned by the skunk, positioned close to the anus. Each about the size of an almond, they are cul-de-sacs of the skin; positioned at 4 and 8 o'clock relative to the bottom, filled with greasy, sticky and smelly cell debris, memorably described by Alexandra Horowitz (2012) as 'dead-fish-in-a-sweatsock' secretions. These sacs open adjacent to the anus through narrow ducts. Secretions from the anal sacs provide each dog's individual scent to their faeces and perineum. They can also sometimes be released explosively when the dog is alarmed. If the ducts that lead into the sacs become blocked, the sacs start to enlarge with retrained secretion and become irritating to the dog. The first thing that occurs to me when a dog presents with a history of 'scooting', rubbing their bottom on the ground, or nibbling around their perineum, is that they might have impacted or inflamed anal sacs. This problem can often be relieved simply by manually expressing the glands (not my favourite job, a disposable glove is essential). Anal sac problems are particularly common in the smaller spaniel breeds and brachycephalic dogs.

Recurrent anal sac problems often accompany other itchy skin conditions, especially atopy or food allergy. The condition can also provoke a 'hot spot' (see below).

'Hot spot' (acute moist dermatitis, aka pyotraumatic dermatitis)

Any itchy skin condition, or another unresolved problem such as pain, can lead a dog to nibble and bite themselves and seriously self-traumatise the skin.

Over a matter of a few hours, typically overnight, a 'hot spot' is created. The most common sites for this lesion are either on the head and neck as a result of an ear problem, or around the thighs, perineum and rump associated with anal sac disease or flea bites. The lesion may not be clearly seen until the hair coat is parted or clipped; the skin is often virtually denuded of hair, red raw with a sharply defined edge, and is usually overlain by a sticky secretion and / or matted hair. Hot spots are more common in warm weather and particularly seen in Labradors, Golden Retrievers, Collies and St Bernard dogs. Although undoubtedly there is bacterial contamination, the condition does not appear to be a primary infection of the skin. Immediate management requires pain relief, local clipping of hair, and wound disinfection / cleansing. Sometimes the patient will need sedation or even general anaesthesia to permit this nursing care. Treatment to break the itch-scratch cycle, particularly with corticosteroids, is necessary. Most lesions respond quickly to treatment. A thorough search for underlying skin disease should be made because if that is not addressed the dog might present recurrently with similar lesions.

THE EAR

The ear is formed of three parts. The outer ear is a long, twisted cone with a flap, the pinna, which has a characteristic shape and appearance in different breeds. So, for instance, Basset hounds have long droopy pinnae, whereas Terriers usually have short pricked-up pinnae. The outer ear canal is continuous with the skin, so diseases of the outer ear are often forms of skin disease. Obviously, the canal is to some extent shielded from the environment but changes in the local micro-environment of humidity and temperature can have an impact on the microbes which reside there. The ear canal is closed at its inner end by the tympanic membrane or 'ear drum'. This membrane is the skin of the drum. Beyond it lies the middle ear cavity, formed by a bony blister on the base of the skull. This is a resonating chamber (the body of the drum) that affects the transmission and perception of sound. Three tiny bones, the ossicles (sometimes coined the hammer, the anvil, and the stirrup), carry the sound impulses across the middle ear cavity from the ear drum to the inner ear. The inner ear itself is the sensory part. It is formed of a series of bony canals and delicate membranous structures housed within a very robust bone. The cochlea is the part concerned with sound perception. Other parts of the inner ear are concerned with balance and orientation of

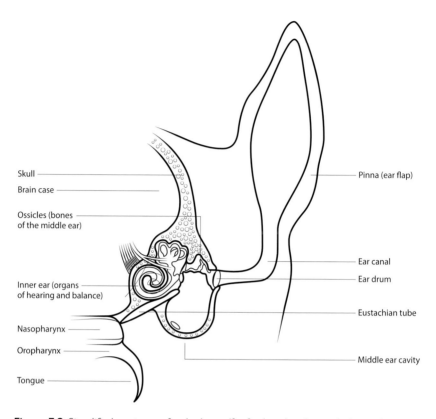

Skull

Brain case

Ossicles (bones
of the middle ear)

Inner ear (organs
of hearing and balance)

Nasopharynx

Oropharynx

Tongue

Pinna (ear flap)

Ear canal

Ear drum

Eustachian tube

Middle ear cavity

Figure 7.2. Simplified anatomy of a dog's ear (for further detail consult the text).

the body in space, an overlooked sixth sense. Messages from the inner ear are carried to the brain via the 8th cranial nerve.

Otitis externa, an inflammatory condition of the ear(s), is a very frequent reason for dogs to attend the vet. The condition is clearly distressing for the patient and the diagnosis is easy to make; typically, the dog will shake their head, attempt to scratch the ear, rub their head on furniture or carpets, and sometimes moan or yelp in pain, especially if the ear is inadvertently touched. Almost always some form of discharge is present in the ear canal and often the skin of the ear flap, the pinna, on its hairless side, and at the opening of the canal, is reddened. *But,* as we've learned from the example of Rosie, the Westie, this is not a simple infection, even though there usually are numerous yeasts or bacteria present in the discharge.

Having made the diagnosis, we need to discover why the otitis has developed. This will be familiar now; we must look again for an ultimate cause. The answer is often complex and not always apparent.

Firstly, many dogs are predisposed to developing otitis; for example, if they have floppy pinnae, or their ear canals are naturally narrow, or particularly hairy, then the microenvironment within the ear tends to be more moist; that predisposes the dog to otitis because microbes tend to thrive in moist environments.

Secondly, most cases of bilateral (both ears) and recurrent otitis occur in dogs who have underlying allergic skin disease (atopy or food allergy). Less frequently ear mites (*Otodectes cynotis*) can cause bilateral otitis (these mites are much more frequent in cats). A thorough clinical history and skin examination is invariably helpful (again, see Rosie's story).

Thirdly, in any dog with otitis there is often a local explanation for this, especially if only one ear is affected. For instance, there might be a foreign body (such as a grass seed) in the ear canal (see later, p. 183) or, there may have been localised trauma (such as a bite wound), which explains the problem, or perhaps there may be some form of growth or tumour in the ear (these are uncommon, but not rare). So, the examination of any dog with otitis should always include 'otoscopy', visual examination of the ear canal using an illuminated ear cone – to look for these problems and assess the skin lining the ear canal. If the ear is very sore the patient might have to be anaesthetised for this.

Fourthly, examination of the discharge under a microscope – cytology – is almost always helpful. This often enables the type of microbes that are present to be identified, which in turn helps the vet to choose the most useful drug(s) for treatment.

Sometimes additional tests are necessary, such as microbial culture and sensitivity testing, or, in advanced / recurrent cases X-rays (radiography) or even CT (computerised tomography). Further skin tests might be required too.

Fifthly, in some cases no explanation is obvious. Treatment is still possible, but the underlying cause is uncertain. These are the cases that trouble me most.

'THE FIVE WHYS': A USEFUL APPROACH TO DIAGNOSIS?

In business and manufacturing a rule of thumb called 'The Five Whys' is sometimes used to get to the root cause of a problem. The concept is that you begin by identifying the problem then keep asking Why? until you get past the proximate cause(s) so that the ultimate cause(s) become clear. This approach could be used in a dog such as Rosie who has otitis as follows:

Rosie has a painful red ear with a discharge; The diagnosis is *otitis externa*.

Why?

She has a yeast infection in the ear which I have found from cytology (see p. 127).

Why?

She gets repeated yeast infections because her skin is abnormal.

Why?

Her recurrent itchy skin problem meets the criteria for a diagnosis of atopy and she belongs to a predisposed breed. She has atopic dermatitis (see p. 129), which is poorly controlled.

Why?

We need to treat her yeast infections in her ears and on her feet and begin long-term treatment of her atopic dermatitis.

Why?

We want to solve her itches and pain so that her quality of life improves. This will also help her owner develop trust in our service.

Since the visit described earlier, Rosie has been treated. Her otitis responded to local topical ear drops that contain a corticosteroid and two different antibiotics, one of which, miconazole, is particularly effective against Malassezia yeasts. She has been regularly shampooed, concentrating particularly on her feet, with a chlorhexidine-based shampoo, which is especially good at controlling opportunist skin infections. For the atopy, she is now on Oclacitinib tablets daily. Response to treatment has been excellent so far, however flare-ups are to be expected.

In some dogs who get repeated episodes of *otitis externa*, the skin of the ear becomes scarred and thickened by these events. Because the ear canal is a tube, inevitably the lumen of the tube becomes narrowed; also, the self-cleaning mechanism of the ear begins to fail. These changes mean the ear often becomes chronically clogged by debris and discharge that creates a medium for further secondary infections with yeast and bacteria. This is a downward spiral that is difficult to reverse. The inflammation sometimes extends through the ear drum into the middle ear cavity beyond.

In such cases, sometimes the only solution is radical surgery to open out the ear canal, or, in the worst cases, to remove the external ear completely. Major surgery. Daunting for most vets and owners too. Usually a job for a specialist. This end result is preventable in most cases by taking ear disease seriously in the first instance, especially if it occurs more than once, or seems to respond incompletely to treatment.

Aural haematoma

A haematoma is a swelling formed of bloody fluid. Aural haematomas, which form within the cartilage of the ear flap, the pinna, occur relatively frequently, affecting about 1 in 400 dogs each year. The condition presents suddenly as a smooth plum-shaped swelling which is most obvious on the hairless, concave, aspect of the ear flap. It may appear warm and quite tense. The swelling seems to be painful; certainly, it provokes many dogs to shake their head. The exact cause of aural haematoma has not been definitively proven. Trauma would seem a likely explanation. In a proportion of cases, about half, the affected ears are also affected by *otitis externa*. There is also good evidence that preceding the haematoma the ear cartilage has undergone a degenerative process affecting

masses, localised pain, fluid, etc. They will be looking to recognise if the cause of the vomiting might be serious. If they think the dog has a mild self-limiting illness, the clinician might simply recommend judicious use of oral fluids and dietary management and will perhaps give your dog an anti-emetic, a drug that should stop the vomiting. However, if they are more concerned, they might recommend blood samples are taken for haematology (examination of the cells) and a biochemistry profile (i.e. a panel of tests which evaluate systemic health). Urine examination is often helpful too. These tests aim to identify infections, inflammation, dehydration, kidney function, liver health and a whole gamut of other abnormalities. Other tests might be recommended. The tests chosen will depend on the clinical suspicions of the vet, which will be influenced by a host of different factors such as the age, breed, weight, body condition and sexual status of the patient and the presence or absence of other clinical signs. So, for instance, in an intact bitch who has recently been in season and who is vomiting and drinking more than usual, the vet will be concerned that she could have womb infection ('pyometra'- see later, p. 187). In that case, the most useful tests include haematology and either an ultrasound or radiographic examination of the abdomen. In an immature dog with a history of sudden onset recent vomiting, a foreign body in the intestine or another form of gut obstruction might come uppermost in a list of potential diagnoses. For this case, radiographic and / or ultrasound imaging studies will be required. To give another example: an adult neutered poodle bitch with vomiting, lethargy and dehydration seemed to respond well to intravenous fluid therapy but then almost immediately relapsed. In this scenario, the clinician might be particularly concerned that the dog could have kidney disease or a rather uncommon hormonal condition called hypoadrenocorticism (aka 'Addison's disease' see p. 223), in which the adrenal glands are not working well. The most useful tests for that patient would be blood biochemistry (including measurements of sodium and potassium) and urinalysis, often with follow-up tests of adrenal function.

Treatment of each of these dogs will depend on the findings from the tests and the diagnosis made, but might involve intravenous fluid therapy, surgery or other interventions that require hospitalisation.

Diarrhoea

Diarrhoea often will accompany vomiting. When these problems coincide then obviously a gut problem is the most likely cause. Diarrhoea is a sign of intestinal disease. The nature of the diarrhoea can help to define the problem. So, your vet is likely to ask you about this. If the diarrhoea is very watery often the problem is located in the upper intestine, whereas lower intestinal disease will frequently manifest as diarrhoea containing mucus or sometimes fresh blood. If your dog seems to need to pass diarrhoea very urgently this too can indicate that the source of the problem is the lower bowel. The colour of the diarrhoea can sometimes be meaningful too. If it is black that could be due to bleeding high up in the gut (called melaena). If the faeces are orange or yellowish that may mean the contents of the gut have passed through rather quickly.

Short-lived diarrhoea, like vomiting, is often treated simply by giving oral fluids and fasting the dog for 12–24 hours, then offering the same sort of plain diet recommended for vomiting. Probiotics might be given in the hope that this will speed recovery by seeding the gut with healthy bacteria. In some cases, drugs are also used.

Parvovirus is an infectious cause of diarrhoea that is very serious indeed, often fatal. The disease, which was new at the time, caused a pandemic in the early 1980s, but following the development of vaccines has become much less common. Any dog who develops sudden onset severe vomiting and diarrhoea accompanied by weakness and lethargy might be suffering from this virus, particularly if they are young, have never been vaccinated, or their vaccines have not been renewed for years. Vets are vigilant against parvovirus. If a vet suspects your dog to have this disease they will recommend immediate hospitalisation, in isolation, and intravenous fluid therapy. Other investigations and supportive treatment will be required too.

There are many, many other causes of vomiting and diarrhoea. A definite diagnosis can be difficult to achieve. Most conditions are short-lived and self-limiting. They are often ascribed to 'dietary indiscretion', bearing in mind the proclivity of dogs to explore the world by eating things that smell interesting. In truth, we rarely identify the cause. However, if a dog becomes very unwell, exhibits pain, or shows recurrent or persistent signs (lasting for more than a few days) then it becomes important to delve more deeply. This may require a gamut of tests, which can seem frustrating and is often expensive.

Chronic or recurrent diarrhoea is rather a common problem in dogs that tends to necessitate an iterative approach. Initially, symptomatic treatment would probably be given including drugs to remove intestinal parasites. Once it is clear that the problem has not resolved then further tests will be required to assess bowel function, the health of the liver, pancreas, etc. *(and possibly new ELIZA tests for IgA markers of inflammation within the bowel wall – not yet widely available – watch this space).* Faecal samples to search for infectious disease might be needed. Once again, abdominal imaging such as radiography and ultrasound examinations might be called for, perhaps followed by endoscopy in which a flexible telescope is passed into the upper and lower gut to examine it from inside. Ultimately, samples of the bowel wall itself (biopsies) might be needed to reach a diagnosis. In some cases, these biopsies can be obtained by endoscopy (but this is quite a demanding procedure); in other cases, they must be obtained by surgery; either way, they will need to be examined by a pathologist.

The results of these procedures may lead to a diagnosis of chronic inflammatory enteropathy (previously called inflammatory bowel disease or IBD). Even then, effective treatment might require further testing. So, for instance, dietary sensitivities can cause chronic inflammation of the gut. Accurate diagnosis might require diet trials. Other cases might respond to corticosteroid drugs, yet others to chronic administration of antibiotics. It might seem surprising that I have mentioned antibiotics last but we have learned over the last half century that antibiotic therapy can often disrupt the healthy microflora of the gut, sometimes doing more harm than good, so we usually avoid giving antibiotics to animals with diarrhoea except in particular circumstances where we have sound evidence that they will not do harm.

Pancreatitis

The pancreas, a small strap-like organ in the abdomen, has dual functions in the body. It is the main source of digestive enzymes, secreted into the small intestine via a duct. The pancreas also supplies insulin, the hormone that controls blood sugar levels (see diabetes mellitus, p. 223).

Some dogs with vomiting, weakness, refusal to eat, and possibly diarrhoea, or very obvious abdominal pain, are suffering from inflammation of the pancreas: 'pancreatitis'. These dogs might have a fever, or jaundice (in which the colour of the gums, the membranes around the eyes and parts of the skin develop a coppery tint). A few might have blood in their poo, or the faeces can be black, like treacle, due to bleeding high in the gut.

It is believed that many cases of pancreatitis are induced by a diet high in fat. This could even be a single very fatty meal or an episode of 'dietary indiscretion' when a dog has got hold of some illicit fatty food. Until fairly recently, this was rather a difficult diagnosis to make, but in the last decade or so several different blood tests have become available that can help in reaching a diagnosis. Imaging studies of the abdomen with ultrasound, radiography or computerised tomography are often done. The main aim of imaging is to make sure the dog does not have a problem that requires surgical treatment, such as a foreign body lodged in the gut. Imaging can also help to clinch the diagnosis of pancreatitis but this does call for a very high degree of skill.

Some breeds of dog seem especially prone to pancreatitis, including miniature Schnauzers and Cocker Spaniels. There is evidence that in Cocker Spaniels at least, this might be an auto-immune disorder, in which the body is attacking its own tissue.

Treatment of pancreatitis when it first occurs as an acute disease, depends on non-specific supportive measures, such as pain relief and intravenous fluid therapy as well as drugs to stop vomiting. This often means that a dog must be hospitalised for a few days. Unfortunately, some dogs with pancreatitis die. When the patient recovers, as a high proportion do, then it is usual to try to prevent further episodes by feeding a diet that has a restricted fat content. Dogs who have had pancreatitis are prone to further acute episodes, or grumbling recurrent episodes of the condition. In Cocker Spaniels, where the disease is thought to have an auto-immune origin, there is interest in using anti-inflammatory drugs in long-term management, although this is by no means standard therapy at present.

It is completely beyond the scope of this book to cover all the many causes of vomiting and diarrhoea from which dogs can suffer. However, I hope the information I have provided gives you some insight and is helpful.

Sometimes you have to be creative. Walking backwards shows you the same world differently.

'Mojito' is a cross-bred dog who looks like she's got collie and German Shepherd in her ancestry. I first saw her at the age of nearly 13 as a second opinion. The history was of long-term diarrhoea, off and on for two years. At one time, apparently, she was very chubby indeed weighing in at 27 kg. Two years ago, when the diarrhoea started, she was 22 kg. By the time I saw her she was only 14.3 kg with a Body Condition Score (BCS) of 1/9 – that is to say, completely emaciated. The owner had noticed severe weight loss in the previous month. Vomiting was absent. The drinking and urination history were unremarkable.

In a dog with severe emaciation and sudden severe weight loss the first thing any experienced clinician would think of is cancer, or another form of organ failure. The answer is usually in the history and physical exam findings. Mojito seemed quite alert and responsive but a bit quiet. Body temperature was normal (38.9°C), heart and pulse rate were fine (100 bpm). She seemed well hydrated but possibly slightly pale. Breathing was fast at 50 brpm, but it was a warm day and Mojito didn't know me. There were no abnormal breath sounds. The teeth showed some tartar but no serious dental disease was found and the gums were not inflamed. On palpation of her abdomen, Mojito showed no discomfort and I didn't feel a mass, an enlarged liver, or spleen, or anything else which worried me. Listening to the gut it was rather quiet, few gurgles.

I went back over the history with her owner. Mojito had always been a bit choosy about her food. In the last two years, the faeces was always soft, frequently watery, often yellowish or pale brown, never bloody. Sometimes there had been a bit of jelly – mucus – in the poo. Often, Mojito produced noxious smelly farts. Sometimes she needed to defecate urgently. Mojito seemed a bit better when fed a special diet. She had remained on that diet because it was one of the few she seemed to enjoy, but the improvement had not been sustained.

This history and the physical findings suggested chronic disease of the large and small intestine. I felt this was likely to be a form of chronic inflammatory enteropathy (previously called inflammatory bowel disease, IBD) but the recent marked deterioration could mean there had been transformation in the gut to cancer; a condition called intestinal lymphoma was at the back of my mind. The vet who had previously been caring for Mojito had done a good thorough job before sending her on to me. This included some blood tests that showed Mojito was a little anaemic with notably low protein levels in the blood. A test of pancreatic function had been done. The result was normal.

The classical diagnostic approach to a case like this is to do some further blood tests and then biopsy the gut wall in several places, either by endoscopy (passing a flexible telescope into the gut from both ends), or by open abdominal surgery ('laparotomy'). However, Mojito was really not a good candidate for this because she was so emaciated that her fitness to survive surgery was highly questionable (gut biopsies are a risky procedure especially if the dog is in poor condition). To cap that, Mojito's owner couldn't afford to pay for biopsies. We would have to find another way.

Mojito's owner loves her. She would not accept that her dog might be at the end of her life. I felt we could approach this by using treatment as an index of diagnosis. I explained my thinking and warned Mojito's owner that I could easily be wrong. We agreed we would treat Mojito as if she had chronic inflammatory enteropathy or possibly lymphoma. I started the dog on a high dose of corticosteroids, antibiotics by mouth, and a vitamin B12 supplement. We didn't change her diet.

Two weeks later Mojito was transformed, she'd gained nearly 2 kg in weight, her coat looked glossy, she was much brighter, and best of all the diarrhoea had completely ceased within 24 hours of starting the new treatment.

So, after some discussion, we decided to withdraw the antibiotic therapy.

Two days later the client rang: the diarrhoea had returned the night before 'with a vengeance' – very liquid, no blood, no mucus. I saw Mojito again the next day. She looked dreadful but we felt it was worth re-starting the antibiotics. This I did. To our delight and relief Mojito improved again. Based on this I felt justified in making a diagnosis of 'antibiotic responsive chronic enteropathy'. Over the following two months, I maintained antibiotic treatment but gradually reduced the corticosteroid dose. Mojito did well. Antibiotic therapy was continued long-term.

Mojito died suddenly seven months later, aged 13 years. A post-mortem examination showed a ruptured splenic tumour that appeared to be of recent origin.

EYES

Dog's vision differs from that of humans. They have much better vision in low intensity light and have a more acute perception of movement than people, but their colour vision is poorer – attuned to yellow or blue but not to red hues. Depth perception in dogs is poorer than that of people. These differences between the species exist because the anatomy of the eyes and brain differ; for instance, dogs have a reflective inner lining in the eye, called the tapetum, which enhances night-vision. Humans don't have a tapetum. The light receptors in the retina differ between the species too. Dogs have a preponderance of rods, but far fewer cones than humans, which enhances their ability to perceive movement but means their colour vision differs. Dogs have a wider field of view than we do, but the area directly in front of the nose, where both eyes share a field of view, is narrower than humans. Because they have a smaller area of binocular vision, dogs' perception of

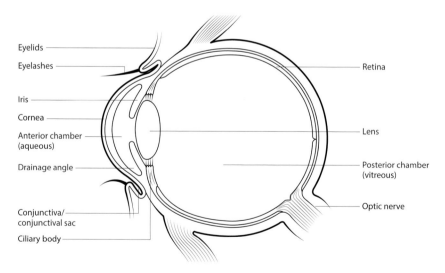

Figure 7.3. Basic anatomy of the dog's eye (see text for further details).

distance is poor compared with us. The shapes of dogs' heads vary, so the visual abilities of different breeds differ substantially.

Problems with the eyes and nearby tissues are common in dogs. The eyes are also often injured in accidents, in disputes with cats (claw wounds), or during dog fights. These traumatic lesions can be very serious. They are covered in the chapter on emergencies (Chapter 8, p. 215). Other common eye conditions are discussed below.

Red, sore, cloudy or runny eyes

The eyelids and eyelashes protect the eye. They ensure the clear cornea is bathed in tears and wiped gently by blinking. Tears are composed of three parts: lipid, mucous and aqueous phases. The aqueous (watery) component is mainly provided by the lacrymal gland hidden below the upper eyelid. Tiny glands at the base of the eyelashes provide the oily lipid, whilst the mucus comes from special cells in the conjunctiva called goblet cells. The tears moisten and nourish the clear surface of the eye, the cornea, which normally has no blood supply. Tears wash away debris. They also contain many different proteins, such as antibodies and lysozyme that fight microbes. The conjunctiva is the membrane around the eye that forms the inner surface of the eyelid, covers the third eyelid (hidden behind the inner corner of the eye close to the nose), and is continuous with the transparent cornea. Tears normally run out of the eyes through a duct into the nose. This is why you snivel when you cry. If this drainage system is overwhelmed – for example, if the eye is inflamed, or these ducts are blocked – tears may spill across the face.

Inflammation of the conjunctiva, 'conjunctivitis', is common in dogs. Conjunctivitis is itchy. Characterised by reddening and increased tear production, it is often seen in dogs who have a respiratory infection, such as 'kennel cough' (see section on Coughing and sneezing, beginning p. 174). Other causes include, allergies, trauma or anything that interferes with the contour and function of the eyelids. In some dogs the eyelids are faulty, so that the shape of the lid does not closely match the contour of the eye, or the lid may be distorted in some other way. A common problem is entropion, in which the eyelid edges are rolled over so that the lashes rub against the eye. This is painful, and often tears spill across the face below the eye. Entropion is usually a condition the dog has been born with ('congenital'), becoming obvious as the head grows and matures in the first few months of life. Treatment is surgical. Several other anatomical faults can cause persistent irritation of the eyes from a young age; for instance, sometimes the eyelashes grow abnormally, or the skin of the face may be excessively folded so that facial hair rubs against the eye(s) leading to pain, and the excessive production of tears. These problems are treatable.

The cornea itself, the clear window of the eye, can also become inflamed. This is called keratitis, which occurs when it is damaged by foreign bodies, infection, or if the tears are faulty in some way. In dogs with prominent bulging eyes, the tear film often fails so that the corneal surface tends to become dried out – desiccated. Persistent low-grade keratitis of this sort often leads to the deposition of pigment in the cornea which gradually spreads across the eye(s). Another cause of keratitis is 'dry eye', kerato-conjunctivitis sicca, in which the patient produces a reduced volume of abnormal tears that are very sticky. Dry eye usually develops because the lacrymal gland is inflamed. Any dog who appears to get repeated episodes of conjunctivitis or keratitis should be tested for this disease, which is common but can be easily recognised and very effectively treated in most cases (see Chapter 9, p. 220).

As a result of conjunctivitis and keratitis the surface of the cornea (the epithelium) might become ulcerated. This is painful. A corneal ulcer might be obvious as a pale grey or white spot towards the centre of the cornea. Those dogs will screw up their eye(s), have an ocular discharge, and obvious discomfort. However, frequently corneal ulceration is more subtle than this and can only be picked up by a clinician using flourescein, a sterile stain, which adheres to and highlights the damaged corneal epithelium. Corneal ulceration can spread and deepen quickly, especially if the eye is infected with bacteria, or the dog persistently rubs at it. Without timely treatment these melting ulcers can ultimately rupture, so that the fluid in the chamber of the eye in front of the lens starts to leak out. Inflammation and infection can quickly spread into the deeper parts. This is an emergency, which if not treated promptly will lead to total loss of the eye. However, when treated appropriately and quickly most corneal ulcers will heal. Often, treatment requires frequent application of several different drugs to the eye as well as the use of systemic painkillers. Because these drugs must be given through the day and night and the eye must be re-examined frequently, it might be necessary to hospitalise your dog.

Occasionally, corneal ulcers persist and fail to heal because the surface cells cannot properly attach to the corneal tissue beneath. These 'indolent' ulcers must first be treated surgically. Healthy corneal epithelium then can spread centripetally across the defect and the ulcer heals.

Sometimes a dog might present with a cloudy eye. This could be due to corneal ulceration and fluid 'water-logging' the cornea, termed 'corneal oedema'. But clouding of the eye can occur for a host of other reasons. For instance, if the deeper structures of the eye are inflamed, 'uveitis', the whole eye might appear cloudy. This can happen in dogs with certain systemic infections, such as canine adenovirus, or if there has been bleeding into the eye as a result of trauma or a problem with the ability of the blood to clot. Sometimes uveitis is caused by a tumour in the eye. Rarely, high blood pressure can lead to retinal detachment and bleeding into one or both eyes. The affected eye becomes functionally blind. This scenario is rather common in cats, but much less common in dogs. Aggressive drug therapy to lower blood pressure sometimes leads to the restoration of sight, which always feels a bit like a miracle. Another very important cause of a cloudy eye is glaucoma (see below).

The lens of the eye itself can become opaque, which is known as cataract. There are several different sorts of cataract. Some cataracts develop in young dogs because of inherited genetic abnormalities; breeds affected include the Belgian Shepherd, German Shepherd, Labrador, Golden Retriever, Staffordshire Bull Terrier, Old English Sheepdog, Miniature and Giant Schnauzers, Welsh Springer Spaniels and the Standard Poodle, as well as several more exotic breeds. In some cases, the precise genetic defect has been identified and can be tested for. In others the inheritance pattern is not yet known. Cataract can also be acquired due to trauma to the lens, in which case it usually only affects one eye (unilateral), or as part of a more generalised eye problem, or associated with a tumour in the eye. One of the most spectacular types of cataract is the dramatic blue-grey opacification that occurs in dogs with diabetes. This cataract often develops quite early on the course of the disease in spite of successful management of the diabetes itself (see Chapter 9, p. 223). Another condition, which is very common in old dogs, is nuclear sclerosis, in which the lens slowly develops a light grey hue. This is not a true cataract and causes little visual impairment.

Glaucoma

The front of the globe of the eye behind the cornea is called the anterior segment. This houses the lens and the iris, which is the pigmented circular curtain surrounding the pupil. The anterior segment is filled with fluid, aqueous humour, which is produced by the ciliary body, a structure behind the edge of the iris. This fluid, which nourishes the lens and the iris, is constantly created, flows through the anterior chamber, then drains away through tiny pores at the periphery of the iris forming a halo deep to the cornea but in front of the lens. This halo of pores is called the drainage angle. Glaucoma is a condition in which the rate of production of aqueous humour exceeds the rate of drainage. This means that the fluid pressure within the eye increases beyond normal. As the intra-ocular pressure increases, so the delicate sensory parts of the eye, the retina and the optic nerve are damaged. Found in association with several different eye diseases, congenital, genetic and acquired, glaucoma is very serious because it can lead to blindness. Sadly, glaucoma is relatively common.

There are many signs that dogs might exhibit if they have glaucoma, such as excessive tears, facial pain, clouding of the cornea, dilation of the pupil and protrusion of the third eyelid. Dogs with ocular pain often screw up their eyelids (called blepharospasm). Sometimes blood vessels overlying the white of the eye become very prominent. As you now know, these clinical signs are also seen with many other eye complaints, which means that most cases of glaucoma cannot be diagnosed on this basis alone. If a vet is concerned that a dog might have glaucoma, they will need to measure the pressure within the eye, which they can do with a sensitive instrument called a tonometer. Several different drugs are usually administered to dogs with glaucoma and where possible the dog will be referred urgently to see an eye specialist. Sometimes, if glaucoma is quite advanced, the eye becomes larger than normal. If this has occurred the eye will usually be completely blind and the prognosis for the return of sight is virtually hopeless. Surgical removal of the eye on welfare grounds is frequently required. In those cases, attention will also turn to the other eye because many dogs who get glaucoma will have a problem that affects both eyes.

It is worth mentioning here that there are lots of dogs who lose their sight, in one or both eyes, and some who have to have both removed, but many dogs who become blind in this way still cope well in the world and seem to have a good quality of life. This is one occasion when you might find it hard to think of the world the way a dog does. For dogs, the senses of smell and hearing are almost certainly more crucial to their lives than their sight. So, if your dog becomes blind that need not be a disaster. More of this in Chapter 8, 'Emergencies'.

THE LAME DOG

Lameness is one of the most common reasons for a dog to be brought to the vet. Most lameness is painful. In many cases the cause is quickly established and easily treated but in others investigation and treatment can be complex and difficult. If your dog becomes suddenly lame whilst out on a walk a traumatic cause is most likely.

The keys to the cause of lameness begin with establishing that the dog is indeed lame and which leg is affected. This can be much more challenging than it might seem. A dog who is very lame will often refuse to weight bear on the affected limb or might hold it up, but when the lameness is more subtle you must carefully watch the animal walking, trotting or running to establish which limb is affected. Whenever I am presented with a lame dog, I always want to watch them move; walking away from me, then across my line of sight, finally back towards me. Dogs who are lame on a forelimb usually show a characteristic gait in which they nod their head down when the good leg meets the ground and raise their head when the painful limb bears weight. For the back legs this rule is reversed; the pelvis and rump of a dog lame on one back leg drops on that side when the lame leg hits the ground.

Sometimes the problem is bilateral, that is both front- or both back-legs, are affected. This most frequently occurs because of an anatomical problem. Such abnormalities of skeletal development are especially common in certain pure-breeds and usually show themselves in youth. Bilateral lamenesses really can be quite tricky to identify but often the dog will take short strides, or they might swing the limbs outward from their body with each step. There are typical gaits associated with some common joint problems, so, for instance, when there is bilateral lameness of the hind limbs the dog might exhibit a 'bunny-hopping' style. Those who have anatomically malformed hip joints, hip dysplasia, tend to wiggle their bum as they walk (see below).

Other forms of lameness that can be awkward to home in on are those that shift from joint to joint, or leg to leg, if the condition involves the back, the pelvis or multiple sites. Nervous disorders also sometimes manifest as lameness.

Once it has been established which limb(s) is / are affected, the next stage should identify where the seat of pain is. Fools rush in. A dog in pain is liable to resent that. I like to establish rapport with the dog before I go further; stroking, moving quietly, speaking softly. I need to assess the affected limb through observation, palpation and manipulation, site by site, joint by joint, progressing in an orderly fashion. As a rule of thumb, if an animal exhibits severe lameness of sudden (acute) onset it is most often due to a problem far down the leg. I like to begin from the paw and work my way up the limb. Other vets will have their own routines.

In the paw, it is essential to examine the claws ('nails'), the claw-beds, each of the black crusty digital pads, the main pad, the 'webs' between each digit and each digit in turn. The dew-claw, which is the equivalent to our thumb-nail, on the inner (medial) aspect of the paw, must not be forgotten. Palpation of each area might disclose the site of pain and there might be swelling or heat. Manipulation of each joint could reveal pain, swelling, instability, a limited range of motion, or crepitus (where joint surfaces are irregular and grate against each other). Sometimes a small area of moist exudate from a claw-bed or a torn claw will become apparent. A foreign body such as a thorn or a grass-seed might reveal itself. A pad might be lacerated or torn or a thorn or a glass splinter might be lodged in one of the pads. When a dog has a wound, they will usually lick the area so this behaviour is a helpful guide. Another tell-tale sign is nibbling with their front teeth, the incisors, which is often provoked by a foreign body such as a burr between the digits or perhaps a tick attached to the skin. For close observation, it might be necessary to shave the paw. A colleague reminded me that sometimes lameness can be due to things which seem absurd, such as chewing gum stuck in the fur of the foot (thanks Niall).

If there's nothing apparent in the paw, then I move up to the carpus (wrist) of the fore leg or the hock (ankle) of the hind limb, again methodically searching for discomfort, swelling, heat, etc., manipulating each joint to assess the range of movement and whether that movement is free and smooth. The carpus is a very lax joint in the dog. Much more than a hinge, it can be twisted a little, around the axis of the leg, so careful assessment must deliberately induce those movements in turn. When this joint has been traumatised, it often shows impressive swelling, or there could be instability if the supporting structures of the joint have been torn or there have been fractures of the smaller bones in the carpus.

It is generally unusual for sudden lameness to be associated with pain in the shafts of long bones, though there are important exceptions. Sometimes, it can be difficult to localise lesions because during examination it is necessary to hold the shafts of the long bones. When you flex or extend one joint there is a tendency for other joints to bend too, so it's important to try to manipulate one joint at a time. To assess the elbow the joint is flexed and extended but, like the carpus, it must also be twisted a little, as if the dog were unscrewing or tightening a jam jar lid. Elbow lameness is rather common in young dogs of medium and large breeds where it is often caused by a serious condition known as elbow dysplasia (see below). Some other developmental conditions, anatomical anomalies, are also particularly associated with certain types or breeds of dog. So, for example, small terriers frequently have a hip joint abnormality from quite a young age that causes them to carry a hind leg, especially when they accelerate to a trot.[1] Small dogs are also prone to a stifle problem in which the knee cap (patella) slides out of the groove on the front of the joint. This might manifest itself as a skipping lameness. When lameness is caused by joint disease higher up the leg it can be difficult to identify exactly where it originates from, except by performing specific tests that are beyond the scope of this book.

If your dog shows a new (acute) lameness, you might immediately identify a traumatic lesion such as a laceration, abrasion or a foreign body (see 'Wounds, p. 180). Depending on the severity you might be able to treat this yourself by simply removing a splinter, bathing the wound warm – NOT HOT! – salted water is the simplest (see p. 225), and resting the dog for a day or two. Don't be tempted to give drugs designed for human sprains and bruises such as ibuprofen – many of these are toxic to dogs. In other cases, a visit to the vet will be necessary. They will probably quiz you carefully about when the lameness began and whether any trauma seemed to precipitate the problem. They will look for generalised disease as well as a localised problem and will be searching for the source of pain. Sometimes, they might immediately be able to identify the cause. In other circumstances they may be sufficiently concerned to suggest X-raying your dog. If the vet finds nothing too serious, they will probably assume the dog has suffered a bump, bruise, strain or sprain, perhaps due to unwitnessed trauma. The usual advice in such cases would be strict rest for a few days. Some form of analgesia, for instance with a non-steroidal anti-inflammatory agent, might be prescribed for a few days, up to two weeks. In the event the lameness fails to resolve, or returns soon after the analgesia has been withdrawn, then further investigation is usually warranted.

---

[1] The condition is called aseptic necrosis of the femoral head, aka Legg-Calve-Perthes disease.

Specific problems

Fractures

Dogs often break their bones during road accidents or as a result of a fall. The technical term for a broken bone is a fracture. Most animals with fractures will be very lame indeed. If a vet suspects a fracture, they will want to take radiographs. The appropriate treatment for each fracture depends on numerous different factors such as the age and general health of the dog, their behaviour, as well as the site and type of fracture. Young animals in good general health tend to heal well, but those who have not yet reached adult body size and maturity are in danger of long-term consequences if fractures are not managed perfectly because when the bones are still growing, deformities could develop, especially if the fracture(s) involve the long bones of the limbs. Older dogs, and those who are in poor general health for other reasons, such as those with a systemic illness, are more challenging to treat.

If the break has occurred in the middle of the shaft of a long bone, there are few fragments, and the parts are not displaced, then it may be possible to treat it by using an external splint and bandaging. If, on the other hand, there are multiple fragments, the fragments are very displaced, there is an open wound, or there is a lot of muscle or other tissue around the fracture site – as with breaks in the upper parts of the limbs – then repair is more likely to require surgical treatment and internal, or external, fixation with bone plates, pins, wires or other devices. When a vet is evaluating your dog's fracture, they will be considering how to get a really stable temporary fix in which the broken fragments are closely apposed to each other. This is known as fracture reduction. It is important to manage each fracture without compromising the health of other parts of the limb; this the clinician will be thinking about the joints above and below the fracture site, not just the break alone. They will try to prevent complications of treatment too, such as bone infections, which are more likely if the break is exposed through an open wound. If fracture fragments are inaccurately opposed then the bone might heal with an angular deformity. If the fragments wobble, then the fracture might not heal at all. Added to all this we must tailor treatment to your dog's lifestyle. Those animals that are extremely boisterous and those who are overweight will subject the lesion to higher forces; they are more likely to disrupt the fracture fragments.

All fractures require several weeks to heal. During the convalescence your dog will be given pain relief and must be rested. Short lead walks only will be permitted, although these should lengthen as your dog improves. Follow-up will inevitably require further radiology.

Cranial cruciate rupture

This is an injury that occurs particularly in middle-aged dogs of the larger breeds, such as Retrievers, Rottweilers and Mastiffs; it is also rather common in terriers. There are two cruciate ligaments (cranial and caudal) inside the knee joint that cross each other running between the femur (the thigh bone) and the tibia (the main bone of the shin). Rupture of these ligaments, especially the cranial ligament, is usually the end-stage of a degenerative process that has gone on for a considerable length of time, but the final rupture is usually sudden, brought on by a twisting movement of the knee. Once this has happened your dog's stance might be telling; a characteristic posture in which the hind paw is slightly flexed over whilst little weight is taken on that limb. The injury is painful, so, if it is suspected, your vet will probably need to examine the dog under anaesthesia. Radiography of the joint will likely be required. Treatment usually necessitates surgery to improve the stability of the stifle. Over the years, the favoured surgical techniques have evolved. Presently, most orthopaedic surgeons choose a procedure called a tibial plateau levelling operation (TPLO) or a tibial tuberosity advancement (TTA). This is advanced surgery, usually must be done by a specialist, and is likely to cost several thousand pounds. In small, lightweight dogs, simpler and cheaper treatment can work well. After surgery every dog will need potent pain-relief and have to be rested. Re-introduction of exercise is done very gradually in a controlled manner over many weeks. Long-term outcomes can be excellent but these dogs are prone to osteoarthritis of the stifle joints in later life. More than half the dogs who rupture a cranial cruciate ligament in one knee will do so in the other knee, often within a year.

Hip dysplasia

Hip dysplasia is an anatomical and conformational problem in which the ball ('head') of the femur, the thigh bone, is not properly seated in the socket, the acetabulum, of the pelvis. This instability allows the femoral head to bounce in and out of the socket, which traumatises the tissues leading to chronic inflammation. Pain inevitably follows. Eventually osteoarthritis develops. Dogs are not born with hip dysplasia, but like many of the conditions we have discussed, this is a condition to which some animals are genetically predisposed. Additional lifestyle

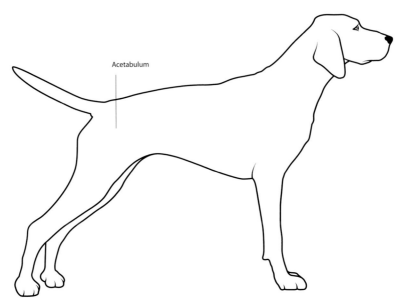

Figure 7.4. The socket joint of the hip, the acetabulum, forms part of the bony pelvis under the gluteal muscles of the rump.

factors may also be important. If young dogs of predisposed breeds are fed to appetite or grow very rapidly, this increases their risk of developing hip dysplasia. Conversely, it has been shown that dogs who are relatively underfed during growth, remaining lean throughout puppyhood, have less hip dysplasia. This is best achieved by feeding a relatively high protein puppy diet. Some authorities suggest that controlled lead-based walking of young dogs can improve the muscle bulk and support structures around the joints, condition the hips, and thus minimise instability, whereas boisterous unrestricted exercise and the rough play young dogs love to indulge in may be more likely to lead to joint damage. Hip dysplasia is particularly common in Retrievers, including Labradors, Border Collies, German Shepherd Dogs, Rottweilers, Mastiffs, Boxers, English Bulldogs and Old English Sheepdogs. Many breeders nowadays screen their dogs for hip dysplasia before breeding (see https://www.bva.co.uk/canine-health-schemes/hip-scheme) and choose not to breed with dogs showing any deformities. Notwithstanding these efforts hip dysplasia remains common and disables many dogs.

Clinical signs of hip dysplasia are often absent until dogs are middle-aged when they begin to develop osteoarthritis and hip pain. You might only notice your dog has become slow to rise in the morning, less interested in walks, or lays down for a rest during exercise. In other cases, there are obvious signs referable to the hind-limbs, including a 'bum-wiggle' best seen as the dog walks away from you. Many dogs with this condition take a lot of their body weight on the forelimbs, which alters their forelimb gait too.

In the early stages of this disease, whilst a dog is young, some orthopaedic specialists recommend ceasing all off-lead activity; replacing it with controlled lead exercise that aims to build up the support structures around the hips, to bulk-up the muscles of the thighs and to improve joint stability. Sometimes specialised surgical procedures are performed at this age which aim to improve hip anatomy. The outcomes can be good but are often less than perfect. Ultimately, many dogs with hip dysplasia develop severe osteoarthritis (which can be treated but not cured, see below). Hip replacement surgery can be performed in dogs. It is often very successful. Unfortunately, only a few talented surgeons have the skill, experience and facilities to do this. You will not be surprised to learn costs of hip replacement are eye-watering.

Elbow dysplasia

Another fairly common cause of lameness in youngish dogs is known as elbow dysplasia. Several different, rather subtle anatomic anomalies comprise this complex of problems, which can be very challenging indeed to diagnose. Often a clinician will be very suspicious of this disease based on the history and clinical findings. Radiography can be helpful but more specialised techniques are sometimes necessary to prove the cause. Arthroscopy, in which the joint is examined with an optical device inserted through a small incision, is helpful. Computerised tomography (CT) or even MRI (magnetic resonance imaging) are sometimes required. Treatment is surgical. On occasion this can be accomplished using 'key-hole' methods. Without treatment osteoarthritis is inevitable.

Osteoarthritis

Osteoarthritis (OA) is an incurable degenerative condition of the joint(s) that occurs as an end result of longstanding injury. In dogs, it most frequently affects the elbows, shoulders, knees (stifles) and hips, but it can affect any joint, including those of the spine and the digits. OA usually results from abnormal wear of a normal joint (for example, caused by obesity) or normal wear on an abnormal joint (such as a dysplastic hip). Dogs that have OA will usually have some pain but it can be difficult to clearly and objectively assess that pain. What's more, pain (which is a sensation) and suffering (which, arguably, is an emotion) are not always directly correlated and this too can make the evaluation of the effects of OA on quality of life challenging. Recently, several different owner questionnaires have been created which have been designed for use in dogs with health problems or OA (see e.g. LOAD – Liverpool OA in Dogs questionnaire (from the University of Liverpool; see Muller et al. (2009) and the Canine Brief Pain Inventory: www.CanineBPI.com). These can help us to understand the effects of this condition on your dog's welfare and quality of life, particularly if they are used before, and after, introducing any change in the management of the problem.

It is said that at least a quarter of dogs aged nine years or above have OA. These dogs may exhibit one or more or a large constellation of clinical signs that include obvious lameness and stiffness (especially on getting to their feet after sleep or rest). The dog might be slower on walks, hesitant to get into or out of the car, unwilling to rise to greet you when you arrive home, reluctant to climb or descend the stairs, no longer jump onto your lap or into a favourite chair, display new or unusual postures when sitting, or simply seem lazy. Some dogs with OA become unsociable and withdraw from company or no longer want to play with other dogs. Some will lick their limb(s) persistently. If a dog is uncomfortable, they might become restless during the night and pace the house persistently when they should be asleep. Others become bad-tempered, or constipated (especially if they have back and / or hip pain). Dogs who are uncomfortable may pant for no very apparent reason (such cases are sometimes mistaken to have respiratory or cardiac disease, or even anxiety). Many dogs with joint disease will alter their gait in such a way that their claws become abnormally worn.

The clinical signs that a vet might find during examination are also quite legion; including pain localised to one or several joints, crepitus (see p. 155) or joint instability, and often restricted range of movement in the joint(s). Some joints will be swollen, possibly warm, or palpably disfigured. Very often there will be muscle loss in the affected limbs ('atrophy'), which is most easily appreciated if the problem is unilateral – affecting one limb of a pair.

Imaging of the joint by X-rays, CT or MRI can disclose remodelling of the joint and the deposition of irregular new bone spurs ('osteophytes') around the joint. Excessive fluid within the joint space might be found in the stifle or either side of the point of the elbow. In some cases the cartilage of the joint is thinned or eroded and bone beneath the joint may be denser than normal (known as sub-chondral sclerosis).

Because OA is so common and other forms of joint disease occur relatively infrequently in dogs, laboratory evaluation of the joint is not commonly done. However, when a joint is clearly hot or swollen, the possibility of an infection should be considered. Septic arthritis of this sort can be evaluated by looking for inflammatory white blood cells under a microscope and bacteria by culture of the joint fluid. Lastly, some dogs who have inflammation of several joints ('polyarthritis') might have an auto-immune condition such as rheumatoid arthritis or an infectious cause such as Lyme disease – which is caused by *Borrelia Burgdorferi,* a bacteria spread by ticks.

The treatment of OA centres around three principles; analgesia, weight management and exercise management. In addition to these, there are things that can be done in the home that might help the dog to live more comfortably with the condition.

Treating osteoarthritis

Analgesia (pain relief)
Most dogs with OA are treated with a non-steroidal anti-inflammatory agent (commonly coined NSAIDs). There are numerous drugs of this sort licensed for veterinary use, meaning that they have been proven to be safe and effective as well as showing relatively few side-effects.[2] This treatment will often dramatically reduce signs of pain and may have some joint-sparing effects too, although this is controversial. Side-effects are not common at the recommended dose rates, but in theory these types of drug can potentiate renal (kidney) diseases and in a few patients NSAIDs definitely do seriously damage the gut wall, even causing vomiting of blood, haemorrhagic diarrhoea, or, very rarely, perforation of a stomach ulcer. Fortunately, many dogs that might not tolerate one NSAID will tolerate an alternative, so, if the first choice causes side-effects, or doesn't work well, experimentation with other drug(s) of the same class is often fruitful. A new

---

[2] Most of the NSAIDs are 'COX inhibitors', that is to say they work by breaking an important link in the inflammatory chain known as the arachidonic acid pathway by inhibition of an enzyme called cyclo-oxygenase.

drug, **grapiprant**, which is a novel type of NSAID has recently become available.[3] Early experience suggests that this drug may be safer than conventional NSAIDs, but it might not be quite so potent and unfortunately gastrointestinal side-effects do occur in a small proportion of dogs.

During the preparation of this book, a fascinating and exciting new treatment has become licensed for the treatment of dogs with OA. The drug, called **Bedinvetmab**, is an injectable monoclonal antibody that acts against a molecule called 'nerve growth factor' (NGF). Monoclonal antibodies are an absolutely transformational form of treatment because they are not drugs in the conventional sense of the word. Monoclonal antibodies are physiological biochemicals and function within the body in a way completely analogous to the natural antibodies that all dogs (and other animals, including people) have. Unlike, for instance, the NSAIDs, they have been shown to have virtually no impact on the liver, the gut, the kidneys or the cardiovascular system. Dogs treated with this drug, which is given by sub-cutaneous injection at four-week intervals, have shown marked reductions in pain, improvements in mobility and quality of life. The treatment is expected to be used instead of NSAIDs in most cases, although in principle, for very severe advanced cases it might be used alongside other treatments. At the time of writing, there have been rather severe supply problems because initial excitement in the veterinary community and amongst owners has been very high.

Multi-drug therapy is necessary in some dogs with OA. Alternative analgesia is certainly warranted in a dog who cannot tolerate NSAIDs. The first alternative or additional drug chosen is often paracetamol (which is tolerated well at low doses). (THIS DRUG IS TOXIC TO CATS). Another drug often used is Tramadol, which is an opiate, rather like morphine or codeine. Tramadol has no anti-inflammatory properties but acts as a painkiller via several different mechanisms. Like paracetamol, this drug is licensed for use in dogs, which means that the safety and efficacy of the drug has been thoroughly studied. However, there are some dogs who do not seem to benefit from Tramadol and indeed a fair amount of anecdote suggests that the analgesic effects of this drug in dogs have been exaggerated. Veterinary anaesthesiologists suggest that there are a number of other painkilling agents

---

[3] Grapiprant acts on the same inflammatory pathway, but this is not a COX inhibitor. Instead it works more specifically as a prostaglandin receptor inhibitor (or 'Piprant') which blocks the effects of a crucial inflammatory and pain mediator called EP4.

we can use in dogs with OA if licensed drugs fail to provide enough relief. These include gabapentin, amantadine and amitriptyline. These drugs are widely used in human medicine but are not licensed for use in dogs in the UK at present. Vets are allowed to use them at their own discretion but they have to obtain a client's permission (see the Prescribing Cascade, p. 301).

Weight management

Some elderly dogs with OA have, severe muscle loss and generalised weight loss. They will have a BCS of 3/9 or less. For those dogs, feeding a highly digestible high protein and high fat diet can help to ameliorate this weight loss. Dogs usually find such diets very attractive. Any new diet should be introduced gradually over several days. If appropriate analgesia is in place the dog's exercise regime should aim to build up muscle mass starting from brief and gentle beginnings (see below). If the weight loss continues it is very likely another illness is responsible.

Any dog who is overweight is likely to suffer if they have OA. Your dog will benefit if they are kept slim. A credible and practical aim in the treatment of dogs with OA is that they should have a body condition score of 5/9 or less. I appreciate most dogs love their grub and it might seem mean to diet a dog who is also challenged by chronic discomfort, but those overweight dogs with arthritis who lose weight really do benefit by being in less pain and by enjoying a longer and happier life. In Chapter 5, I covered the subject of feeding dogs and also addressed how to diet a dog who is overweight (see pp. 95–99). It is often helpful if you see a vet or a veterinary nurse at the outset to plan a weight reduction programme. Most practices will be very happy to help and often will arrange regular re-visits to monitor your success. There are specific diets formulated to aid you in this process. They are helpful but not mandatory.

Here is a simple approach: never feed a dog to appetite. Feed a dog to achieve and maintain healthy body weight, which is a body condition score of 4 or 5/9. Sensible and easy first steps are to limit the number of feeds to one per day and buy a smaller dog-food bowl. Weigh out what you are currently feeding per day (all of it, including 'dental-treats' and other rewards) and initially reduce the amount you feed to 4/5ths (80%). Feed this amount for the first 4 weeks. Weigh your dog once a week. Aim to lose 1–2% of body weight per week. Re-adjust the volume of food as necessary. Continue until your dog reaches your target weight and BCS. This can take many months. If this approach doesn't seem to be working, don't give up – go back to your vet for more help.

about these products is wrapped in marketing hype but cuts no mustard as scientific proof. Client testimonials are not a reliable way to make judgements. On the other hand, some proper peer-reviewed scientific evidence does show that omega III polyunsaturated fatty acid (PUFA) supplements, often based on cod liver oil or diets rich in these agents, have a beneficial effect in mild to moderate arthritis.[5] Moreover, it has been clearly established that they can modify a crucial inflammatory pathway known as the arachidonic acid cascade; a mode of action has been proven. This intervention usually should be trialled for 4–6 weeks before concluding if it has helped a particular dog, or not. Green-lipped mussels and oil derived from them, which contain omega IIIs and other constituents, have also been shown to help dogs with this condition, although not all products claiming to be composed from this mollusc are likely to be of equal value. There is little convincing evidence that glucosamine sulphate, or chondroitin are helpful, although these products seem to be popular and are very widely available. Other products derived from turmeric, cannabis, or chilli oil are also being sold with the implication that they help but as yet I can find no convincing scientific evidence of efficacy. That doesn't necessarily mean they are ineffective but does mean you should be wary.

For a long time, acupuncture was regarded with suspicion by mainstream clinicians but it is now irrefutable that the technique can work well to manage chronic pain. It is recognised in human medicine and by the NHS as useful in people with chronic OA of the knees and hips. Unfortunately, few veterinary clinicians have the requisite training and experience to deliver acupuncture effectively. If you and your vet agree that acupuncture therapy might help your dog the best way forward is probably to be referred to a vet who is a member of the Association of Veterinary Acupuncturists, or at least one who has had training from them.

Several other new forms of treatment for OA show promise but are not yet widely available or clinically proven. These approaches are aimed at improving joint health directly by manipulating joint biology. They include various forms of stem cell therapy, the intra-articular injections of platelet rich plasma, or a blood product, serum, derived from the patient themselves. It is conjectured that treatments of this sort might promote recovery of healthy tissue within the joints. The background cell biology to these approaches has involved colossal efforts and huge

---

[5] Particularly those containing high concentrations of DHA (docosahexaenoic acid) and EPA (eicosapentaenoic acid).

sums of money. One day, this research will probably pay huge dividends, but it is unlikely to be mainstream therapy for some time yet.

> I have known Zip for almost his entire life. I vaccinated him as a pup. A tri-colour collie with a mad obsession for chasing balls and a complete disdain for other dogs, Zip was always slim, muscular and active. He aged well. But over the last two years or so he has become disabled by arthritis. Drugs have helped him but over time it has become increasingly more difficult to keep him mobile and comfortable. Until a month ago, he still enjoyed two short walks every day. Now, he's hardly able to get up. Last week he reached the grand old age of 16.
>
> I've been asked to put him to sleep tomorrow, at home.

THE SUDDENLY DULL, LETHARGIC AND DEJECTED DOG

One of the common presentations at our practice is the dog who suddenly seems dejected and lethargic; 'going down ill', as one of my French colleagues used to put it. Anorexia, refusal to go for a walk, withdrawal to a quiet place in the house, sleeping longer. These are the sorts of signs clients often mention. Don't ignore this behaviour but don't panic either. Make an appointment to see your vet in the next 24 hours. Meanwhile, think carefully about what your dog's been doing, and not doing, in the previous day or two. Here are some issues to consider:

- Are they eating and drinking normally?
  - If not, are they completely refusing food (anorexia) and /or drink (adipsia). Have they been seen to drink excessively?
- Have they been sick?
  - If so, when, in relation to feeding? How often?
- Have they passed faeces (poo) and urine?
  - Was that unusual in any way (colour, consistency, volume, frequency, smell)?
- Have they been sleeping normally, excessively, or have they been restless?

- Have you noticed abnormal or noisy breathing?

    ○ It can be useful to measure the breathing rate but this is best done whilst the dog is asleep. Dogs should normally breathe quietly, with only gentle chest movements, at between 20 to 30 breaths per minute whilst asleep. If they breathe more slowly, that is not a reason to worry. All dogs sigh occasionally when asleep.

- Has your dog been coughing? If so, how frequently?

- Has your dog been sneezing? If so, how often?

- Have you noticed any bleeding? If so, where from?

- Have you noticed any new lameness, new swellings, new smells, new sounds or new behaviours?

Over the previous couple of days, it's worth thinking about where your dog has been, what he has eaten, whether she has met other dogs, and if there was anything they have done out of the ordinary, such as a long walk, scavenging, drinking from a slime-covered lake or an oily puddle, etc.

It can also be very helpful to make notes about what you've noticed so you can answer your vet's questions when you see them. Sometimes a short video clip on your phone can be useful too.

If the dog seems to be getting worse very quickly then you should get to the vet as soon as possible.

Faced with a dog with this history, your vet will want to make a very careful examination that, as usual, will start from the general and move on to be more specific and targeted as the history becomes clear and clinical findings unfold. Invariably, they will begin by measuring vital signs as well as an evaluation of the level of consciousness and evidence of pain. A dog that is exhibiting very obvious neurological signs will receive a different examination to one that has an abnormal heart rhythm. Similarly, a dog who is very weak or collapsed will receive a different approach to one who is principally showing breathing difficulties. However, the aim is always to get as much relevant information as possible whilst minimising the patient's distress and avoiding harm.

In this kind of case your vet is very likely to want to take some blood and /or urine from your dog for a profile of tests. Testing of this sort is sometimes derided as 'fishing' for a problem, but the approach is justified because if all the results are normal then many questions have been answered, whilst on the other hand, frequently some of these data stick out like the cartoon sore thumb, pointing the clinician's gaze in a useful direction.

It is completely beyond the scope of this book to list and discuss all the different problems that could present in this way. That would not be very helpful to you either, but once your vet has examined your dog and has a more focused idea of what is wrong then they ought to be able to talk to you about what they've found and the next steps. This is when a good rapport between client and vet is so important.

URINARY INCONTINENCE, URINARY ACCIDENTS, EXCESSIVE URINATION AND OTHER SIGNS OF URINARY DYSFUNCTION

Incontinence

If a dog has incontinence, they will pee where they are lying without being aware they have done so. Often, they wake up and give you a look that seems to say: 'Someone has pissed in my bed, I really don't think it was me.' Urinary incontinence is highly uncommon (though not rare) in male dogs, but common in bitches, especially those who have been neutered. There is general agreement that bitches who are neutered young are more likely to become incontinent than those who are neutered at a year of age or more. Often urinary incontinence is a problem of the elderly, particularly bitches in their teens. Certainly, the onset of incontinence frequently doesn't occur until years after neutering. The onset of incontinence is often sudden but sometimes rather subtle. You might simply notice the dog's bedding or the dog herself becoming smelly with the acrid tang of ammonia. Many owners are a bit embarrassed if their dog has become incontinent but it is usually easily treated. Without treatment the dog will suffer urine scalding of the skin and become liable to urinary tract infections that can be dangerous as well as uncomfortable for the sufferer.

When you see a vet for this issue, they will ask about general health, appetite, thirst and defecation as well as urination. They will probably weigh your dog and check their BCS. They might want to watch your dog walking and trotting to ascertain if they have any evidence of a neurologic problem, arthritis, or back pain. They will probably want to discuss your dog's ability to exercise and when/how they urinate. Abdominal palpation and a rectal examination will be done in a search for pelvic diseases, masses, etc. Tests of nerve function might be done too. In some circumstances the vet might want to do laboratory testing such as the examination of blood samples, especially to look for renal (kidney) disease, diabetes, liver problems, anaemia, or a raised white blood cell count. Sometimes urine examination and urine culture (searching for infection) might be deemed helpful and abdominal imaging to look at the bladder, kidneys, etc., might be recommended too. Remember, if you are in any doubt, always ask the clinician why they wish to do these tests and also what these will cost.

Urinary incontinence is usually treated medically. There are two different medications that are widely used, namely, phenylpropanolamine (also called diphenylhiramine) and oestriol (also called estriol). Both drugs can work well, but like all drugs there can be side-effects or other issues to consider.

Phenylpropanolamine comes as a liquid. It is usually given three times a day (i.e. ideally every eight hours), although in my experience many clients discover it works adequately given twice, or even once, daily. The drug works by gently constricting the urethra, the tube carrying the urine out from the bladder. In this way, the normal valvular function of the urethra is restored. Unfortunately, this drug, which is a catecholamine (similar to the fight or flight hormone adrenalin), can cause constriction of blood vessels too, which can raise the blood pressure. This can be troublesome. So, if your dog has heart disease, kidney problems or some other conditions, your vet might prefer to avoid this drug.

Oestriol is given as a tablet once daily, or every other day. This drug, which also improves the sphincter mechanism of the urethra, works very well too in many cases. Oestriol is an oestrogen, a hormone, and as such it should be handled carefully, because all hormone therapies potentially carry slight risks to the person who administers the drug (wear disposable drugs or wash hands thoroughly after handling). In a few dogs, this drug can suppress the bone marrow that could lead to anaemia.

In a few incontinent dogs, adequate control of the problem is only achieved by using both drugs. Some dogs do not respond to medical therapy at all. This used to be a more common problem in the days when tail-docking was permitted. That mutilation alters the anatomy and functioning of the perineum, particularly if the tail is docked very close to the bottom, which can cause, or exacerbate, urinary incontinence. There are surgical treatments that can help such cases, but the details are beyond the scope of this text.

'Accidents' and excessive urination (polyuria)

Some dogs urinate indoors on occasion. If that is happening with your dog then you should see the vet. Dogs who urinate indoors might do so for behavioural reasons; 'marking their territory' because they are anxious or upset by something, such as a new baby in the household, or a dominant dog who has moved in next door. So, the consultation with your vet should examine this possibility. Behavioural treatment might be required, but there are many other issues that can lead to urination in the wrong spot. One possibility would be that your dog has a disease that is causing them to pass a lot of urine (called polyuria) or to pass urine more frequently (termed pollakiuria). The vet will quiz you carefully to try to understand your dog's problem.

Many conditions cause polyuria. In these diseases, the dog will also be thirsty. Examples include diabetes mellitus (see p. 223), kidney failure (see p. 236), womb infections ('pyometra', see p. 187), a hormone disease termed hyperadrenocorticism (or 'Cushing's syndrome', see p. 221), certain liver disorders, and more. Any dog who has excessive thirst and is passing more urine than normal must usually have urine and blood tests to begin to untangle the problem. A word of warning here: most cases of 'PUPD' – polyuria / polydipsia – will need quite a lot of testing to get to the final diagnosis. Treatments are often really successful – see Chapter 9 – but of course this will depend on the diagnosis.

Other signs of urinary dysfunction:

Conditions that make a dog pass urine very frequently (pollakiuria) are usually those associated with inflammation involving, or close to, the lower urinary tract, such as inflammation of the bladder (cystitis), bladder stones (uroliths), inflammation of the prostate (prostatitis), or other pelvic diseases (for instance, a tumour in the bladder, or of the prostate). Dogs who have pollakiuria often also have discomfort during urination. They may strain to pass urine, the urine stream might be thin, or intermittent, also the urine may be bloody or otherwise discoloured. To work out the cause of the signs, again blood and urine testing are likely to be necessary as well as imaging studies of the pelvis and abdomen and frequently cytology of tissue samples to determine precisely which tissues are involved, and how. Cystitis might be treated with antibiotics – chosen after samples of urine have been cultured to grow and identify any bacteria that are present and tested to see which antibiotics are most likely to be effective. Prostate infections too might be treated in this way, but for serious prostatic infections or abscesses it is sometimes necessary to resort to surgical treatment. Urinary stones can sometimes be dissolved by feeding special diets but to choose the appropriate diet your vet will need to determine exactly what type of stones they are. Often this means bladder stones must be removed surgically then sent off for definitive analysis.

There are times when the signs might suggest urinary disease but in fact the seat of disease is elsewhere. For instance, sometimes discoloured urine is a sign of muscle damage. That might sound daft! In such cases, there is muscle pigment in the urine, myoglobinuria, due to muscle cell death. Myoglobinuria can also damage the kidneys; an example of a problem in one body system causing disease elsewhere. Another cause of discoloured urine is haemoglobinuria, when blood pigment is contaminating the urine. This can occur for a variety of reasons if the circulating red blood cells (erythrocytes) are being destroyed (e.g. Immune Mediated Haemolytic Anaemia – IMHA). Complete urinary obstruction is rather uncommon in dogs (cf. cats) but can be caused by a bladder stone obstructing the urethra (urolithiasis). A colleague (you again, H) pointed me to several cases where dogs seemed unable to urinate freely or were straining to urinate. These dogs were all suffering from constipation. The urinary obstruction was secondary to this.

COUGHING, SNEEZING, CHOKING AND RESPIRATORY NOISE

Sneezing and coughing are reflexes that move or remove matter from the airways. Sneezing is due to nasal irritation or disease, whereas coughing occurs when the cause lies somewhere further back – between the throat and the smallest airways deep in the lungs. Lung and chest diseases that do not involve the airways probably rarely cause coughing; although many dogs with heart diseases do cough, the exact mechanism for this is controversial.

The type of cough is rarely of much help in deciding its cause. However, there are exceptions. A persistent very loud honking cough in an older small dog such as a Yorkshire terrier or Pomeranian is usually caused by collapse of the trachea (the windpipe). A difficult problem to treat. Spasms of soft weak huffing coughs in elderly dogs are often due to heart disease. Sometimes a cough will be very loud and explosive. Indeed, clients often feel convinced that their dog has something stuck in the throat. In reality, choking is rather rare. When it does occur, it can be an acute emergency, usually caused by a foreign body such as a ball, a piece of food, a bone or vomit lodged in the throat or windpipe. Dogs who are choking are prevented by the obstruction from inspiring quickly or deeply so they cannot develop the explosive force to cough a foreign body out. If a dog is choking you must try to remove the obstruction manually or perform the Heimlich manoeuvre (see p. 197).

Loud respiratory noises such as snoring and grunting are generated by the vibration of tissue in the throat obstructing the free movement of air. In an awake dog these noises should never be considered normal. Make no mistake, those dogs who make these sounds with every breath all their lives are chronically disabled.

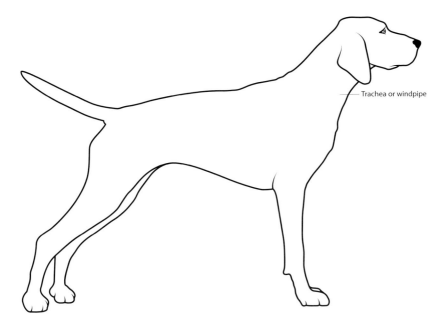

Trachea or windpipe

Figure 7.5. The trachea or windpipe is the tube which carries gases from the throat to and from the lungs.

If a dog who previously breathed silently develops loud breathing this demands veterinary attention. High pitched sounds during inspiration are almost always caused by obstructions high up in the airways. This is called stridor. When a dog's breathing is obstructed in this way the inspiratory phase of the breathing cycle will be prolonged. Low-pitched sounds occurring during either phase of the breathing cycle also usually come from the throat. This is called stertor. Many different conditions could be the cause of these noises. A common cause in older dogs is laryngeal paralysis. The voice box, or larynx, is the apparatus which generates the dog's bark. It also serves as a valve that directs the breath in and out the windpipe, whereas food and water are sent down the gullet (oesophagus), thus preventing these from being inhaled. Large dogs, such as Labradors, Setters and Afghan hounds, sometimes develop laryngeal paralysis as they get older. The first indication might be that they find exercise increasingly difficult. This can be misinterpreted as arthritis, or another musculoskeletal problem. Frequently, the sound of their bark alters, or they may go on to lose their bark completely. They start to make characteristic hee-hawing respiratory sounds, like someone sawing wood; in-and-out with each breath, especially if they become excited or exercise. Eventually, they develop an almost complete obstruction of their airway. Laryngeal paralysis can be quite effectively treated but the treatment requires a highly skilled surgeon; referral to a specialist is usually required.

The commonest causes of coughing and sneezing in dogs are infectious diseases. 'Kennel cough' denotes any infectious canine respiratory disease, usually caused by a virus or bacteria. It is very common, and certainly not limited to dogs which have been recently kennelled. It can occur in any dog but is more common in those who are young and who mix frequently with other dogs. The infectious agents can survive for some time in the environment so direct dog to dog contact is not necessary for the condition to spread. Faced with a dog with suspected kennel cough, your vet will carefully examine the upper airway and the chest and check the dog's temperature. Most dogs with kennel cough, just like most people with a cold, are not seriously ill. Some will show conjunctivitis and ocular discharge, their tonsils might be enlarged and red too, but most exhibit no additional clinical signs.

Vaccinations against 'kennel cough' do provide some protection against the two most frequent causes, namely; *Bordetella bronchiseptica* (a bacteria) and parainfluenza (a virus), but that protection is far from completely secure (see Chapter 4, p. 50). Also, there are many other agents, both bacterial and viral, which can cause infectious respiratory disease. Fortunately, the horrible distemper virus, which formerly killed many dogs, is now very uncommon indeed.

The majority of dogs who get kennel cough recover within 2–3 weeks. If they are not systemically unwell, treatment is considered to be unnecessary. However, your vet will advise you to keep the dog isolated away from other dogs and to avoid very vigorous exercise. If your dog has a high temperature, seems to be systemically unwell, or exhibits other clinical signs such as rapid or noisy breathing, lack of appetite, an altered bark, etc., then the vet might decide to give antibiotic therapy, or to investigate the patient more thoroughly.

If the cough persists for more than a month, or there are other clinical signs that are not typical of kennel cough, then further investigation is called for. For example, if a dog with a cough has a history of tiring during walks, refusing exercise, weakness, fainting, a fast or irregular heart rate, then the vet will be suspicious that heart disease could be a cause. Most dogs with heart disease will also have a heart murmur, which is an abnormal sound occurring as the heart beats. Heart murmurs vary in intensity. Loud heart murmurs are generally more serious than soft heart murmurs, but this depends on the underlying disease (see Chapter 9, p. 226). If a vet suspects heart disease, then further tests, especially echocardiography (an ultrasound examination of the heart), and chest X-rays, will usually be advised.

Unfortunately, some dogs with a cough are actually very unwell, perhaps because of pneumonia, bronchial or tracheal collapse, severe laryngeal paralysis, some form of allergic airway disease, lungworm (*Angiostrongylus vasorum*), or a lung tumour. Very few clinicians are able to make an accurate diagnosis from the clinical picture alone, but there are some signs that are helpful. So, for instance, if a dog's respiratory rate and depth increase but neither seems to require marked effort, and the dog seems to tire quickly, then a lung mass or fluid in the chest might explain these signs. In parts of the country where lungworm are common, younger dogs with a cough should be tested for this parasite (blood tests or faecal analysis are both helpful, but neither are infallible). To reach a diagnosis in other cases imaging of the airway and / or chest; by X-rays, ultrasonography, direct examination of the upper airway, endoscopy, CT (computerised tomography), or a range of these techniques, might be necessary.

Some respiratory diseases are curable, others are very responsive to treatment but unfortunately some have a very poor outcome.

DENTAL DISEASE AND RELATED PROBLEMS

If your dog has very smelly breath, seems to have pain around the mouth, or appears to have difficulty eating, then you will be worried that they may have dental disease. Certainly, dental problems and inflammation of the gums, gingivitis, are common in dogs and definitely under-diagnosed, but there are other conditions which affect the mouth or the jaws which must be ruled out. These include abscesses, trauma, foreign bodies, and oral tumours. Sometimes ear disease, a dislocated jaw, a mass behind an eye, or another condition is the source of the problem. Bad breath doesn't always signify disease of the mouth, sometimes it can come from the gut, the kidneys, or elsewhere, and it doesn't always indicate ill health at all. It's best to start with an open mind.

When questioning you about the problem, your vet will want to establish how long it has been present, whether the clinical signs are constant or intermittent, whether the dog seems otherwise well, and if they have any history of eating, chewing, chasing or playing with sticks, stones, balls or bones. Many dogs are head-shy. They resent close examination of their head. If anyone tries to open a dog's mouth that is painful they might see nothing, just anger the dog and get bitten. So, before trying to examine the mouth the vet will want to get to know the dog and to learn as much as they can from observation and touch. They will look carefully at the shape of your dog's head, looking for asymmetry, or swellings, and, after stroking them gently to establish rapport, will cautiously palpate and manipulate the facial structures including the eyes and ears to see if these are normal. They will then probably want to feel the glands high in the neck just below the corners of the jaw to discover if they are enlarged or painful.

Moving on to the mouth itself; I personally begin by looking at the lips, gums and teeth from each side, to see if the teeth meet in a normal fashion and whether any teeth appear to be loose, broken, out of position, covered in tartar, or fringed by pus. Healthy gums are smooth, light pink and glistening. If the gums are red raw, irregular, swollen, or bleeding, these findings are important. Next, I like to open the mouth to inspect all the teeth; incisors, canines, pre-molars and molars, top and bottom, looking at orientation, shape and colour of the crowns, which are the visible part of the tooth above the gum, and to establish if any are broken. I also like to look at the palate, the tongue, under the tongue, inside the cheeks, at the back of the mouth (the pharynx), and the folds of the lips. However, this calls for honesty; it is really difficult to make a complete and thorough examination of a dog's mouth whilst they are conscious, especially if the mouth is painful. Having been caught-out in the past more than once, nowadays I like to warn my clients that a conscious oral exam can never be completely relied upon.

In respect of the teeth themselves, experience – and veterinary dentists – tell us that it is very difficult to make a proper evaluation of the health of the tooth by looking at the crown alone. A detailed dental examination requires that the gingival sulcus, the narrow groove between each tooth and the gum, be probed, to see if it is deeper than normal. Deep gingival pockets reveal that the perio-dontal ligament, which holds the tooth in the jaw is diseased. Most veterinary dentists say that dental X-rays (radiographs) are an invaluable part of a dental examination.

This whole process must be done under general anaesthesia for it to be safe, effective and tolerable to the dog. Clients are understandably nervous about this because we all know that general anaesthesia is potentially hazardous and can be expensive. To minimise risk, your vet will carefully examine your dog before the anaesthetic is given. During anaesthesia a soft tube will be inserted into the windpipe to act as a temporary airway. This tube has an inflatable cuff that gently seals the tube into the throat to prevent fluids and debris in the mouth being inhaled.

It may be that the examination shows that some teeth must be removed. This can be a difficult and time-consuming procedure especially if some of the largest teeth are diseased. Teeth with multiple roots must be sectioned before removal. Fortunately, the tissues of the mouth usually heal very rapidly after extractions. If a tooth is fractured then sometimes it can be saved. Root canal treatment is a specialist procedure but can be done.

Dental scaling, and polishing of the teeth helps to arrest or at least slow down the development of dental disease. Scaling is usually done with the aid of an ultra-sonic probe that removes the tartar with minimal damage to the surface of the tooth. Hand-scaling curettes are also used, especially to clean out the crucial cal-culus lurking in the gingival sulcus. After scaling, the teeth are polished, which aims to remove micro-abrasions of the enamel surface.

When your dog recovers from the anaesthetic they will be given pain relief and your vet or veterinary nurse will discuss with you how brushing of the teeth can help to maintain good oral health. Without the introduction of a long-term preventative program the benefits of descaling are very short-lived indeed.

A task force of dental experts who recently drew up guidelines for The American Animal Hospital Association has recommended that all adult dogs should have a complete dental examination and dental radiographs by the age of two years! (see Bellows et al., 2019). If you are thinking what I am thinking . . . there is a serious mismatch here between what veterinary dentists advise and practical reality. If a proper dental examination must involve examination of each tooth under anaesthesia and a set of dental radiographs then it is completely impractical to expect that every dog should have a full dental evaluation regularly. I believe such an approach would in fact constitute over-investigation, over-treatment and bad medicine, but I have no claim to be a veterinary dentist. I'd love to get a frank response to this conundrum from one of them.

Recently, a handy and practical test has been developed to identify chemicals in dogs' saliva called thiols. Most dogs with dental disease show high concentrations of thiols in the saliva so it seems that this test might be a very useful one. The test is supported by some good science and has become commercially available.

WOUNDS

To a dog every walk is an adventure. Every dog is liable to get wounded occasionally. Sometimes a dog will come to you apologetically holding up a limb dripping blood. You might find them casually licking a paw that has been sliced or discover an unexplained gaping wound. The backstory behind such trauma is often a mystery.

There are few golden rules in veterinary medicine, but here's one: NEVER THROW STICKS FOR YOUR DOG TO CHASE. Once in a while, a dog chasing a stick will impale themselves. At the very least, this is painful and messy, but in a substantial fraction of cases a bit of the stick will break off inside the dog. Such injuries are extremely difficult to treat because the broken piece of wood will be carrying a profusion of bacteria and other microbes. Wood is generally invisible on X ray pictures. What's more, such fragments can wander hither and thither through the body spreading infection as they travel. Solving such cases can be very difficult, necessitate CT imaging, multiple anaesthetics and repeated surgical explorations. Troubling. Very expensive.

Most wounds should receive veterinary attention soon after they're discovered because they are liable to be contaminated; however, first aid should be given. If there is profuse bleeding apply pressure over the site with a clean cloth. Wait for at least four minutes before looking to see if the bleeding has stopped. If the haemorrhage continues despite this, emergency treatment is necessary. Where profuse bleeding is absent the wound should be bathed in copious amounts of clean water or an isotonic solution to remove contamination. A simple isotonic solution can be made at home; one teaspoon of salt to about 500ml of tap-water (see p. 255). Antiseptic solutions are controversial (see p. 255) so, if in any doubt take your dog to the vet.

When you see the vet, they will decide how the wound is best treated but it can be challenging to establish the extent of an injury if the dog is in a lot of discomfort. Often a thorough examination cannot be made whilst the patient is conscious. Puncture wounds may look innocuous but can be serious if a projectile, a stick or another sharp object has penetrated deeply into the body. Clean lacerations may often be amenable to stitching, ragged wounds might need to be handled differently. Wounds in the pads of the paws are sometimes not stitched because they often heal more successfully when left open. Aftercare of the wound might include the use of antibiotics and analgesic drugs. A head collar and / or bandages are often required.

When Tullulah, our Lurcher, was young she threw herself willy-nilly into every experience. It often ended badly. One Christmas Eve she went to Blean Woods near our home for a walk with my partner. After an hour or so, back at the car-park, Denise noticed Tally was lame on a foreleg with blood on her foot. Tally seemed unconcerned. Hoping to avoid too much mess in the car, Denise put a stout carrier bag over the foot. She tied it in place with a shoelace wrapped round Tally's wrist (carpus). Ten minutes later, back home, I found the bag was filled with bright red blood. Tally had severed the deep arteries to the paw. Spurts of scarlet haemorrhage continued with every beat of her heart. I took her straight to the practice . . .

Dear . . .,

I hope you can help this dog, 'Button', who was chasing a stick last Friday. Exactly what happened is a bit hazy, but the dog suddenly cried out in pain and has been rather miserable ever since. She has eaten nothing in the last three days. I suspect she ran onto the stick but there doesn't seem to be a wound in her mouth. I know stick injuries can be difficult to treat, so I've down-played the outlook. The clients have a life-time insurance policy and are very keen to solve this.

Thanks for taking on this referral.

Alf

Dear Alf,

Thank you for referring this middle-aged Labrador to see me as an emergency. You suspected a stick injury. On examination Button was quiet and dull but responsive. She was running a fever (40.2°C), showed forelimb lameness, and had very smelly breath. Manipulation of her neck caused Button discomfort.

Given the history and your suspicions Button was anaesthetised for a CT examination which showed pneumomediastinum [gas around the soft-tissues in the chest], enlarged local lymph nodes [glands], and a linear pointed foreign body towards the RHS of midline extending from the larynx [voice box] to the level of the shoulder. This foreign body, which was a stick about 20 cm in length, was surgically removed via a ventral approach. A tear was present in the oesophagus [gullet] measuring about 3 cm in length. Haematology from Button indicated neutrophilic leukocytosis [a high white blood cell count] consistent with the fever.

Even following successful removal of this sort of foreign body the prognosis is guarded especially since the stick had been in situ for several days. Button is hospitalised at present on intravenous antibiotics and fluid therapy. She has a gastrotomy feeding tube in place to allow the oesophagus to heal. A surgical drain is in place too. She is on regular analgesia with injectable methadone. We expect Button to remain hospitalised for several days.

Thanks again for referring this dog.

Mike . . . (RCVS Advanced Practitioner in Soft Tissue Surgery).

Dear Alf,

I'm pleased to let you know that 'Button', the Labrador who had the stick injury, was discharged from our hospital after eight days. The surgical drain was kept in place for four days, the gastrotomy tube was removed after six days. She had been eating for herself for the last two days before discharge. Her pyrexia resolved.

I saw Button again this morning (day 14) when I removed all the sutures. Her stoma from the feeding tube has healed nicely too. I'm pleased to say there have been no obvious complications. The owners will not be throwing sticks for her in future.

Regards, Mike . . .

Grass seeds

Every vet will have an anecdote to warn you about the dangers of grass-seed foreign bodies that can lodge in many parts of the body, especially the ears and between the toes. If the seed is in the ear canal the dog will shake their head, paw at the ear and often howl in misery. If the paw is the site, they will lick it incessantly. When you look at the shape of these seeds it's not hard to understand how this comes about. When grasses reach maturation in summer and early autumn, the seed heads dry, shrink and harden. The seeds then break off to attach to the coat of a passing dog. At one end of the seed is a sharp hard spike, at the other end a quill formed from short stiff bristles or barbs. The whole seed has an arrow-head shape, sometimes referred to as a 'flea dart'. Americans call them 'foxtails'. The shape of the seeds means they tend to migrate one way, deep into the coat, the sharp spike leading driven forward by the orientation of the barbs, to reach and then penetrate the skin. When one of these seeds punctures the skin, it carries with it a plethora of bacteria and other microbes. Every grass-seed foreign body will cause intense irritation and pain. If they are not swiftly removed infection follows. Many cases become extremely challenging to treat, especially if a few days elapse before being seen by a vet. I have found grass seeds in many different places including in the ears, the eyes, the nose, the lungs, the 'arm-pit' (axillae), the prepuce and the vulva. Removal always requires anaesthesia. On one occasion, I removed seven grass seeds from the feet of a Spaniel one evening only to discover a couple of additional ones embedded in the skin of the back a few days later. When a dog presents to a vet with an unexplained fever and evidence of a systemic infection then a wandering grass-seed foreign body will always be somewhere on the list of possible causes. It goes without saying that such cases can be very difficult and expensive to solve.

If you have a long-haired dog, you can go some way to preventing this problem by getting your dog clipped, or stripped, in the warmer months of the year, paying particular attention to the feet and around the ears. You can also try to avoid fields and heaths abundant in tall dry grass. It pays when you get home from a walk to seek-out flea darts in the coat and to look between the toes. Also, remember sudden-onset irritation of an ear might be due to a grass seed. Like most hazards it is impossible to remove all risk so you should be vigilant.

Freda is a loud, tall, young woman with blue hair in braids and a nose ring. Her dog, by contrast, is a quiet, unassuming Cavalier King Charles Spaniel, 6 years old, called Pip. I saw the pair a couple of weeks ago, early September, because Pip had a sore right ear that had 'started a few days previously'. She'd never had an ear problem before. Her skin was unremarkable. The other ear was fine. It was impossible to get a good look down Pip's ear because there was a discharge and she was uncomfortable. Freda was in a hurry. So was I, it was after seven, last consultation, Friday evening. I gave out some topical treatment, said I was unsure the cause of this, so if Pip's ear was no better by Monday she ought to bring her back.

On Monday and Tuesday, I saw no sign of Freda or Pip. By Wednesday Pip's problem had slipped from my radar. I took a few days off. On the following Wednesday, last consultation of the day, there was Pip again. Her ear had improved a bit for a few days but now it was worse. Still unilateral. I felt guilty. Her ear was certainly really sore. More discharge than before. Quite smelly. Conscious examination was impossible.

Freda agreed to an anaesthetic for Pip, though she was pretty unhappy about it. Once Pip was asleep the task became easier. Mmmmm . . . There seemed to be a tiny little fragment of something deep in that ear canal, probably nothing, worth a check . . . Long crocodile forceps . . . I pulled out not one, but TWO grass seeds from deep in her ear. Problem solved.

Hair shirt donned, I went to see Freda . . .

LUMPS AND BUMPS

Many different conditions present as lumps or bumps in or under the skin. They are often found fortuitously. Some will be tumours, others might be abscesses, cysts or bruises. It is foolish to ignore them, especially if they grow quickly or seem painful. By far the most common lumps are lipomas, which are soft, painless, benign (non-cancerous) fatty tumours, but there are some serious and malignant 'cancerous' skin tumours. A few masses have an almost diagnostic appearance and character, but most cannot be diagnosed with certainty without tissue samples, such as a fine needle aspirate or a larger biopsy sample. Vets have a saying: 'A lump, is a lump, is a lump, until a pathologist tells you what it is.' If you find any form of lump in the skin then you should probably get a veterinary opinion. Here are a few things that might help you to decide if the problem needs immediate attention.

- Is the lump causing pain or receiving a lot of attention from the dog?

- Is it growing quickly?

- Is the mass interfering with function? For example, masses on the eyelids often distort the lid and usually lead to excessive tears; lumps in the groin or the axillae ('arm-pits') can lead to an altered gait or frank lameness.

- Is there a discharge, or is the mass hot?

- Has the hair over the lump fallen out or does the skin seem ulcerated, discoloured, crusty or moist?

If the answer to any of these questions is yes, I recommend you see your vet promptly.

Let me tell you about Tam, a black and tan cross-bred terrier of mine. Tam was a typical terrier; he loved hunting smells, very inquisitive, a bit bossy, always the dominant one when meeting other dogs; loyal, scruffy, greedy, joyful; an undiluted enthusiast. One morning, when he had just turned six, on a walk he jumped up to me for a tickle. I caressed him under the ear just about the angle of the jaw. My heart stopped. There are very few signs in veterinary medicine which are unambiguous. I felt again, at either corner of the jaw. Then I felt behind Tam's stifles and into the axillae close to the point of the elbow. 'Bugger!' Tam had firm, swollen, painless 'glands' (lymph nodes) at each of these places. There is only one disease in the UK that commonly causes this 'disseminated lymphadenopathy', a tumour called lymphoma. It is invariably fatal, though it can be treated. I treated Tam. He responded well, but was dead within 14 months. He broke my heart.

CONSTIPATION

Constipation is not a common sign in dogs despite the nature of their diet that is typically rather low in fibre. Dogs who develop constipation have often been eating an unusual diet. An example would be the dog who has been gnawing bones that splinter and break so that the faeces is largely composed of bone fragments. If a dog's diet has not changed but they start to strain to defecate, I worry that they might have an undisclosed problem in their pelvis (such as a mass of some sort, or distortion of the course of the lower bowel). Another primary cause of constipation is back pain, in which the dog has discomfort adopting the normal posture to poo. A third possibility might be disease of the tissues around the anus itself. So, when the anal sacs are painful a dog might resist the urge to poo because it is sore to do so. A fourth possible cause can be dehydration in which virtually all the liquid within the diet has been absorbed so that the faeces that arrives in the rectum is particularly dry.

If your dog seems to be constipated, occasionally the opposite is true. Dogs who strain to defecate might have a persistent urge to do so because of diarrhoea not constipation. It is a common mistake.

Constipation is easily confirmed by your vet by rectal examination and is usually quite treatable. Sometimes a change of management is all that is required.

In other cases, enemas might be necessary. It is always wise to try to identify if there is a primary cause.

FALSE PREGNANCY ('PSEUDOPREGNANCY')

If you have a female dog who is not neutered then this is a condition you might see.

In Chapter 5, I described the normal sexual cycle of female dogs (see pp. 87–88). After a bitch has been in heat, if she does not become pregnant then she goes through a period known as dioestrus, which typically lasts for two months. Towards the end of that period bitches often show changes in behaviour and biology that mimic pregnancy. So, they might become especially interested in their toys, show nesting behaviour, seem more territorial than normal and become rather moody. Often their appetite declines. Some bitches actually start to produce milk in their teats. Although this condition – termed false pregnancy – is not dangerous, I think the bitches who develop it do suffer.

This condition is treatable with drugs and usually easily cured but those bitches who show false pregnancy tend to do so repeatedly after each season. They are also especially liable to develop womb infections (pyometra – see below). Surgical treatment, neutering, might be necessary, or advisable.

WOMB INFECTIONS (PYOMETRA)

In the past, female dogs were neutered less frequently than they are in Britain today. In some parts of the world, neutering is frowned upon (or even illegal). Bitches who are 'entire', not neutered, are prone to develop womb infections, technically called pyometritis, or simply 'a pyo'. This is especially true for bitches who never experience pregnancy. The risk of developing a womb infection increases with each sexual cycle. Risks are higher in those bitches who have previously had a false pregnancy.

There is a constellation of clinical signs that a bitch might show if she is developing pyometra. These signs classically occur from two to five weeks after being 'in heat'. Dullness, lethargy, a vulval discharge, poor appetite, increased thirst, a slightly elevated body temperature and vomiting. A few bitches show all these signs and in such cases diagnosis is easy, but more often a bitch will only show some of these signs, especially if they are presented to the vet early in the course of the disease. When you see your vet, they might be suspicious but uncertain. In such an event during the consultation they will palpate the abdomen to feel for an enlarged womb and look closely for any signs of a discharge from the vulva. They will probably want to do some lab tests too, especially haematology and / or cytology of any discharge. Other tests that are often done are ultrasound or X-ray imaging to examine the womb and biochemistry to understand if there are other explanations and if there are complications, such as dehydration.

Untreated pyometra is usually fatal. Once a diagnosis has been reached, treatment should be performed quickly by surgical neutering under general anaesthesia. This is not without risk, especially in those bitches who are particularly ill, but the success rate of treatment is high. Hospitalisation, administration of intravenous fluids guided by biochemistry testing, and antibiotic therapy are usually necessary. Non-surgical treatment of pyometra is feasible, using hormones and antibiotics, but outcomes from that approach are not usually as good as from surgery. When treated medically in this way, there is also a substantial risk the condition will recur after the next season.

8

EMERGENCIES

This chapter is devoted to veterinary emergencies such as road accidents, poisoning, dog-fights, 'bloat' (gastric-dilatation-volvulus), choking, collapse, fainting, seizures, emergencies involving the eyes, severe breathing difficulties and heat-stroke. First aid for these problems will be discussed. Emergency facilities and treatments will be explained.

The old Boy Scout's motto, 'Be Prepared', is no doubt useful advice, but exquisitely non-specific. How can you prepare for veterinary emergencies? There are a few practical things. Firstly, make sure your dog wears a collar and tag with your name, address and phone number on it. Some people put their vet's phone number on the tag too. Don't have the dog's name engraved on the tag because that could make it easier for someone to kidnap your dog. A microchip is a legal requirement for all dogs too. I.D. is essential because one of the most likely emergencies is that your dog goes missing – escapes from your garden, runs off on a walk after a squirrel or a cat, or bolts when a lorry back-fires. Secondly, make sure you have your vet's phone number on your mobile and/or stuck to the fridge with a magnet. Thirdly, read this chapter. It'll give you some ideas what you might need to face so that you can 'Be Prepared'.

Many vets provide their own 24-hour services, but in cities and urban areas nowadays there are often dedicated out-of-hours emergency clinics. If you live in one of these zones, it is highly likely that your vet's practice will subscribe to an emergency service so that during unsociable hours your emergency call will be diverted. The vets and nurses who work in these emergency practices are usually especially skilled in dealing with these cases. Such services are often pricey because they are dedicated to the management of seriously ill animals during the night, at weekends and during public holidays. This type of work also requires a high staff to patient ratio, which is expensive.

LOST DOG

If your dog goes missing, don't panic. If you are missing your dog, they are probably missing you too. Most dogs have at least as good a sense of direction as their owners.

1. Begin by recalling exactly when and where he/she was last time you saw them. Quite often if you return there, you'll find your dog is waiting for you.

2. If you are somewhere unfamiliar but there are other dogs and owners about, ask them if they've seen your dog. Describe the dog simply: size, colour and breed or type, including the appearance of their collar or harness. Give them your dog's name. Exchange mobile numbers so that you can communicate if the dog is found.

3. If you're somewhere familiar it might be your dog has gone looking for you; for instance, where you began your walk in the car park. If you've come from home on foot the dog might have gone back there.

4. Phone local veterinary practices, the RSPCA and the police. Give them a thumbnail sketch of your dog, where they went missing and when.

5. Contact social media, local residents' groups, the local paper and radio station.

6. Make some simple fliers/posters and offer a reward. A picture of the dog is really helpful. Print these and display them near where the dog went missing. Ask local shops to display these. Push them through letter boxes. Stick them to lamp-posts. Think saturation advertising.

7. When you get your dog back, as you almost certainly will, make sure you tell people you've been reunited, using the same media. It's a great way of spreading happiness.

FOUND DOG

If you find a dog who seems to be lost, you can try cautiously and quietly to approach it. Patience often will pay off. If you have dog treats on you then use these to get the dog's confidence. Your aim should be to lure the dog onto a lead so that you can read their tag. However, you must use circumspection here. A dog who is lost will be nervous and a frightened dog can be aggressive (especially if they feel cornered). Do not deliberately put yourself in harm's way. It is also senseless to try to grab the dog's collar or to run after a lost dog because it will almost certainly be quick to bolt and then become even more difficult to capture. Be aware the dog might be injured, and this might not be immediately obvious. An injured dog can also be aggressive. Provided you do manage to look at the dog's tag, ring the owner. Reuniting a lost dog and their owner is enormously rewarding.

If there's no tag, or you can't catch the dog, the next best thing is to ring local vets, the RSPCA, the local dog warden (if there is one) and the police. Explain exactly where the dog has been found (use the location facility on your smart phone if you have one) and give a simple clear description: colour, size, sex and breed or type. If the animal is injured take them to a vet. Vets have microchip readers that ought to enable them to locate the dog's owner. They will have protocols for dealing with lost dogs.

ROAD ACCIDENTS

Roads are dangerous places. Road traffic injuries are the among the most common causes of dog trauma. If a dog is hit by a car, it will likely be badly injured. Also frightened and in pain. Some are killed outright. Some are unable to walk. Some are unconscious. Some will be bleeding heavily.

Be careful, because any dog in this situation might bite. This advice even applies to your own dog. If the dog is able to move, they must be caught and restrained in some way so that they don't run back into traffic or try to run off. If you have help, delegate one person to control the traffic (without putting themselves in danger) and one person to contact a vet, whilst you attempt to control the dog. Hysterical screaming is unhelpful. Noisy, gawping onlookers should be asked to help or to leave.

Try to speak calmly and clearly to the dog to reassure them, move slowly but deliberately to gain their confidence and enable you to get a lead, a belt, or a rope noosed around them or their collar/harness. If the dog cannot be caught and is causing, or liable to cause, a further traffic hazard, inform the police of the accident. In some instances, such as a dog on a motorway or a busy urban junction, where the dog could cause a pile-up, a 999 call would be completely appropriate. Use your judgement.

Once a vet has been alerted, they will help you to work out what to do and how the dog should be transported. Sometimes the vet or veterinary nurse might come out to you, but that's rarely practical. Heavy bleeding can be stopped with a pressure bandage. Any clean cloth will do. If the dog cannot move it should be handled VERY carefully. Some form of rudimentary stretcher might be required. If a dog is in severe discomfort, it is sometimes impossible to help them because they have become intensely fearful and dangerous. In such an instance, it is reasonable to muzzle them to prevent people being hurt and enable assistance to the dog. On page ... I describe, and illustrate, how to fashion a secure muzzle from a rope, a tie or a similar piece of cord.

Initial assessment of emergency patients is known as 'Triage' ('sorting out'). It tends to follow a set protocol, ABCD: Airway, Breathing, Circulation and Consciousness, Dysfunction. First assessment might be done by a nurse, time being of the essence. This approach enables the most life-threatening crises to be identified first and will ignore superficial injuries even if they look spectacular. First aid might begin then if required. The vet will repeat this brief examination of vital signs: heart rate and pulse, breathing rate and effort, colour, body temperature and level of consciousness. Neurologic deficits (such as lack of sensation or movement in part of the body) will be sought, life-threatening injuries such as spinal fractures, arterial bleeding or open chest wounds will be identified, and the extent of your dog's pain will be assessed. Once this has been done, a plan for pain-management and further assessment will emerge. At this point the vet or nurse should be able to give you some guidance. Very often, after providing pain relief and obtaining intravenous access for fluids and drugs, imaging studies will be necessary, using radiography, ultrasonography or possibly other methods. These studies should help to reveal hidden injuries such as rupture of the urinary bladder or leakage of air into the chest from a punctured lung. They will also provide more information about skeletal injuries such as fractures and dislocations. This phase of trauma management is crucial. Perhaps to your surprise many very obvious injuries such as fractures of the long bones do not need to be repaired immediately, whereas some invisible injuries such as a ruptured spleen or urinary bladder are potentially far more serious and require immediate attention.

Road accidents are a significant cause of death, euthanasia or life-changing injury to dogs. An extremely obedient dog might nevertheless run into the road if they see a cat, a squirrel or a belligerent dog. All dogs should be kept on a lead near roads.

DOG FIGHTS

Dog fights happen. They are not common but even the most benign and polite dog can get into a fight. Fights sometimes lead to serious injuries, especially if a small dog is picked on by a much bigger one. If your dog gets into a fight, you need to separate the dogs as soon as possible. The best way to do this is by throwing a bucket of cold water over them. Unfortunately, few of us will have a bucket of water handy; however, the same principal might be successfully applied in another way. You will need to startle the dogs. You might be able do this by making an unusual noise loudly. If the dogs have leashes and collars, or harnesses, you might be able to grab them by this. Usually, this takes at least two people. Don't put yourself into danger.

Once the dogs have been separated the extent of the wounding must be assessed. Bite wounds most commonly occur on the limbs, head and neck. The severity is not always plain to see because subcutaneous structures have often been traumatised. This can extend to a ripped windpipe (trachea), fractured ribs, a punctured lung, severe nerve trauma or a broken neck. Dogs' mouths are full of bacteria. Bite wounds will be contaminated. For all these reasons, virtually every dog who has been in a serious fight should be examined soon afterwards by a vet. Pain relief and cleansing of wounds and possibly antibiotic treatment might be all that's required. Delay of a day or two can lead to much worse outcomes if abscesses develop or infection tracks deeper into the body.

These attempts fail. Soon they become distressed with rapid painful breathing. Within a short time, they appear profoundly unwell, often weak. Distension and discomfort are quickly followed by profound depression and collapse. Dogs with GDV die if they are not swiftly treated.

This dog will need emergency treatment immediately. If you ring your vet and explain the signs, they will want you to come in as soon as possible. Quite often the vet you see will be able to make a diagnosis immediately, but they will usually take an X-ray to confirm it. Treatment usually necessitates surgery, although in a small percentage of cases (when volvulus has not yet occurred), the problem can be relieved by passing a wide-bore flexible tube into the stomach to release gas.

No dog with GDV is an ideal subject for surgery because profound changes will be occurring in multiple organ systems including the liver, kidneys, heart and lungs. These derangements affect key functions such as the delivery of oxygen to the tissues and the removal of wastes, carbon dioxide and acids, via the circulation and kidneys. Intravenous fluid therapy is usually initiated immediately to treat shock. Drugs to suppress heart rhythm abnormalities and treat other metabolic crises may be required.

The dog is anaesthetised. The abdomen is opened. The stomach is decompressed and untwisted. Then the stomach is sutured to the body wall, a procedure known as gastropexy. Treatment with painkillers, drugs and fluids to correct the systemic crises are usually necessary in hospital for 24–48 hours after the surgery, sometimes longer. Future management should include small frequent meals usually of canned wet food. Exercise after eating should be avoided.

CHOKING

Choking is an uncommon emergency that most often occurs if a dog tries to swallow something in a hurry, or inhales whilst vomiting. Initially, the dog might seem able to inhale but unable to exhale and unable to cough effectively. Whatever the antecedence there will be an obstruction in the throat. This obstruction must be dislodged quickly. Prompt action by those immediately on hand is essential.

If possible, the mouth should be opened, but this can be hazardous because dogs who are choking are liable to panic and might bite. Ideally, this is a two-person job.

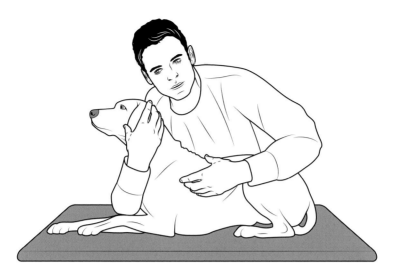

Figure 8.1. Secure restraint of a dog on a table (see text for details).

One person holds the dog firmly to their chest with one arm wrapped around the torso and the second arm cradling the neck (see Figure 8.1). The second person opens the mouth by gripping the upper jaw from above with one hand whilst pressing in on the lips and pushing their thumb into the space behind the upper long canine teeth to rest on the hard palate (see Figure 8.2). The application of firm pressure to the hard palate invokes a reflex that inhibits the dog from biting. The other hand is used to hook the obstruction out from the back of the mouth. If this fails, sometimes it might be possible to hook out the obstruction with some form of blunt lever such as the handle of a long spoon. If the dog continues to choke, they might lose consciousness.

If this method proves impossible, an alternative is to try some form of Heimlich manoeuvre. A small dog can be picked up so that they are 'wheelbarrowing' on their front legs or are completely suspended vertically. A large dog must stay stand-ing. The handler grasps the dog's body behind the chest in a tight hug with their hands clasped at the level of the bellybutton (umbilicus) and delivers a series of sharp squeezes or blows to the back of the chest where the ribs meet. This sudden increase in abdominal pressure should forcibly dislodge the obstruction. Again, in some cases the obstruction will not shift, and the patient might lose consciousness.

If a dog who has been choking loses consciousness, all is not lost. Deprived of oxygen, the brain does not immediately and irreversibly stop functioning. In this

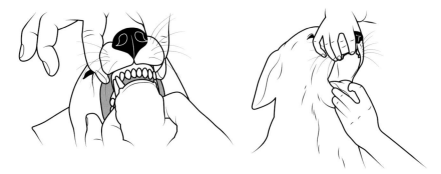

Figure 8.2. Opening a dog's mouth. This requires two people. The first person should securely restrain the dog, as shown in the previous illustration. Use both hands to open the dog's mouth (see text for details).

state they will be floppy and it should be much easier to dislodge the obstruction, so further attempts should be made both by applying sharp sudden pressure to the back of the thorax, by hooking the obstruction out through the mouth, or by delivering sharp claps to the back. Once the obstruction has been dislodged, chest compressions can be used to stimulate the dog to begin breathing again. Take the dog to a vet immediately.

I was at a veterinary conference in Malta where, as usual, when not listening to lectures, I hung out with my colleagues and friends interested in cardiology. We were on the seafront one evening yarning together, drinking beer.

Lamb kebabs were on the menu. I was hungry. I tucked in.

The chunk I was trying to swallow was quite big. I tried again, again. It wouldn't go down. The others were chatting away, oblivious. I tried to swallow once again, hard. My ears popped. Nope, I couldn't swallow. Nor, I suddenly realised, could I bring the chunk back up, or speak . . . It was a long moment of pure dread. I started to wave my arms and look piercingly at my friends. Dave got up, realising my distress. He grabbed me from behind, wrapped his arms around my chest, hugged me suddenly and fiercely. Once. Twice. On the third time, a hunk of lamb shot from my mouth like a cork from a bottle. I could breathe. Thank you, Dave, and of course the wonderful Dr Heimlich, for the Heimlich manoeuvre!

HINDLIMB WEAKNESS: 'GOING OFF THE BACK LEGS'

There are many different problems that can hamper the conduction of nervous messages up and down the spine. Some have a slow and insidious onset and these are often degenerative conditions. However, those that are acute (sudden) in onset must be evaluated swiftly because some of these must have decisive early treatment. So, if a dog suddenly becomes weak, wobbly or unable to use their hind-limbs, this necessitates urgent veterinary attention.

Here are some important questions you are likely to be asked:

- Has there been any known trauma; a slip, a fall, a road accident, a kick, a dog-fight?

- If so, were signs of a problem immediately obvious or have they developed progressively since the incident?

- Has your dog voluntarily urinated or defecated since the onset of the problem?

- Can your dog wag his tail?

When the vet examines your dog, they will especially want to know if any nervous messages at all are travelling up and down the spine, because if not then emergency surgery will offer the only hope of preventing complete permanent paralysis. To do so, they need to establish if your dog can appreciate a painful stimulus applied to the foot or the tail. This is usually done by grasping a claw tightly with forceps. If your dog howls that is good news. To an observer this test can appear crude and brutal but it really is essential.

POISONING

When a dog becomes suddenly ill people can suspect poisoning. In truth, deliberate malicious poisoning of dogs is very rarely proven and probably very uncommon indeed, but dogs can be accidentally poisoned, usually by eating a toxic food or plant, by getting access to human drugs, slug bait, rat poisons or chewing-gum sweetened with xylitol. Poisoning from chemicals on the paws, skin and fur, such as paint, oils, petrol, cement, tar or an agrochemical, which a dog might attempt to lick off, is less common.

Be aware that many things we wouldn't eat, a dog might. Most cases of accidental poisoning occur in young dogs up to about three years old, especially puppies, who are inquisitive and curious. If you have a garden DO NOT USE SLUG-BAIT (metaldehyde). It KILLS MANY DOGS (see below) and is a nasty environmental toxin. Its use is now illegal anyway. Be very careful to keep all garage and garden chemicals stored where dogs cannot get access. When do you use these, keep the dogs away. Also, keep all drugs (human and veterinary) out of the reach of canine mouths. If you carry these with you in a handbag or a pocket be vigilant. Some human foods, including many different chewing-gums, some cakes, ketchups, peanut-butters and anything that is described as 'sugar-free' might contain the sweetener xylitol (sometimes called sugar alcohol), which is perfectly safe for humans but can be fatal for dogs.

Sometimes dogs are given toxins inadvertently or as pranks. For instance, a former colleague (you know who you are) used to regularly feed her Doberman grapes, before it became widely known that vine fruits (grapes, raisins, sultanas and currants) can be toxic to dogs. Her dog seemed to show no ill effects (see later). I have seen cases of dogs fed Cannabis in brownies or given chocolate-coated coffee beans without malicious intent. The effects can be serious.

When you're out walking your dogs, be prepared that they might come across something toxic. Mouldy vegetation and composts, for instance, sometimes contain mycotoxins that can cause seizures. Fungi, mushrooms and toadstools, grow in damp woods in the autumn. Many are completely safe but a few are deadly. Blue-green algae growing in lakes, lochs and reservoirs in hot summer weather can proliferate to create toxic cocktails, and scum, which a dog might drink or get on their fur. Severe vomiting, diarrhoea and bleeding might follow and sometimes result in death. I was once involved with a case where two dogs were poisoned by paraquat from eating a deer carcass illegally laced with it. The perpetrators were aiming to kill eagles (sometimes I despair of the human race). Paraquat damages the lungs irreversibly. The dogs died.

In summary: for poisons, prevention of access is key.

When a dog has been exposed to a toxic substance it might deteriorate very quickly, so it is crucial that veterinary assistance is sought swiftly. One of your first steps should be to contact the Animal Poison Line (https://www.animalpoisonline. co.uk or phone 01202 509000). This is a dedicated 24/7 amenity run by vets and toxicologists from the Veterinary Poisons Information Service. They have a database of something like a quarter of a million previous cases to call on. Following their advice, around three-quarters of clients find they do not need to immediately visit their vets. The service will cost you about the price of a takeaway meal for two. It might save you the price of an out-of-hours visit to the vet. If they do advise you to go to the vet, you would do well to follow their recommendation because it could save your dog's life.

Colleagues at the Animal Poison Line tell me that almost one-third of the phone-calls they receive from the public are about animals that have managed to get hold of medicines, especially human drugs. In many instances these involve bored dogs left alone with an accessible packet of pills. In other cases, people have given their dogs a human drug with the best of intentions and then thought the better of it, or been shocked to discover it has made their beloved pet ill. **As a rule, you should never give a dog a drug prescribed for a person, or another animal, unless a vet has specifically advised you this is safe and called for**. Drugs that are safe for one species may not be safe for another (penicillin can kill guinea pigs, ibuprofen can kill dogs, aspirin can kill cats). There are also a few instances where a drug that is safe for most dogs is unsafe in a few specific breeds (e.g. Ivermectin, a drug that is safe and very effective against many parasites of the dog, can be fatal in Collies).

When you contact your veterinary practice, do so by telephone in the first instance. Provide details of the dog (age, breed, weight (if known), sex and name) as well as your own name and address. Also, make certain that you confirm your phone number so that the practice can contact you if you get cut off. If you know what the dog has had access to, try to provide precise details of the product and manufacturer from the wrapper, package insert or product label. Read out and spell chemical names and give the details of the strength or concentration of the active ingredients, if listed. If the dog has eaten a plant that you know is toxic, please try to accurately identify it. Next, explain exactly how the dog might have been poisoned. It is important to say if the poisoning has been definitely witnessed rather than merely suspected, but where there is doubt it is wise to assume poisoning has occurred.

If there has been a delay in contacting the practice, or the time that the poisoning occurred is not known, this might have a bearing on what is done. So, for instance, if a dog was seen to eat some fruit cake within the last hour, then your vet will probably want to make the dog sick as soon as possible, whereas, if you have returned home after being out for four hours, to discover a package of pills has been eaten by the dog, then there might be little point in trying to empty the dog's stomach. If it's obvious to you that your dog is ill, again try to give an accurate description of what you see. A video clip on a smart phone might be helpful, but don't waste time if you can't organise this immediately.

Sometimes, based on this information, it is quite easy to say that the dog has not ingested a toxic dose. With chocolate for example, depending on the type of chocolate and the size of dog, it is often clear that the amount of coco solids and theobromine (the chocolate toxin) that has been eaten is safe (see below). However, if there is a shred of doubt, the vet will almost certainly want to see the dog as soon as possible. If you have it, take the product packaging with you, which should enable the clinician to establish exactly what the toxin is, and estimate the dose the dog has had. If the packet itself has been eaten or destroyed, you might have another identical box or packet in the household – take that instead. If the dog has eaten a plant, some compost, or another ill-defined substance then take a piece of it with you, or, if that's impractical, a photo.

Sadly, contrary to the expectations of some clients, there are very few specific antidotes for toxins. Nevertheless, a lot of experience has been gained over the years in dealing with pet poisoning. If the poison has been swallowed, which is by far the most common route, and this has happened recently, within 2 hours, then emptying the stomach by induction of vomiting is often useful (but not if the toxin is caustic or the dog is very depressed, collapsed or seizing). Activated charcoal, a substance that sequesters poisons in the gut to prevent them being adsorbed, given by mouth can be helpful. Other supportive measures, such as IV fluid therapy, are useful too.

SPECIFIC POISONS

Here are some examples of a few more commonly asked about, or serious, causes of canine poisoning.

Rat poison

Many different poisons are used to kill rats and mice added to a bait that attracts the rodent to feed. The classic example of these is Warfarin, an anticoagulant (it prevents the blood from clotting) from a chemical series known as Coumarins, but many others exist. The Coumarin toxins all interfere with the ability of the liver to make the blood clotting factors. The effect is to cause bleeding. Sometimes a dog will get access to the poisoned bait itself, but knowledge of that danger, especially in the pest control business, has meant that usually careful steps are taken to prevent that. For instance, bait might be hidden in some piping giving the rodent access but not a dog. Unfortunately, the doomed rat or mouse, carrying a heavy dose of the poison, often will become slow and weakened before dying. It can then be preyed upon by a dog. This means that sometimes a dog will be poisoned with no known immediate access to the poison, sometimes days or a week or two, after the rat-bait was laid.

You might be aware your dog has had access to rat-bait, or that they have killed and eaten a rat, but often you will not have this knowledge. Recent ingestion of the bait or a poisoned rat can be treated first by inducing vomiting and giving activated charcoal to inhibit absorption of the poison from the gut. Your vet will also want to do blood tests to establish if your dog's blood clots normally. Often this test will not be available in-house so blood samples will have to be sent away. Treatment may have to begin presumptively. Vitamin K can be given as an antidote, initially by injection, then by mouth. But some of the coumarins are very potent and long-lasting, which means some dogs have to be treated with this vitamin repeatedly for weeks. The costs of this can be high but the success rate is good.

Chocolate

Most people know chocolate is poisonous for dogs. What really matters is how much of the chocolate toxin(s), theobromine, (and caffeine) has been ingested and the weight of the dog. White chocolate contains virtually no theobromine and is harmless. 'Sugar-free' chocolate could contain Xylitol (see below), which is extremely toxic to dogs. The most popular brands of milk chocolate in the UK contain about 20–26% cocoa solids, which means that a dog would need to eat around 10g of the chocolate per kilogram of body weight to develop even mild signs of toxicity. On the other hand, dark chocolates contain a much higher concentration of cocoa solids than milk chocolate (from 35% up to 75% or even higher); these products are much more likely to cause toxic signs. Obviously, there are other sources of chocolate, from cakes to Easter eggs. Cocoa powder, cocoa beans and cacao nibs are the most concentrated dangerous sources. If a dog ingests more than 2 g/kg of the darkest chocolate, or above about 15–20 mg/kg of theobromine, they are at some danger of developing signs of illness which typically begin with vomiting and / or diarrhoea. Signs can take 4–6 hours to develop. Other signs can include an increase in thirst, restlessness, excitability, rapid breathing, muscle tremors, seizures, rapid heart rate, coma and death. The lethal dose is said to be around 100–200 mg of theobromine per kilogram of body weight, but some dogs are more sensitive than others. There are chocolate toxicity calculators on the internet to enable you to work out if your dog might have eaten a dangerous amount. If in any doubt ring the Animal Poison Line or visit your vet. If your vet concludes that your dog might have ingested a toxic amount of chocolate then they will want to make the dog sick and probably also give activated charcoal. Monitoring for 6–24 hours is required.

Adder bite

Adders are the only venomous snakes found in the UK. They have a striking dark zig-zag pattern on their upper surface, and vary from grey or green to dark brown. Adders are shy so they are not often encountered but may sometimes be disturbed sun-bathing on heaths, sand-dunes or moors. Inquisitive dogs can be bitten if they surprise or provoke these reptiles. The bites most commonly occur on the head and forelimbs, are extremely painful, swell, bruise, then swiftly cause other signs such as lethargy, loss of consciousness and sometimes palpitations of the heart. Treatment with the specific antidote, 'anti-venom', is often necessary and must be done as soon as possible because this can be fatal.

Alliums (onions, garlic, leeks, chives)

These foods are somewhat toxic to dogs. Few dogs will deliberately choose to eat them; cooked human table-scraps are the usual source of poisoning. A few pure-breeds, such as the Japanese Akita, appear to be predisposed. Onions and their relatives contain organo-sulphoxides that can cause vomiting, diarrhoea and abdominal pain. They also damage haemoglobin, the red cell pigment, which carries oxygen in the blood. This can lead on to anaemia. If a dog ingests these foods, treatment can include the use of emetics, drugs that induce vomiting to empty the stomach, and activated charcoal. Other supportive treatment such as intravenous fluid therapy is sometimes given. The outcome is usually favourable.

Slug bait – metaldehyde

This toxin can rapidly cause severe neurologic signs within less than an hour of being ingested. By the time you see a vet your dog might be exhibiting twitches, muscle tremors, hyper-excitability, respiratory distress and convulsions. Metaldehyde is rapidly absorbed from the stomach, so usually it is too late or too risky to make the dogs sick. The vet will give sedative or anaesthetic drugs to control the neurologic signs. Some dogs will have hyperthermia (high body temperature) because of the excessive muscular activity and will need to be cooled. Full recovery is possible because the poison is broken down within the body, but that can take three days or more.

STOP PRESS: Sales and use of metaldehyde slug pellets are now illegal.

Vine fruits (grapes, raisins, sultanas, fruit cake, chocolate raisins, hot-cross buns, etc.)

Why grapes and raisins can be toxic to dogs is not known. Various theories exist but none are proven. A current theory is that the toxin is tartaric acid, which has a variable concentration in grapes, and that some dogs are genetically sensitive to this toxin. It appears that more than half of dogs exposed to these fruits show no signs of ill health at all, but even very small amounts can cause serious illness in some dogs. What is certain is that a proportion of dogs who ingest them can develop severe vomiting, diarrhoea, kidney failure and die. Signs usually develop a few hours after the fruit has been eaten. The accepted and prudent strategy is that all dogs who are known to have been exposed should be treated. In cases where ingestion was recent, the vet will want to make the dog sick to empty the stomach. Then, activated charcoal will be given and intravenous fluid therapy. Outcome is good in most cases, but tends to be much worse if treatment is delayed, especially if signs of kidney dysfunction develop.

Mycotoxins

Mouldy cheese, silage, compost, even windfall mouldy fruit can sometimes cause illness in dogs soon after ingestion. The agents seem to act on the nervous system but the signs of toxicity vary hugely, and are similar to those seen with slug bait;

for example, vomiting, excitement, rapid breathing, rapid heart-rate, tremors, giddiness and 'drunken' behaviour (ataxia), seizures and coma. Treatment early on to induce vomiting might be chosen but if tremors and seizures have developed that will not be safe. Some dogs will develop high temperatures if the muscle tremors are severe. Sedatives and anaesthetics may be required. Recently, the use of an intravenous lipid emulsion has become commonplace in treating dogs with these signs and seems to be helpful. This treatment is costly.

Ethylene glycol

This is an antifreeze used in screen wash, car radiators and brake fluids. It tastes sweet and as a result may be swallowed by dogs. It is converted in the liver to toxic metabolites that can damage the brain, heart, lungs and kidneys. There are typically three phases of toxicity. The first phase is characterised by vomiting, 'drunken' behaviour (technically called ataxia), weakness and convulsions. Phase two is typified by signs affecting breathing and the heart. The final phase is due to kidney failure. Recognition of this poisoning is very difficult unless the dog has been witnessed to drink the liquid, although there are some characteristic findings from urinalysis in certain cases. However, where this poison is known to be the culprit, ethanol (i.e. alcohol) is a specific antidote that should be given as soon as possible. Mortality in confirmed cases is high (up to 70% or more), especially once signs of kidney involvement occur. Cases that recover tend to show improvement within 24 hours.

Xylitol

This is most commonly found in chewing-gum. It is an artificial sweetener, safe for people, but even very small amounts can be fatal to dogs. When a dog swallows xylitol it is rapidly absorbed from the gut, within half-an-hour. It fools the pancreas to release a huge pulse of the hormone insulin, which in turn swiftly lowers blood glucose to dangerous levels. Treatment must be given urgently to prevent blood glucose falling dangerously low. High doses of xylitol can also cause liver failure, which might develop up to three days after the xylitol was swallowed. Provided signs of liver failure are avoided many dogs fully recover.

Batteries

There are lots of different types of battery that might be chewed, swallowed, or both. Leakage of alkali or toxic metals can occur leading to chemical burns in the mouth, the gullet, the stomach or further down the gut. On the other hand, some batteries that are swallowed can pass all the way through without causing any damage. This is a case where your vet should advise you on a case-by-case basis. Various forms of imaging, such as radiography or endoscopy, might be required. In a few cases, surgical treatment will be necessary.

When a vet has strong evidence that a dog of a certain weight has swallowed a known amount of a known toxin, they can usually determine a treatment plan with a good chance of the dog recovering. On the other hand, it is nearly impossible to effectively treat a dog for suspected poisoning if the toxin is unknown and the time of ingestion or exposure is also clouded in mystery.

However, there are exceptions.

> Years ago, I saw a huge hairy German Shepherd Dog, Mister Bojangles, who had some very strange angry-looking ulcerated patches on his scrotum. These lesions had worsened over a few weeks. A biopsy sample, examined under a microscope, showed a very characteristic pattern to the skin known technically as necrotic migratory erythema (NME). NME is sometimes coined 'Hepatocutaneous Syndrome' because the skin condition is linked to dysfunction of the liver. I took a blood sample from Mr B for biochemistry which showed that he did indeed have rather serious liver damage. The owner had told me, in passing, that the big bag of dog food he had been feeding had got damp, but the dog was still happily eating it. He brought a sample of the food in a jam jar. It smelled musty. At a loose end to establish what was causing the skin disease, I decided to follow this up. I found an academic with a particular expertise with fungi. She was interested and volunteered to screen the food for hepatotoxins. Low and behold it turned out that there were several different mycotoxins in the food. Withdrawal of the food and symptomatic treatment lead to a complete recovery. (Little et al., 1991)

COLLAPSE

I forget. It's a skill. When I move on from one patient to the next, I swiftly forget the first one. This helps me focus on the new patient. It means I have to keep absolutely thorough case notes, so, when I read them they jog my memory of each particular animal. However, 30 years on I still remember the unusual history of Gerty, a brindled wire-haired pointer aged eight. She used to go running with her master in the hills every day, no lead, same route, five miles. She loved it. Then an odd thing; she'd go for the run but discovered a short cut; after a couple of miles she'd peel off and reappear half a mile from home. It seemed she'd become lazy, suddenly. Gerty began to get a little fatter too. Then another oddity, when they were on the run Gerty began to sing; an off-key vibrato howling, especially on the way home. Then trouble. One day out running, Gerty began her howl early, slowed down for a few hundred metres, wobbled a bit, collapsed like a tree being felled, more than a mile from home. No joke in the Scottish hills. Before mobile phones. Thirty kilos of dog, still breathing, collapsed in a heap . . .

Collapse should always be taken very seriously. Urgent veterinary attention is usually necessary. Collapse can occur for a wide variety of reasons, which include sudden disturbances to the rhythm of the heart, anaemia, especially that caused by internal blood loss (haemorrhage), heat stroke (see pp. 194–195), an obstruction in the windpipe, a fall in the concentration of glucose in the body, various nervous diseases, pain, and certain other musculoskeletal problems too. Sometimes a dog will collapse like a ragdoll then recover almost immediately – this is fainting (technically called syncope) – most often due to heart disease (see p. 226). Sometimes a dog collapses only on the back legs. In those cases, spinal disease or possibly an interruption in the blood supply to the rear-end of the body are the most likely causes. When collapse does occur, in most cases, with the benefit of hindsight, it has not come entirely out of the blue. So, if your dog ever does this it is worthwhile turning over in your mind what hints there might have been in the days or weeks before that might have warned you there was something amiss. A change in behaviour, appetite, or thirst? Reluctance to go for a walk or to climb stairs? Tiring during a walk? Stiffness, lameness, limping? Heavy or loud breathing? Coughing?

When a vet is presented with a dog who has collapsed, they will begin by checking all the vital signs I've mentioned before: heart and pulse rate, breathing rate and effort, body temperature, the level of consciousness. They'll also search for evidence of pain. Systematically, they will try to establish if there is an underlying problem with the brain, the circulation, the breathing, the muscles, the bones or joints, and the rest of the nervous system. When your vet interviews you, they will quiz you in detail about the time leading up to the collapse and what exactly happened at the time. Did your dog seem bewildered or crazy in the minutes before the collapse? Did the dog howl or whimper, urinate or defecate, when they collapsed? Was there gasping or other abnormal sounds? Were there any convulsions or seizures, or did your dog seem completely floppy? How long did the collapse last – seconds, minutes, or longer? Did you notice if the gums or the tongue were pale or blueish?

Often, by the time the vet sees the patient the dog will have improved or even seem to be completely normal. This can be frustrating for you, the client, and for the vet too (believe me). So, if you have a smart phone on you when the event occurs, it's a really good idea to make a video recording of your pet. There might be vital clues which a vet or a specialist neurologist will find useful in the search for a diagnosis.

Sometimes it will be very obvious why a dog has collapsed, especially if they have choked, or the body temperature is very high, but in many cases there will be few clues. In dogs with serious heart disease or breathing problems, the clinical examination will usually provide strong hints to the problem, such as an irregular heart rhythm, a heart murmur, or abnormal breath sounds. In other cases, there might be very little to go on. The next stage your vet will advise will be blood tests to look for anaemia or some biochemical disturbances within the body. If they are concerned about the heart then they might want to record the heart rhythm – an electrocardiogram (ECG) – and to examine the heart by ultrasound, or to get chest X-ray pictures. Sometimes a time-lapse study of the heart rhythm is required; your dog will wear a device about the size of a mobile phone, in a jacket, with sticky electrodes on the chest. This is a Holter monitor that can record the ECG for hours, or even days, if necessary. Interpretation and effective treatment of heart problems might require a specialist. Similarly, many biochemical or neurologic problems are best handled by specialised clinicians who have particular knowledge of internal medicine or neurology. This can be expensive. Multiple tests are often necessary. However, without a definitive diagnosis, treatment of dogs who collapse might be impossible.

On the other hand, there are many dogs who only ever exhibit one event of this type or perhaps two episodes of brief collapse with very long periods of normality in between. Bearing in mind that it can be frustratingly difficult to find an explanation, if your vet examines your dog and is unable to find anything, there are certainly occasions when multiple investigations really may not be justified. This is a situation where careful discussions with your vet should help you to decide what is the most appropriate course for you and your dog.

> . . . Gerty's owner managed to carry her to a farmhouse. She was seen by a vet and referred to me at the veterinary school in Glasgow where I worked at the time. There were no signs of heart disease. The clues were in her history; odd behaviour and weight gain preceded the collapse. After an array of expensive tests, it turned out she had a tumour in her pancreas that was secreting large amounts of insulin. She had collapsed because the excessive insulin had caused dangerously low blood sugar levels (hypoglycaemia). Insulin also stimulates fat deposition. The professor of surgery, Mr Gorman, removed the tumour. A tricky procedure. Gerty recovered. In veterinary medicine, just as in many walks of life, you often need a team effort.

FAINTING (SYNCOPE – SUDDEN, TRANSIENT, LOSS OF CONSCIOUSNESS)

Dogs faint just as people do, often with little warning. They tend to recover very quickly too, though they might seem quite bewildered immediately after the event. A single event might never be repeated and might be quickly forgotten if the dog seems perfectly normal afterwards, but if a pattern of repeated syncope becomes established, or other clinical signs are present, a diagnostic investigation is definitely called for.

Syncope in dogs typically occurs when the blood-pressure suddenly drops and blood-flow to the brain is interrupted. This usually happens during exercise, on rising after rest, or sometimes immediately after coughing, urinating or having a poo. The usual causes are perturbations to the rhythmic beating of the heart such as a burst of very fast beats, or a period during which the heartbeat temporarily ceases completely. Many other forms of rhythm disturbance can occur and might cause syncope. These are often due to intrinsic heart disease but can be caused by diseases elsewhere in the body too.

Here's something you've probably never thought about; contrary to what you might believe, the heart is not a regular pump. It beats intermittently. In most dogs the rhythm of the heart is actually not very regular at all, instead it varies many times every minute being readjusted beat-by-beat due to nervous messages between the brain and the heart itself. For instance, most dogs when they are resting exhibit a heart rate that speeds up slightly every time they breathe in and slows down as they breathe out. This is called respiratory sinus arrhythmia. Another example: during sleep, normal dogs will sometimes have pauses between heartbeats lasting for two or three seconds. These pauses are infrequent, but if the heart rhythm is monitored for hours at a time they show up.

When a dog is active or excited their heart rate increases. Indeed, a normal dog can show a heart rate of 250 beats per minute, or more, when they are chasing a squirrel, swimming, or playing with another dog! Dogs' heart rates are much more variable than humans, which is one reason why they are such astonishing athletes.

Dogs who faint most frequently do so due to abnormalities of heart rate, or irregularities of the rhythm. Your vet might detect these when they listen to the heart and feel your dog's pulse. However, even dogs with serious rhythm disturbances can have long periods during which their heart rate and rhythm seems normal, so the brief 'snap-shot' of a clinical examination cannot be relied on to indicate what the rhythm and rate is at other times. This is another situation when a much longer recording of the heart rhythm, a Holter study, might be useful. Other diagnostic tests, such as the measurement of your dog's blood pressure and imaging procedures such as echocardiography (ultrasound examination of the heart), might be necessary too.

SEIZURES (CONVULSIONS, FITS) AND OTHER BRIEF EVENTS AFFECTING CONSCIOUSNESS AND BEHAVIOUR

A seizure, convulsion or 'fit' is an episode of repetitive involuntary movement caused by abnormal electrical activity in the brain. Seizures are relatively common. During the most typical seizures (called 'generalised' or Grand Mal) dogs fall to their side, lose consciousness, and rhythmically paddle their limbs as if trying to swim. Often, they howl, salivate profusely and pass urine or faeces.

During a seizure, the eyes are normally open, although the dog will not be really conscious. Sometimes seizures are much more subtle ('partial' seizures, Petit Mal); for instance, a dog might simply show repeated rhythmic muscle twitches of one leg or facial muscle(s). Sometimes such 'focal seizures' then become 'generalised' into a more severe event. Most seizures start suddenly out-of-the-blue, last for two or three minutes, or less, then quickly resolve. There are other episodic events during which a dog's consciousness is disturbed that resemble seizures, so when you see a vet it is important to try to describe exactly what happened.

Seizures can occur due to poisoning, head-trauma, fever, oxygen deprivation, low blood sugar (glucose), systemic illness, inflammation of the brain, or even a brain tumour. However, in most cases the exact cause of a seizure is not immediately obvious and must be searched for.

Epilepsy is a term used to describe repeated seizures, but there is more than one form of epilepsy. Idiopathic epilepsy, which is thought to be a genetically programmed disorder, has some peculiar features, which vets have come to recognise as typical. This condition is said to be the most common persistent brain disorder of dogs and seems to occur in around one dog in every 150.

If your dog exhibits a seizure, or similar event, don't panic. Human experience suggests seizures are not painful. Move obvious hazards, such as furniture from nearby. Don't allow the dog to fall downstairs. Talk quietly to your dog in re-assuring tones. Carefully observe what is happening, and the order in which events unfold, because your vet will want to quiz you thoroughly about this. A video-recording might be helpful. The duration of the seizure is a key factor to understanding the cause and best treatment, so, time it if you can.

Some dogs experience cluster seizures (two or more in 24 hours). This can be quite distressing. In other cases, a syndrome called status epilepticus occurs in which either a seizure extends for more than five minutes, or one seizure seems to begin to resolve but before the dog has fully recovered then another seizure occurs. Status epilepticus can be very serious indeed, even fatal. So, if your dog shows this prolonged convulsive activity, emergency treatment is essential.

A single seizure that resolves need not necessarily require you to visit your vet immediately as an emergency because these can sometimes be 'one-off' events. However, you should definitely arrange to see your vet soon. The vet will take a thorough history. They will want to know what your dog was doing before the seizure, what exactly happened during and after the seizure, and also how long it lasted. In many cases, a seizure first occurs when a dog is asleep, resting, or waking early in the morning. Some dogs show abnormal behaviour and anxiety in the hours or minutes before a seizure. After an event, which is known as the post-ictal phase, dogs are often rather confused and might seem blind. Aimless wandering is common during recovery. Frequently, the dog might seem to be very thirsty or very hungry. This phase can be as short as 15 minutes or last as long as 24 hours.

Because seizures and other brief signs of disturbed consciousness can be a manifestation of systemic disease, or another brain disorder, your dog will be examined carefully. The vet will assess the vital signs and try to establish if your dog is fully aware. They will want to see your dog walking and interacting with you and will do a comprehensive neurologic examination to test various nerve reflexes and so on. They will also ask you further questions about your dog's health and wellbeing in the previous few weeks. If you are giving your dog any drugs or food-supplements, or the diet has changed, this might be relevant, so make sure you tell your vet about these. Frequently, your vet will advise blood or urine tests to seek any evidence of systemic disease. In some cases, they might want to record the rhythm and electrical behaviour of the heart with an ECG.

If all these clinical findings and laboratory tests are normal, it is highly unlikely your vet will prescribe any treatment for a dog who has had only one short seizure because this event might never be repeated. Dogs who have several seizures spaced out over a period of years may also not be candidates for treatment, because the drugs used can have problematic side-effects. On the other hand, a dog that has two or more seizures within a couple of months, or has clusters (more than two in 24 hours), or has a seizure lasting more than 5 minutes, will probably require treatment. If the first seizure occurs between 6 months and three or four years of age, and no systemic illness or other explanation is found, the most likely diagnosis is 'Idiopathic Epilepsy' for which lifelong drug therapy is usually necessary. The management of that problem is considered in detail in the next chapter (p. 234). Older dogs who develop seizures and other similar events usually either have a systemic problem, or a brain disorder. Such patients might need further investigations, including MRI or other complex and expensive tests, frequently under the guidance of a neurology specialist.

I was asked to see Hogarth by my colleague Don. The dog, a 12-year-old male Lakeland Terrier, had experienced many, perhaps up to 20 brief seizure (?) episodes, lasting for as little as 20 seconds or up to three minutes, over a period of about six months. All these events occurred during the night, invariably beginning whilst asleep. Hogarth's owner, a science teacher with a matter-of-fact manner, explained that she did not think the seizures were epileptic fits: '... because I had a dog with epilepsy ... these "fits" are completely different.' Apparently, Hogarth slept in the teacher's bed. In the middle of the night, he would suddenly howl, stretch his forelegs forwards, arch his back and throw his head backwards in tension. This whilst completely unconscious, apparently not breathing at all. Within a minute or so he would relax from this spasm and begin to breathe, but it would be three minutes, or more, before he would seem properly conscious. Hogarth would be weak, wobbly and 'a bit drunk', for up to an hour afterwards.

Don had seen Hogarth several times and examined him repeatedly. At each examination Hogarth was bright and alert. Neurologic examinations, in between events – evaluating consciousness, behaviour, ambulation and nervous reflexes – were unremarkable. There were no respiratory or cardiovascular abnormalities picked up. Hogarth was eating well and his thirst was normal. Blood biochemistry, haematology and routine urinalysis tests were also normal. The teacher was not keen for Hogarth to see a neurologist, so we decided between us that a time-lapse examination of the heart rhythm, a Holter study, might be useful.

It was.

Most of the recording was normal. The heart rate would increase when Hogarth was barking at a neighbour, anticipating a meal, or enjoying a walk. The heart would slow up when he was resting or asleep. This is entirely expected. However, during the night Hogarth's heart sometimes ceased beating completely – asystole – for 5 seconds or more. One period of asystole lasted for nearly eight seconds. During another period, 16 seconds long, only three heartbeats occurred. Thirty-seven pauses of more than four seconds were recorded during a night's sleep. These unusual findings seemed to suggest the nocturnal 'fits' were caused by interruptions in blood and oxygen delivery to the brain.

Sometimes rhythm disturbances of this kind can only be treated using expensive technology; fitting a pacemaker into the heart. In other cases, drugs can be given to improve the regularity of the heart. Hogarth was treated with a human drug, probanthine, which helps to uncouple the heart from braking effects driven by the brain. I am pleased to say that since we started Hogarth on treatment, more than 30 months ago, he has had few 'fits'. Now elderly, aged nearly 15, he is blind and in failing health, but for the time being he still has a good quality of life.

EMERGENCIES INVOLVING THE EYES

Three types of eye problem typically require emergency treatment.

The first is trauma – from a fall, a road accident, a fight with a dog or cat, or perhaps a foreign-body, such as a thorn piercing the eye. The eye is normally protected from injury by the bony socket of the skull, the orbit and the eyelids. Dogs have three lids – the third lid is normally hidden out of sight at the inner corner of the eye. Our canine friends have very fast reaction-times compared with people and this helps them defend their eyes. However, accidents do happen.

Sometimes an eye can be completely displaced from its normal housing so that it is prolapsed in front of the eyelids. This is called proptosis. It looks awful! Proptosis more commonly happens to those dogs with flat faces (brachycephalics, such as pugs). If this emergency affects your dog take them to a vet immediately. In the meantime, it can be a good idea to protect the surface of the eye with a clean cloth soaked in water. A prolapsed eye can sometimes be saved, especially if seen promptly by an eye specialist.

On other occasions, when an eye is damaged the cornea, the clear 'window' at the front, might be torn by a claw or lacerated by a sharp object. This too is an emergency. An important factor here is the depth of the penetration into the eye. If the cornea is deeply pierced and the lens or the iris is wounded then the prospects for return of sight are much worse than when the damage is superficial. If the wounding object is still in the eye leave it there, but get to a vet as soon as you can.

After a dog fight or another accident one of the eyelids might be ripped or grazed. This type of wound tends to bleed profusely, but the good news is that eyelids tend to heal very well. If the lid requires stitching this calls for general anaesthesia and very precise surgery. Again, it might pay to see an eye specialist vet.

Another ocular emergency you might see is glaucoma – in which the fluid pressure within the eye increases and the whole globe swells. This subject is dealt with in Chapter 7 (pp. 153–154).

Corneal ulcers, if they deteriorate quickly, may also necessitate emergency treatment (see pp. 152–153).

DYSPNOEA (DIFFICULT OR PAINFUL BREATHING)

Like people, dogs can get respiratory diseases of various kinds (see Chapter 6, p. 174). The usual signs might be a cough, sneeze, snore, heavy breathing or panting. If your dog seems to be having serious difficulty or discomfort breathing then you ought to see a vet promptly, especially if they are making a lot of noise when they breathe or seem unable to rest. Dogs with dyspnoea can die quickly. Sometimes a dog with breathing difficulties will start to show signs suddenly in the middle of the night. This is a particularly frequent story in dogs with heart failure. However, it is practically impossible for a vet to make a definitive diagnosis of the cause of dyspnoea from the clinical history and examination alone, so expect that your dog will require emergency treatment and further investigations to run concurrently.

Dogs who make a lot of respiratory noise, such as many of the flat-faced breeds – for instance, bulldogs – sometimes develop heat-stroke and breathing difficulties concurrently, especially if they exercise vigorously in hot and humid weather. This can also happen to older dogs with acquired breathing difficulties, such as those with tracheal collapse (seen especially in small dogs) and older large-breed dogs who are developing laryngeal paralysis. If you think your dog is very hot and distressed with noisy breathing then you might be able to help immediately by swiftly cooling them. Whole body immersion in a pond, a stream, or the sea, is probably the best first aid. If you can't achieve that, it would still help if you soak them with cold water. **This is another case where your dog should be seen by a vet as quickly as possible.** (More information on heat stroke is provided on pages 194–195).

I can hardly stress this enough. I have seen several dogs with this problem who died on the way to our practice simply because action was taken too late.

A local practice contacted me; they had a middle-aged Maltese terrier who was collapsed with serious breathing problems. Topaz arrived soon after. She looked exhausted, couldn't stand, was breathing deeply, noisily and very quickly. The thermometer registered 40.4°C. Loud crackles, squeaks and wheezes were present in her chest, so that even with a good stethoscope, it was impossible to hear her heart at all. Her gums were a deep pink colour, almost purple.

These ominous signs had all developed quickly.

Three days before, Topaz had had an anaesthetic to extract some teeth and clean the others. Afterwards she recovered well and had gone home. That evening she ate. She had breakfast the next morning, but that afternoon she had a sudden coughing spell that was protracted, continuing off and on for an hour or more. She improved, ate dinner and seemed fine again next day. The coughing was forgotten. Until the third morning, when Topaz was struggling for breath.

We immediately started Topaz on two different intravenous antibiotics and oxygen delivered by a soft catheter in her nose (nasal prongs). A blood sample showed Topaz had a low white blood cell count with lots of immature cells, known as band neutrophils. This blood picture is typical of overwhelming infection. Chest radiographs showed a pattern suggestive of pneumonia caused by inhalation. This had probably happened at the time of the coughing fit a couple of days previously.

With careful nursing, ongoing oxygen therapy and pain relief, Topaz struggled on, but a few hours later she began to cough up blood. When a case is hopeless sometimes the kindest thing that we can do is end the suffering by injecting an overdose of anaesthetic – euthanasia – providing a good death where otherwise a painful and distressing death is inevitable.

Miss Gordon, an elderly lady rang us; she had been looking after her neighbours' dog whilst they were spending a few days away. He had been for a walk that morning and run around without any signs of distress but now he seemed to be breathing very hard.

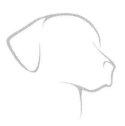

9

CHRONIC
DISEASES

We all would like to lead healthy lives and want the same thing for our dogs, but nature doesn't always allow us this luxury. Some serious or disabling diseases might be fatal. Other conditions might be so nasty that the dog's life becomes intolerable. But there are many diseases that, though they might be incurable, can be successfully treated and managed with modern medicine. This chapter highlights some of these. I will focus on a small number of important medical problems that require careful evaluation and very intensive treatments: dry eye, Cushing's disease, diabetes mellitus, heart disease and failure, hypothyroidism, epilepsy, Addison's disease, hypertension and renal failure. These are serious conditions that can be extremely rewarding to treat and where the outcome is highly dependent on close cooperation between the veterinary team and the dog's carers.

'DRY EYE': KERATOCONJUNCTIVITIS SICCA

The tear film that covers the surface of the eye provides that lovely smooth glistening surface, the glint. It keeps the eye healthy. Tears are not simple, made up from several different components (see p. 151). Whenever a dog has discomfort of the eyes your vet will probably want to measure the tear production with a procedure called the Schirmer tear test. This involves placing a specially calibrated strip of absorbent paper into the puddle of tears behind the lower eyelid then measuring the distance along the strip that becomes wet after 60 seconds. Additional tests are sometimes performed.

If your dog doesn't produce enough tears the eyes will become inflamed and soon the surface of the cornea, the clear window into the eye, will become irregular, and painful. This is called 'dry eye', more technically keratoconjunctivitis sicca, or just KCS. Dogs with this disease often show sticky stringy discharge across the surface of the cornea that might appear opaque and irregular. Any dog who seems to get repeated episodes of conjuctivitis or discomfort of the eyes ought to be checked to look for this condition. KCS is particularly seen in some common breeds of dog such as the West Highland White Terrier, Cocker and Springer Spaniels, Bulldog, Toy Poodle and Lhasa Apso. KCS is also sometimes found in association with some hormonal problems; namely, diabetes mellitus (see p. 223), Cushing's disease (see p. 221) and hypothyroidism (see p. 231).

In most cases of KCS, treatment should be instituted immediately it is recognised, and continued for life. A drug called ciclosporin in an ointment form is the treatment of choice. This is an immunosuppressive drug that also stimulates tear production. Ciclosporin ointment is expensive. Fortunately, in most cases it works brilliantly. Sometimes, especially if the condition is severe, additional lubricants, tear substitutes and antibiotic drops are also employed, especially in the early stages before the ciclosporin has really begun to work.

In a few cases, ciclosporin treatment seems to be ineffective, perhaps because the disease had become too advanced before it was recognised. Less frequently, there could be an alternative explanation, because there are dogs who have a similar disease that is congenital, present from birth. Occasionally, KCS occurs in one eye only due to a nervous disorder called Horner's Syndrome. Other drug therapy might be used; for example, a higher concentration of ciclosporin might be prescribed, or another immunomodulatory drug called tacrolimus. If these fail, there is a surgical procedure that is sometimes the last resort; a duct from a salivary gland is transplanted from the mouth to the eye that irrigates the eye with spit. Far from ideal, but better than constant discomfort and eventual blindness.

CUSHING'S DISEASE (HYPERADRENOCORTICISM)

Cushing's disease, also known as hyperadrenocorticism (HAC) is one of the more common diseases that cause dogs to drink and pee a lot. It is most frequently caused by a tumour in the pituitary gland (~85% of cases). The tumour secretes a hormone, ACTH. This hormone causes the adrenal glands that lie just in front of the kidneys to enlarge and secrete large amounts of cortisol. The cortisol (another hormone) makes the dog hungry and thirsty. Cortisol has other effects, which take some months to become obvious, but include muscular weakness, thinning of the skin and loss of hair – often in a symmetrical pattern either side of the back. Infrequently, dogs with this disease also start to show patches of mineralisation in the skin. This is called 'calcinosis cutis'. Cortisol excess in the body suppresses the immune system, which can render the patient at risk from infection. Sometimes, though this is rare, dogs afflicted with Cushing's disease can get blood clots in the lung. This leads to sudden severe breathing problems and may be fatal.

For the owners of most dogs with Cushing's disease, the condition is highly inconvenient because the dogs are so hungry, so thirsty, and pee such a lot. However, for many dogs the disease is not life-threatening, at least in the medium term.

Eventually, if the Cushing's disease is caused by a pituitary tumour, that tumour grows larger and starts to cause other problems. This can take years. The pituitary gland sits under the brain connected to it by a stalk. The gland itself lies in a little cul-de-sac of the skull, called the pituitary fossa. At the point where the stalk of the pituitary attaches to the brain, the two optic nerves, from the eyes, meet. This is called the optic chiasma. If the pituitary gland enlarges sufficiently this optic chiasma can be damaged. Then the dog will go partially, or completely, blind. Another, eventual, consequence of a pituitary tumour can be neurological signs caused by the tumour pressing on the brain itself.

A proportion of dogs with this disease (the other ~15%) actually have an adrenal tumour. The clinical signs of an adrenal tumour don't differ from those dogs with a pituitary tumour. However adrenal tumours sometimes 'dissect' into the adjacent blood vessels. This can lead to sudden fatal haemorrhage into the abdomen.

Reaching a definite diagnosis of Cushing's disease can be challenging and frustrating for owners and vets. There is a suite of laboratory tests that are required, sometimes backed up by other investigations, such as abdominal ultrasound imaging. It is crucial that a correct and definitive diagnosis is made because treatment is not without risk.

Cushing's disease can be effectively treated using a drug called trilostane that is given every day (sometimes twice), for life. Like many veterinary drugs this is expensive. Drug monitoring must be done, which adds to the costs, because over-dose can have fatal consequences. That said, treatment can be very rewarding indeed.

DIABETES MELLITUS ('SUGAR DIABETES')

This is another disease that can make your dog hungry, excessively thirsty and pass large volumes of urine frequently. Sugar diabetes is a very important disease that can be fatal if not carefully treated. There are other hazards of the disease too such as urinary infections, kidney failure, blindness and disorders of nerve function. In spite of this the vast majority of dogs with this disease can be treated and many will live long, happy and fulfilled lives.

It is essential to understand a little bit about the normal workings of the body, and the basics of this disease, in order to treat and manage diabetes mellitus successfully.

As you will know, food, composed from carbohydrates, fats and proteins, is digested in the gut, broken down by enzymes into smaller molecules; amino acids (from proteins), fatty acids and other lipids and various sugars. These are absorbed from the gut into the bloodstream. Then the liver and the pancreas work together to adjust the levels of fats, amino acids and sugars in the blood. The principle energy source of the body, blood sugar, is glucose. When glucose levels in the bloodstream are high, the body tends to store this, in the form of glycogen, in the liver, and also in longer-term fat deposits. When glucose levels are low the liver converts glycogen back to glucose. Fats too are released from storage.

Normally, in healthy mammals, including dogs and people, the pancreas secretes a small protein hormone molecule, insulin, into the blood. Insulin is released in response to glucose entering the bloodstream from the carbohydrates digested and absorbed from the gut. It acts as a 'key' to open pores in the cells of the body that allows glucose to enter the cells.

Dogs with diabetes mellitus either don't produce insulin from their pancreas, or there is some other fault in the body that makes the insulin they do secrete less effective than it should be. So, in dogs with this disease the cells of the body don't receive enough glucose to work properly. On the other hand, since the insulin is not there to enable cells to take up glucose, the amount of glucose in the circulation and fluids of the body climbs way above normal. This 'extra-cellular' glucose escapes from the circulation, via the kidneys, into the urine and drags large amounts of body water with it. Diabetes mellitus literally means 'sweet urine'. Lots of this urine is formed. Consequently, the affected dog passes great lakes of glucose-rich urine. To replace this large volume of fluid the pet must drink a great deal. Because the cells of the body are starved of energy the dog feels especially hungry much of the time and because their body is unable to use their food properly the dog often loses weight. So, there are four classic clinical signs that are found in canine diabetes mellitus; increased thirst, increased urination, hunger and weight loss.

If your dog presents to a vet with this set of clinical signs, the vet will almost certainly look for the diagnosis by measuring blood and urine glucose as well as other tests to ascertain exactly what is going on.

In the healthy body, when a meal is digested the levels of fats, amino acids and sugars in the circulation increase. The high glucose level stimulates the pancreas to secrete insulin that causes glucose levels to begin to fall. As blood glucose levels decline, insulin release slows down, then stops and blood glucose levels rise again. If the dog is on a diet that is rich in carbohydrates, glucose levels tend to yo-yo up and down after a meal, whereas if the pet is eating a low-carbohydrate diet, rich in protein and fat, the blood glucose levels tend to vary less and to change more slowly too. Very often, as part of the management of canine diabetes, your vet will recommend a prescription diet that has been formulated to avoid large oscillations in blood glucose.

Our aim, as vets and clients faced with a dog with diabetes, is to give the correct amount of insulin for the food intake so that blood glucose levels never get too high or fall too low. It is for this reason that we might need to adjust the food intake and the insulin dose in step. Insulin is normally given by sub-cutaneous injection once or twice a day. Usually, the insulin injection is given just after a meal. Insulin itself is quite fragile. It must be kept in a fridge and handled very gently. Different insulin preparations exist that release this hormone into the body at different rates. Most dogs with sugar diabetes must be treated with insulin designed specifically for use in dogs.

When your dog has high blood glucose levels this tends to cause the pet to be thirsty, hungry and to urinate a lot. If the condition continues your dog will often lose weight. High blood glucose levels, 'hyperglycaemia', can also lead to a dangerous state where the body starts to produce unusual chemicals called ketones. The acidity of the body can also increase. Hyperglycaemia is present for part of the day in virtually all dogs who have diabetes but, provided the hyperglycaemia is mild and of short duration, it will not be a serious danger to your dog. When hyperglycaemia is present there will usually be some glucose in the urine.

If your pet has normal levels of glucose in the blood – this is called 'euglycaemia' – the dog should have no signs of diabetes. When treating a dog with diabetes, we aim to achieve long periods of euglycaemia throughout the day. Finding the appropriate diet and insulin dosing regime takes time and effort.

When a dog has blood glucose levels that are subnormal this is termed 'hypoglycaemia' – a hypo. A dog who has hypoglycaemia is in a fragile state. This can sometimes manifest itself as weakness, confusion, 'drunken' behaviour or sometimes seizures are seen ('fitting'). It is extremely important to avoid serious or prolonged hypoglycaemia because this can be fatal.

Once we have made a diagnosis of diabetes mellitus, we usually need to monitor dogs with this condition very carefully, especially initially. Some of that monitoring can be based around simple observations: body weight, appetite, thirst, urine volume, urine glucose concentrations, etc. In addition, especially as we adjust the treatment regimen, we might want to measure blood glucose concentrations, sometimes every hour or two for 12–24 hours, or more. This is called a glucose curve. This assessment can help us to see if the insulin dose is correct and to get some idea if the blood glucose is falling too fast or too far after the insulin has been given, or if the blood glucose is remaining high for too long a period. Recently, devices have become available that can measure blood glucose continuously. These are increasingly being used to monitor diabetic dogs. Another test vets like to do is to measure a blood chemical called fructosamine. This wonderful test helps us to judge the average blood glucose level over the past two or three weeks.

I have mentioned that poorly controlled sugar diabetes can on occasion lead to other problems. This it is worth a little explanation. Dogs who have a lot of glucose in the urine are prone to infections in the kidneys and the bladder. Urine is normally virtually sterile. But when the urine is full of glucose this can encourage the development of bacterial urinary infections. These are usually highly treatable with antibiotics but if they become long-standing ('chronic') serious kidney damage can result. Persistent high blood sugar levels can lead to a form of lens cataract in the eyes (see p. 153). Occasionally, dogs with diabetes mellitus can also develop degenerative changes in some of their nerves leading; for instance, to deterioration in the co-ordination of their movements.

A fascinating study was published whilst this book was being written. A form of insulin therapy has been formulated for use in dogs that does not need to be given daily. In that study, dogs were given that preparation once every week. The small study that has been published is intriguing but the treatment is experimental at present; it will be at least several years before this type of treatment becomes mainstream (if ever).

I hope you can see that managing diabetes can be quite challenging. However, my experience is that most owners soon get to understand their dog's disease. By working together, vets, veterinary nurses and owners can often manage canine sugar diabetes very well; indeed, I have been delighted to see that this condition sometimes brings people to develop a closer bond with their dog.

HEART DISEASE AND HEART FAILURE

Heart disease

Heart disease is fairly common in dogs. I'll start with a short lesson. Please don't feel patronised. Forgive me.

The heart is a bag of muscle divided into two sides and four chambers. It's a pump, actually two sister pumps, that beat in synchrony, relaxing and contracting time and again, minute by minute, day after day. During the relaxation phase of the heart, called diastole, the venous blood that has just been around the body pours into the right atrium, the first chamber. Venous blood is a deep burgundy colour. It carries carbon dioxide but is depleted of oxygen. This blood traverses the right atrium, passes through a narrowing, the tricuspid valve, into the second right heart chamber, the right ventricle. Towards the end of diastole, the relaxation phase, the right atrium contracts. This pushes additional venous blood into the right ventricle, priming the ventricular pump. The next phase of the cardiac cycle then begins; the right ventricle contracts: 'systole'. This muscular contraction causes that one-way tricuspid valve between the two chambers of the right heart to close, preventing blood returning to the atrium. Pressure within the right ventricle increases, which causes the exit valve from the right ventricle to be flung open. Blood leaves the right ventricle via the pulmonary artery to perfuse the lungs. Here, the venous blood gives up the carbon dioxide it has been carrying. Oxygen is taken up from the lungs into the blood, carried within the red blood cells by the pigment haemoglobin. This blood has now become scarlet in colour, highly nutritious for the cells of the body.

Having travelled through the lungs the oxygenated blood now courses through the pulmonary veins into the left atrium. Here, during cardiac relaxation, the blood is directed from the left atrium into the left ventricle, again crossing through a one-way valve, the mitral valve. As for the right, the left atrium contracts when diastole draws to an end, augmenting the filling of the left ventricular chamber. Again, when systole occurs the left ventricle contracts, the mitral valve closes, pressure within the ventricle increases and a dollop of blood is pushed out through the last heart valve into that great artery of the body, the aorta. The pressure developed within the left ventricle drives the arterial blood around the body carrying oxygen, heat and nutrients to the tissues.

Heart rate is controlled by the brain. Dogs' hearts beat slowly and rather irregularly when they are resting or asleep. This irregularity is not random but arises as a result of a continuous 'conversation' between the heart and the brain. During vigorous exercise or excitement altered nervous discharges from the brain cause the heart to beat much more quickly so that blood can be fed around the body speedily. Healthy dogs are born athletes.

A few dogs are born with anatomic defects affecting the heart. Some of these puppies may not grow well and thrive in the first few months of life. In most cases, a problem is recognised when they are first seen by a vet and examined thoroughly with a stethoscope because the heart sounds abnormal. A murmur is present. Healthy hearts produce a pair of sounds with every beat. These sounds – 'lub-dup, lub-dup, lub-dup' – indicate the closing of the heart valves at the beginning and end of every systolic contraction of the heart. If a systolic murmur is present this usually indicates there is something wrong, blood is flowing irregularly during cardiac contraction. Diastolic murmurs, heard during the relaxation phase of the heartbeat, are less common but they too can be ominous. The precise cause of a heart murmur is difficult to ascertain by auscultation, using a stethoscope, alone. It is a specialist investigation that usually necessitates cardiac ultrasound and other techniques such as electrocardiograms (ECGs) and radiography. I spend much of my life doing these sorts of investigations, but congenital heart disease forms a tiny part of most vets' work and it is not really appropriate to spend much time on this here.

Aside from congenital anatomic problems the most common forms of heart disease in the dog are acquired and usually do not present until middle age or later in life. There are two dominant problems, namely: acquired valvular incompetence and dilated cardiomyopathy.

Valvular incompetence usually develops slowly. It most frequently affects the valve on the left side of the heart between the left atrium and left ventricle. This is the mitral valve. The condition has a variety of names, including 'endocardiosis' and 'myxomatous mitral valve disease'. It is most common in small dogs less than 20 kg body weight. It is particularly frequent in a few breeds, including Cavalier King Charles Spaniels, Maltese Terriers, Norfolk Terriers, Yorkshire Terriers, Dachshunds and Cocker Spaniels. However, the disease is certainly not limited to these breeds and is often found in cross-bred dogs.

Dilated cardiomyopathy, or DCM, just as it says on the tin, is a muscular dysfunction of the heart, a diagnosis made when cavities of the heart are swollen but failing to contract properly. This condition tends to affect large breeds of dog and is especially common in a few, such as the Doberman, Irish Wolfhound, Great Dane, Weimaraner and Springer Spaniel. A variant of this condition is seen quite often in Labrador Retrievers. Another condition, in Boxers, resembles DCM, but has special features that set it apart. In all these breeds there is rather good circumstantial evidence that these conditions are genetic disorders but, in most cases, the precise defect(s) in the DNA are not yet known.

Dogs who have these conditions can sometimes be identified long before they become ill. This is especially true for acquired valvular incompetence because these dogs will usually first develop a systolic heart murmur. Most often a heart murmur is recognised when a dog is being examined for another reason, such as a routine check-up prior to receiving a booster vaccination. Heart murmurs can also develop for non-cardiac reasons, such as anaemia, in which the turbulent irregular blood-flow within the heart occurs simply because the blood is thinner and less viscous than normal. So, if a vet discovers a heart murmur in your dog, they might first ask themselves: 'Is this dog anaemic?'

Vets classify heart murmurs based on their loudness, their timing, and where on the chest the murmur is most easily heard. As a general rule, loud heart murmurs TEND to be associated with more serious disease, but this is not always the case. When your vet examines your dog's circulation, they will assess a variety of features such as the heart rate, the pulse rate, the regularity of both, the colour of the gums and whether the breathing is normal. They also will probably ask you questions about your dog's willingness and ability to exercise and how tired the dog gets.

If a vet is worried that your dog might have significant heart disease, even if the dog seems completely well, they will often want to arrange further investigations. This is because, for some diseases, especially if the heart is obviously enlarged or the heart rhythm is abnormal, drug therapy has been shown to prolong a healthy lifespan significantly. Frequently, these investigations would be done by a heart specialist, like myself.

In small dogs with proven valvular incompetence if the heart is definitely enlarged beyond certain limits, but the dog seems perfectly well, a drug called Pimobendan has been proven to prolong life (when compared with a placebo in a randomised blinded clinical trial) by more than a year on average. Similarly, in dogs with DCM that are clinically well, this drug has been shown to prolong life in a similar blinded and randomised clinical trial.

Other causes of heart disease in the dog are relatively uncommon; however, there are some infrequent problems. These include an accumulation of fluid around the heart, called a pericardial effusion, and tumours of the heart.

Heart failure

This describes the point at which the pumping of the heart is no longer sufficient to fully meet all the needs of the body. Many dogs with heart disease never develop heart failure but all those with heart failure must have heart disease. Dogs with heart failure usually develop characteristic clinical signs. They tend to become tired at exercise or are unwilling to exercise to the extent that they did. Often these dogs breathe more quickly than normal and are prone to develop breathing abnormalities. They may also cough. Dogs with heart failure sometimes collapse or show fainting spells, become lethargic or show generalised weakness.

Veterinary examinations often reveal a heart murmur, and a fast or chaotic heart rate, accompanied by weak, quick or chaotic pulses. Other signs relating to the breathing, the colour of the gums, and the warmth of the tissues are occasionally seen. Sometimes dogs with heart failure develop a swollen abdomen due to the accumulation of fluid. This is called ascites. Heart failure signs can develop quite slowly but might come on very abruptly, especially if the heart rhythm has suddenly deteriorated.

You will realise these signs are not all specific to the heart so the diagnosis of heart failure might not be easy to make. Often it is the total clinical picture, the dog's history and the constellation of clinical signs, which together provide clues. Confirmation of the diagnosis usually requires additional testing.

Veterinary cardiology has developed tremendously during the last 40 years. This is especially through the development of cardiac ultrasound ('echocardiography'), which enables a skilled operator to examine the heart in detail completely non-invasively. Using this technique, the sizes of the cardiac chambers can be measured, the contractility of the heart can be assessed, the source(s) of murmurs can be established and the pressures within the different parts of the heart can be evaluated. The speed of blood flow through each heart valve can be accurately measured and even the cardiac output, the volume of blood being pumped by the heart minute by minute, can be estimated. This sort of information can help a clinician to reach a definitive diagnosis, but it does take much time and effort to develop this skill. A high-quality ultrasound machine is invaluable. Costly kit.

Echocardiography is the cornerstone of modern veterinary cardiology but other tests are needed to complement it, especially if drugs are to be used. Cardiac drugs like all pharmaceuticals can have side-effects or might not always be safe to administer. So, alongside 'echo', we might wish to record an ECG to more precisely understand the heart rhythm, take blood tests to evaluate kidney function, to measure your dog's blood pressure, or radiograph the chest for detailed assessment of the lungs.

Many dogs with heart failure develop pooling of blood in the lungs because the left heart is not functioning well. This congestion can lead to a form of waterlogging of the lung tissue, called pulmonary oedema. Pulmonary oedema hampers normal lung function, which can lead to breathlessness, coughing, severe anxiety and even death. There are drugs that can help to treat this, diuretics, that dry the lungs and make the kidneys produce more urine. Correctly used, diuretics, such as furosemide, are often lifesavers for dogs with heart failure. However, the drugs are not entirely safe in all patients and the dose of these drugs must be carefully titrated to get maximum benefit with minimal side effects.

Some other drugs are often used to treat heart failure. Pimobendan has already been mentioned. This drug, specifically developed for canine heart disease, is classed as an 'inodilator', meaning it makes the heart muscle contract more forcefully (this is called inotropism) whilst also dilating the arterioles, the small arteries which feed the tissues. Vasodilators of various hues have become the mainstay of the treatment of heart failure in people. If the blood vessels are dilated, blood can flow through the vessels under lower pressure. In other words, the heart can work more efficiently with less effort. Vasodilator drugs called ACE Inhibitors (several are marketed) and Spironolactone form some of the other drugs that are often also used to treat heart failure in dogs.

If your dog has heart failure, you might have to reduce their exercise. Dogs with heart failure often lose weight as part of the heart failure syndrome. Evidence shows that this weight loss tends to be accompanied by a worse outlook.

Some interesting recent work suggests that dietary therapy might be helpful for dogs with some heart diseases. For more on this, see Chapter 10.

Successful long-term management of heart failure crucially depends on a dedicated owner, an interested and able vet, vigilance on behalf of both parties, strategic use of further tests, and a willingness to finesse drug treatment as the condition develops. I have spent the best years of my life working on this. It has been a pleasure and an honour to have developed very close relationships with lots of dogs and their families over the years. Science has driven an improvement in the prognosis; love and dedication has played a big role too.

HYPOTHYROIDISM

A series of glands within the body interact to maintain the balance of metabolism. They control an array of functions such as appetite, sleep, body temperature, blood pressure, the response to stress, sexual state, the fine control of blood sugar, salts, etc. These are the endocrine organs that elaborate and secrete specific chemical messengers, hormones, into the blood-stream. Endocrine diseases are fairly frequently diagnosed in dogs. We have already come across two, diabetes mellitus and hyperadrenocorticism. There are others.

> Duchess was found wandering the streets of Glasgow, picked up by a rescue service, and, when nobody claimed her, re-homed to a family in Wishaw. Soon she was devoted to Alan and Fiona who became besotted with her. She was a Doberman, a muscular, sleek energetic black and tan bitch, who loved to go rabbiting in Strathclyde park.
>
> I met her a couple of years after she'd found this home. Over a period of about six months, Duchess had become lethargic and dull. Her appetite was good but she'd put on weight. She weighed 47 kg. More than 10 kg above her prime. She no longer wanted walks. Her coat had lost its lustre; it had become scurfy and greasy to touch. The skin around her face and trunk seemed thick. Her heart rate was slow; 66 bpm, it was also almost inaudible, even with a good stethoscope in a quiet room. When I palpated for the femoral arteries, I found the pulses were weak. Her gums looked a bit pale too and her skin felt cold. Her body temperature was subnormal: 36.8°C.

This cadre of clinical signs arose because Duchess had severe hypothyroidism. Thyroid hormones are intimately involved in the control of metabolic rate, which, in essence, is the speed at which body's organs work. Hypothyroidism, in which organ functions become sluggish, is not actually very common but it is highly treatable. It occurs most often when the thyroid gland has been damaged by the body reacting against its own tissue; an auto-immune disorder. The condition might be suspected from the clinical signs but is not always easily recognised. Diagnosis depends on measuring the levels of two different hormones, namely the active thyroid hormone (T4) and the hormone which triggers the thyroid gland to secrete T4, thyroid stimulating hormone (TSH). If the T4 is low and the TSH is high the diagnosis is confirmed.

When a dog has this condition, thyroid supplementation is necessary for life.

> I started Duchess on a supplementary thyroid hormone at the usual initial dose. It usually takes a few weeks before the clinical signs begin to improve, but within a few days Duchess became nervous, started panting frequently, to vomit occasionally and to drink more. Inevitably, she also started to pass

more urine, which led to her wetting the kitchen floor overnight. Her owners were very disappointed. I was baffled.

I'd thought the diagnosis was secure and the hard part of this case was over. But veterinary medicine is nothing if not humbling. I went over all the history and the clinical findings and talked to the clinical pathologist from the lab. Then I got out my textbooks and read.

It turned out that Duchess was now showing signs of excessive thryroid function, or thyrotoxicosis. These side-effects are uncommon but occur in a small fraction of dogs who seem to be particularly sensitive to the thyroid hormone. The problem was solved by stopping the drug for a few days then re-starting treatment at a lower dose.

Most dogs with this condition are monitored by regular clinical examinations and measuring the levels of thyroid hormones in blood. Once we found the appropriate drug dose for Duchess, she improved. Initially, her heart rate increased and her body temperature rose. Then she started to become more interactive at home and to want to exercise. However, it took several months before her coat improved and her body weight returned to normal. When it did, Fiona and Alan were ecstatic.

I was delighted by a bottle of malt that Christmas, signed with a Doberman paw-print.

HYPOADRENOCORTICISM – 'ADDISON'S DISEASE'

This is another endocrine disorder. It is a condition in which the body has an inadequate supply of steroid hormones, which are normally produced by the adrenal glands, two small organs lying close to the kidneys. We met these glands earlier when I discussed hyperadrenocorticism (see p. 221). The hormones, called mineralocorticoids and corticosteroids, play crucial roles in controlling the water and salt balance within the body, as well as the ability of the dog to cope with stressful situations. Lack of these hormones leads to loss of fluids from the body, diminished kidney function, and to imbalances in the concentration of body salts. When hypoadrenocorticism is severe, dogs can suddenly develop a very low heart rate, weakness and a form of shock that is known as an 'Addisonian crisis', named after the physician who first understood this problem in people. Hypoadrenocorticism is important to recognise because if the diagnosis is missed or delayed the disease is frequently fatal.

We are fortunate that many companion animal practices in the UK have on-site laboratories and are able to swiftly analyse blood samples to pick up some of the tell-tale signs of hypoadrenocorticism. This can expedite the recognition and emergency treatment of these dogs. But, the definitive diagnosis of the disease ultimately requires measurement of a specific hormone, cortisol, before and after stimulating the adrenal glands with a synthetic version of another hormone, ACTH, which originates in the pituitary gland in the skull.

Hypoadrenocorticism is not a common disease. It features here because it can be spectacularly serious but responds very well to treatment, provided it is recognised early enough. It is around three times more common in bitches than dogs. A few breeds, the Poodles and West Highland White Terriers, as well some more exotic ones, are much more prone to this disease than others. Once the disease has been spotted it must be treated for life using replacement hormones. These drugs are given by injection every few weeks and / or tablets every day. Treatment has to be very closely monitored with frequent blood tests, especially early in the course of the disease, to avoid side-effects or repeated crises. For dogs that are well con-trolled the long-term outlook is excellent.

EPILEPSY

Epilepsy simply means recurrent seizures, which can be caused by a variety of problems. The most common form is idiopathic epilepsy, which is believed to have a genetic cause. Epileptic seizures can arise for other reasons, so if your dog has these, diagnostic tests are called for (see Chapter 8, p. 221). Many dogs who have infrequent seizures will not benefit from treatment, which should be avoided if possible because it carries some risks. Treatment is usually begun only after a dog has more than one seizure a month, clusters of seizures (more than one in 24 hours), or seizures that persist for more than 5 minutes.

The most commonly used medications to treat seizures in dogs are phenobarbital, potassium bromide and imepitoin. These drugs are licensed for treating canine epilepsy in the UK, which means they are first-choice agents. Unfortunately, the drugs can sometimes have quite profound side-effects, such as sedation, excessive thirst, an increased appetite and weight gain.

Phenobarbital is a barbiturate medication, related to many anaesthetics, which with long-term use can damage the liver, so vets are encouraged to regularly re-evaluate their patients, do blood tests to check their liver enzymes, and to confirm the drugs have reached therapeutic concentrations in the blood. Good seizure control, which can take some weeks to achieve, is seen in only about two-thirds of dogs treated with Phenobarbital, even when the blood-levels of the drug appear to be adequate.

Potassium bromide can be used on its own but more frequently is used in combination with Phenobarbital. This drug is usually given at a very high dose initially over several days, then the daily dose is gradually reduced. This is because without such a 'loading dose' approach it can take many weeks before adequate drug levels are reached in the body.

Imepitoin became available for treating dogs with epilepsy about a decade ago. The drug has a quicker onset of action and better side-effect profile than phenobarbital or potassium bromide; it also requires less regular monitoring, but unfortunately it is less often effective in seizure control.

Research into the use of other anticonvulsants is ongoing, and newer anticonvulsants such as levetiracetam, a human drug, are sometimes used. These are reserved for dogs that have not responded well to licensed medications because there is less objective safety and efficacy data for these drugs. Some recent work suggests that a diet rich in medium-chain triglycerides (classified as those with carbon chain of 8–10 carbon atoms), which are found particularly in coconut oil, can help to improve seizure control in dogs with idiopathic epilepsy. I would be careful about giving this to your dog because some dogs develop diarrhoea. It would be wise to discuss this first with your vet.

Once anticonvulsant drugs are started, therapy must normally be given for life. It seems that, if anticonvulsant medication is started and then discontinued, the dog has a greater risk of developing more severe seizures in the future. Abrupt withdrawal of these drugs seems to be particularly risky. If anticonvulsant medication must be discontinued or changed for some reason, your veterinarian will guide you through this.

Even with drug therapy most dogs who suffer from epilepsy will still have occasional seizures. If your dog has epilepsy, it can be useful to keep a seizure diary to record frequency of seizures and their length, as well as what medications are being given, and perhaps other information such as diet and activity. This record can be very useful to you, your vet and your veterinary nurse, particularly if the underlying diagnosis is uncertain, drug doses are adjusted, or seizure frequency seems to change.

KIDNEY FAILURE

The elegant, complex and extraordinary soft machinery of the body exists to create an environment in which all the cells in the different tissues are bathed in an almost miraculously stable fluid with precisely controlled levels of salts, glucose, gases, fats, amino acids, temperature and acidity. This environment results from the combined efforts of the organs. The lungs absorb oxygen and release carbon dioxide. The gut, the liver and the pancreas digest, absorb and modify food and fluid into appropriate constituent molecules, providing nourishment. The circulation transports these materials around the body, whilst the nervous and endocrine systems co-ordinate all these activities. This is the essence of metabolism, but metabolism creates waste. Much of this waste is toxic.

When people mention dog waste, they usually mean poo. But the kidneys actually provide the principle cleaning and waste disposal system of the body. A high proportion of all the blood pumped through the heart is directed straight to the kidneys where it is filtered. Only the lungs and brain are more liberally supplied with blood. As the filtered fluid percolates through the kidneys, it is heavily modified to remove acid, wastes and toxins; the product, urine, is then concentrated before leaving the kidneys to be stored in the bladder until released. In essence, if the kidneys begin to fail, these substances accumulate, the fluid surrounding the cells is polluted and normal bodily processes become poisoned. The kidneys take part in several other physiological processes of the body, such as regulation of the blood pressure. They also produce a hormone that stimulates the bone marrow to produce red blood cells. If this process fails it can lead to a form of anaemia. The normal healthy dog has a lot of renal reserve. In other words, they have more functional capacity within the kidneys than necessary to survive under normal circumstances. This is important because a dog can have quite marked loss of kidney function and yet appear to be perfectly healthy.

Kidney disease is common in dogs. If that disease hampers function then kidney failure is developing. Failure of the kidneys, also called renal failure, comes in two general types: acute and chronic. 'Acute' means a disease that is sudden in onset, rapidly progressive and in need of immediate treatment. Acute renal failure is uncommon in dogs. It is nearly always the result of another disease such as an infection, bladder stones, cancer, a genetic fault or poisoning. These dogs are often very ill indeed and deteriorate rapidly, but, depending on the original insult, the condition can sometimes be treated and resolved.

Chronic renal disease and failure, by contrast, is an irreversible, slowly progressive long-term problem. A variety of insults to the kidney can cause chronic renal disease and lead to renal failure. Acute renal failure sometimes develops into a chronic renal failure. Although the disease itself is chronic, it might appear to begin suddenly because signs of illness may have been hidden as the dog's renal reserve has slowly, gradually been eaten into. There is no cure for chronic renal disease; however, early intervention can sometimes limit the damage done to the kidneys and slow the progression of the disease.

The signs of kidney failure can be extremely variable because the kidneys are responsible for so many different processes. Signs can appear suddenly or progressively, and might include the following.

- An increase in thirst and urination, the frequency and volume of both.
- Sometimes dogs who were well house-trained start to urinate indoors and / or at night.
- Loss of appetite, apparent nausea, vomiting and (less frequently) diarrhoea.
- Weight loss.
- Pallor, often first noticed around the eyes and the gums (caused by anaemia).
- Lethargy and weakness.
- Mouth ulcers and bad breath.
- Sudden blindness, caused by high blood pressure.

As you will realise by now if you have read this far, none of these signs are specific to kidney disease. If your dog exhibits some of these then you ought to take them to your vet.

If a vet is concerned a dog might have kidney disease, they will take a detailed history and often ask you about these and other signs. They will examine your dog paying particular attention to their weight, alertness and attitude, colour, heart rate, the health of the mouth, etc. They are likely to palpate the abdomen, to evaluate the kidneys and bladder. They might do a rectal examination. Next, they will usually want to take blood and urine samples. Most dogs with acute kidney disease and all those with chronic renal failure will show changes in their urine. Certain chemicals in the blood, such as urea, creatinine and phosphate, which are often part of a biochemical 'profile' used by vets to screen for disease, tend to increase in dogs with kidney disease. Some of these tests are not particularly sensitive but newer tests are now appearing that offer the chance of earlier detection. Hypertension, increased blood pressure, is often found in dogs with chronic kidney disease, so it is often useful to measure this too. There are, of course, other causes of altered blood pressure. Ultrasound or X-ray imaging may be used to evaluate the size, shape and appearance of the kidneys. Sometimes biopsy of the organs might be helpful.

Once a dog is diagnosed with kidney disease it can be classified according to severity. The International Renal Interest Society (IRIS), a specialist veterinary group, classifies canine renal disease from stage I, where the dog has evidence of disease but no change in kidney function, to stage IV, where the condition is very serious and advanced. Further details on this can be found online.

Treating dogs with chronic kidney disease

Treatment will depend on how advanced your dog's kidney disease is.

Diet

Diet is the cornerstone in managing chronic kidney disease. A specially formulated food, which tends to be especially restricted in phosphates, relatively low in protein, calcium and sodium, but high in omega-3 fatty acids, can help to slow the progression of kidney dysfunction through the stages from I to IV. Diet cannot undo damage that has already been done. There is no perfect diet, and the most appropriate food will depend on the stage of renal disease in your dog, so you'll need advice from your vet before making any adjustments. Unfortunately, many renal diets can be rather unappetising for dogs. When I first qualified, I was dismayed that many dogs with kidney disease refused to eat these. Fortunately, the palatability of the commercial and prescription diets for this condition has improved immensely over the course of the last few decades.

It is essential that any dog with kidney disease is kept well hydrated. Dogs who are peeing more than normal are compelled to do so by their illness. NEVER limit a dog's access to water in the mistaken belief that it will prevent them peeing indoors or at night. This would be very dangerous to their health. It's best to have several water bowls in different parts of your house.

Medication

Renal disease can affect many different bodily functions, so a variety of medications are sometimes used to treat a dog with kidney disease. For instance, if your dog has an elevated blood pressure, drugs can be used to reduce this. If they have vomiting, anti-emetic drugs might prove helpful. For those dogs that are anaemic, sometimes injections of a synthetic hormone, erythropoetin (or analogues of it), can be given to stimulate the bone marrow to produce more red blood cells. In some dogs with kidney disease and a lot of protein in the urine, certain drugs can prove useful to reduce this protein loss. Nutritional supplements might also be used to replace water soluble vitamins lost in the urine of kidney disease patients, but these are only necessary in a minority of dogs. Phosphate binders and vitamin D supplements can be used to try to reduce some of the secondary effects of renal disease by improving calcium and phosphorus balance, especially if your dog refuses to eat a well formulated renal diet. It can be tempting for clients who have a sick dog to ply them with multiple supplements but sometimes the wrong supplement can actually be harmful. So, I urge you to discuss this frankly with your vet.

Fluid therapy

If a dog has advanced kidney failure, they accumulate toxins and at the same time often become dehydrated. I know that many of my clients are puzzled by this because their dogs often seem to be drinking and peeing volumes, but in these instances, the dog is compelled to pee out fluid because the kidneys are unable to concentrate their urine. The dog drinks to try to replace this lost fluid, but eventually they cannot keep up with the deficit. Fluid therapy can be enormously helpful to replace depleted body fluid levels and help the kidneys flush out the toxins in the body. This fluid must usually be given through an intravenous drip whilst the dog is hospitalised. Unfortunately, the efficacy of this sort of treatment is often short-lived.

Kidney dialysis

In cases where all other treatment options have been exhausted, a vet may recommend kidney dialysis, using a special machine to cleanse the blood of toxins to prolong your dog's life. The ethics of doing this can provoke strong sentiments. This costly treatment is available in only a few very specialised centres.

VESTIBULAR SYNDROME

Co-ordination and balance involve a gamut of different parts of the nervous system acting in concert. Sensors in the inner ears provide raw information concerning the position of the head in space and how it is moving through space. Meanwhile related information is provided from the eyes, the spine, the joints and muscles of the body, the paws and even the whiskers. All this information is co-ordinated in the brain. The key elements of this network, the inner ears, their nerves and the cerebellum at the back of the brain, which looks a bit like a small cauliflower, is known as the vestibular system.

'Hello, Barton Veterinary Hospital, Nina speaking. How can I help you?'

'Something awful has happened to my dog! She was alright this morning but she's just tried to get up and can't seem to stand. Her head is all twisted and she's been sick. It's like she's drunk. I think she's had a stroke. What do I do?

'You'll need to bring her in straight away. What's your name and what's your dog called?'

. . .

'Alright Mrs Murphy, bring Cara in. Dr Little will see you when you get here.'

We get a call like this at our practice several times a year.

Sudden and profound disturbances to a dog's sense of balance and equilibrium usually occur because something has gone awry with signalling in the brain or the inner ear. Dogs are brought to us typically showing disorientation and distress. Often, they have a tilt of the head to one side, are unable to walk, or have a very hesitant wobbly gait. Sometimes they walk in circles. Frequently, their eyes seems to rattle from side-to-side, a condition called nystagmus. Careful examination might reveal other nerve deficits; for example, the dog's eyebrows might, be twitching regularly, or the mouth may droop at one corner. This constellation of clinical signs is known as 'vestibular syndrome'.

Syndromes are conditions that are incompletely understood. Vestibular syndrome is sometimes caused by lesions in the brain or infections afflicting the inner ear; for example, as a result of serious external ear disease that has progressed, but most dogs with vestibular syndrome have neither of these problems. More commonly the problem is not an infection, but it does involve the inner ear and its nerve. It is rarely caused by a stroke.

It is sometimes hard to see things from a dog's perspective.

Try this:

When you feel sea-sick, or vertigo, it is because your vestibular system is getting messages which don't add up. It's confused.

Imagine being drunk. You close your eyes, the room spins . . . your vestibular system is confused.

No wonder dogs with vestibular syndrome seem anxious, hesitant, clumsy and nauseous!

Fortunately, most dogs with the common form of this syndrome recover. Tender loving care and treatment to manage nausea and vomiting seems to be helpful. Recovery often begins within about three days, but can take a fortnight or more. Some dogs have a residual tilt of the head and faulty balance long-term. Where there is good reason to suppose the fault lies centrally within the brain, or is due to an ear infection, then further investigations might be necessary. Specialist referral might be advised. The outcome for this group of patients is more uncertain.

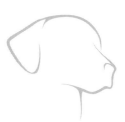

10

PRACTICAL HOME NURSING OF YOUR DOG

This chapter is designed to help you treat your dog when she or he is ill. I will begin by showing how you, often with a friend or a family member, can hold your dog to allow you to examine parts of their body, or to medicate them. I will lay out some biology to explain what common drugs, fluids, etc., can and can't do. This chapter will explain how to collect urine samples, how to give tablets easily, and how to administer other types of drug into the eyes, ears, by mouth and other routes. The value of specific diets for gastrointestinal problems, skin conditions, heart diseases, renal disease and bladder stones will be covered.

HANDLING YOUR DOG

When you are asked to medicate your dog, if you are uncertain how, ask your vet or veterinary nurse to demonstrate. Lots of dogs will happily take tablets concealed in food treats. Favourites with mine are chorizo sausage or cheese.

In the references / bibliography section for this chapter, I have listed some videos you might like to look at online that might help you when you want to restrain your dog for various reasons. Some of these show different techniques from those I recommend, but all are worth a gander if you are unsure. The web is a resource worth looking at for pictures and demonstrations whenever you need to restrain your dog.

Below are some techniques to give drugs directly that I have found work well.

To hold a dog securely, to give medication by mouth, for instance (see Figure 10.1) requires two people. If your dog is small this might best be done on a table.

(a)

(b)

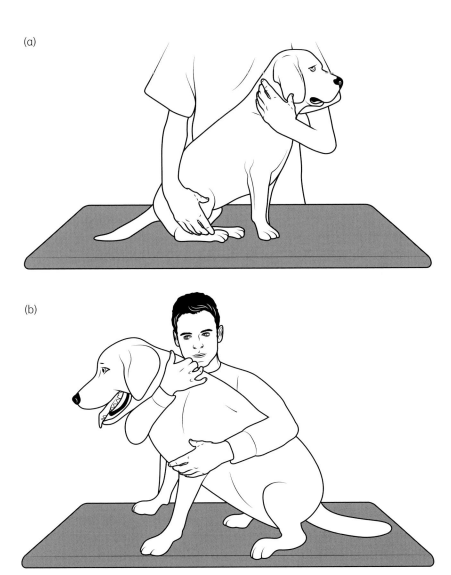

Figure 10.1. (a) Restraining a small/medium dog on a table (see text for details) and (b) large dog being restrained on a table. Notice that one arm is over the back pulling the dog's chest towards the handler. The other arm passes in front of the chest and across the neck, which draws the dog's neck close to the handler. This hand might also grasp the dog's collar.

For larger dogs this should be done on the floor. The dog can assume either a standing or a sitting posture. The best way to give medicine will depend on the dominant hand of the person who is giving the drug. For left-handers, it is easiest to give drugs with the dog on your right; for right-handers, the dog should be on your left. One person should hug the dog close to their chest with one arm clasped around the front of the chest. This hand can grasp the collar. If this is you, then you might find it's a good idea to pull the dog's head in towards your shoulder because dogs are less able to struggle when their head is held close. The other hand clasps either over the back, or under the tum, depending on the size of the dog and what feels most secure. The second person gives the treatment. This method of restraint works well for giving tablets or liquids by mouth, for putting drops or ointment into the eyes and for treating external ear disease. This method can also be used to bathe a paw or as part of the method to examine the mouth (see below).

When you need to open the mouth itself a little care is needed because if a dog feels anxious and threatened then they might just decide to bite you. Even the quietest most benign dog can display aggression on occasion.

Look at Figure 10.2. One person is holding the dog as in Figure 10.1. The second person should put their non-dominant hand across the muzzle of the dog and peel the dog's upper lip upward at the side to reveal the big canine ('eye') teeth of the upper jaw. Just behind this tooth on each side there is a space in the gum before the first cheek tooth. When a little pressure is applied to the sides of the upper jaw at this level most dogs will naturally open their mouths slightly. Swiftly this second person might find it helpful to slide the thumb of their non-dominant hand through this space in the gum and onto the hard palate behind the canine teeth whilst continuing to hold the upper jaw. When this is done your dog experiences a nervous reflex that tends to prevent them biting down and it becomes much easier to give drugs or examine the mouth. To give a tablet, or to look into the mouth, raise the head with the first hand. With the other hand, hold the tablet between index finger and thumb, use the other three fingers to push the lower jaw downwards. Pop the tablet as far back onto the tongue as possible.

To examine a paw, again tends to require two people. The dog is restrained as in Figure 10.1. Many dogs seem to resent people touching their feet, so again be careful when you do this. For the forepaw, the second person should extend the limb by lifting it at the carpus ('wrist') and moving the paw forwards and upwards. See Figure 10.3. It might be necessary to examine each digit individually from

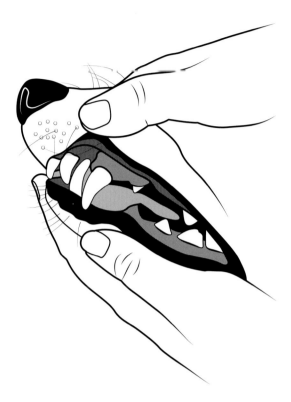

Figure 10.2. Opening a dog's mouth.

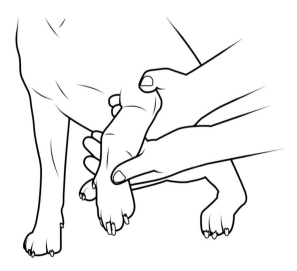

Figure 10.3. Examining a dog's paw from above.

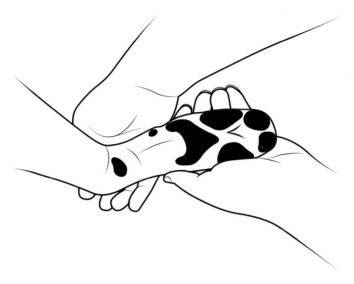

Figure 10.4. Examining the underside of a dog's paw.

above, below and the sides. This tends to be particularly difficult in terriers, spaniels and other long-haired dogs, whereas in Labradors and other short-haired breeds the process is simpler. To look at the claws ('nails'), do so from above, the sides and below. Also look at the claw bed – that recess around each claw where the claw emerges through the skin. This area is particularly prone to infections, which can be quite sore for the dog but where visible signs tend to be subtle. To examine the underside of the paw, flex the leg at the carpus and cup a hand around the paw (Figure 10.4). For the hind paws, use the same technique but grasp the hock or the metatarsus, that part below the hock, to do so.

To examine a dog's skin for fleas or flea dirt ideally again requires two people and a specially designed flea comb with narrow closely arranged tines (see Figure 4.1 and Figure 10.5). Ideally, have a pledget of damp cotton wool or some moist white toilet tissue handy. The dog can be held on a short lead or as in Figure 10.1. The best places to look for fleas and flea dirt are the lower back and around the neck region. Enter the hair-coat with the comb deeply so that the tips of the comb tines reach the skin. Pass the flea comb through the coat from front to back 'with the grain', following the way the hairs are aligned in a gentle but firm action. Repeat several times. Then look at the combings that have lifted off. Do this on the back and around the neck to get a good yield of loose hair and dander. If your dog has fleas, you might just see one – a swiftly moving dark brown insect about

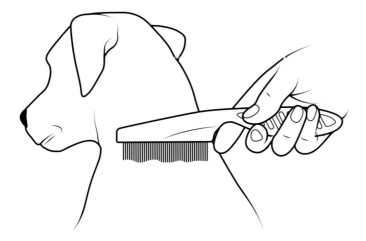

Figure 10.5. Using a flea comb. The tines of the comb are inserted deep into the coat to reach the surface of the skin. The comb is drawn through the coat, with the 'grain', repeatedly, then the combings are examined. Flea dirt is dark brown, almost black, rather granular and often has a slight comma-shape, around 1–2 mm. If placed on damp cotton-wool or tissue it dissolves to a reddish-brown stain. Fleas themselves are small, dark brown and flattened side-to-side, they scurry through the coat or can jump huge distances.

2–3 mm in length. If you don't see any you might still make the diagnosis from the combings. 'Flea dirt', which is flea poo composed of partly digested blood, is dark and granular. Each speck is around 1 mm in size and tends to have a comma shape. If this material is placed on your damp tissue or cotton wool it dissolves into a reddish or brown stain due to the blood fleas feed upon. You might also come across white sandy material – which are flea eggs.

To give tablets, the easiest way is to secrete them in a treat. Cheese, pieces of sausage, chicken or ham are all popular. You can also buy treats designed for the purpose. If you want to give a tablet directly open the mouth using the method shown above (Figure 10.2). Push the tablet as far back as you can toward the throat on the centre of the tongue then firmly close the mouth. Holding the mouth shut, gently massage the throat from below with your other hand. When your dog swallows this should be obvious. On swallowing, a dog often will press their tongue against their front teeth or lick the tip of their nose.

To give liquids or pastes by mouth use a syringe or dropper. Hold the dog as in Figures 10.1 (various) and 10.6, but don't actually open the mouth. Slide the

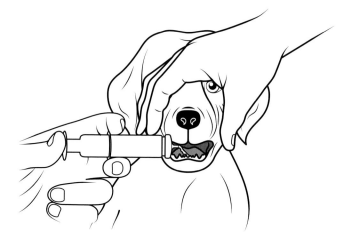

Figure 10.6. Giving liquid medication by mouth using a syringe.

nozzle of the syringe into the mouth through the gap behind the eye tooth. Tilt the head up. Then slowly squeeze the liquid or paste into the mouth. When the dog starts to swallow, they will tend to push the tongue forwards and open the mouth slightly. Allow this but don't let the head completely free. Gradually continue until the medicine has gone down.

If you need to give drops or ointment into the eyes again it is best to have two people. Restrain the patient as in Figure 10.1. There are two alternative ways to get medication into the eye. Firstly, you can try to apply the medication directly onto the cornea – the clear window of the eyeball. Do this by holding the head with one hand – tilting the head up then give the drug with the other hand (Figure 10.7). Alternatively, with one hand, depress the eye back into its socket with a finger or thumb applied to the closed upper eyelid. This tends to open the 'envelope' behind the lower lid so creating a pocket into which you can then introduce the ointment or liquid.

Sometimes dogs with ear disease need to be treated with drops. The dog should be held by one person as in Figure 10.1. The second person should gently grasp the flap of the ear, the pinna, and smoothly draw the pinna backwards and upwards so that the opening of the ear canal is clearly exposed. Medication can then be applied to the hairless surface of the pinna and around the opening of the ear canal (Figure 10.8). Then, turn the ear flap back over and gently, methodically, massage the ear. As the liquid warms, it ought to seep deeper into the ear.

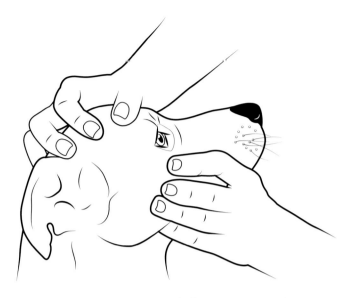

Figure 10.7. Exposing the eye in order to apply drops or an ointment.

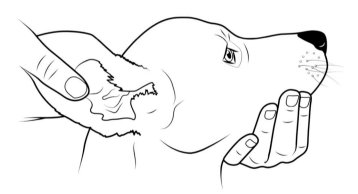

Figure 10.8. Holding a dog in order to allow the application of medication to the ear. The dog must be held on a table or the floor depending on the size of dog (see previous figures). A second person gently grasps the flap of the ear, the pinna, and smoothly draws the pinna backwards and upwards so that the opening of the ear canal is clearly exposed. Medication can then be applied as necessary to the hairless surface of the pinna and around the opening of the ear canal.

When you do this, the dog often will groan with the pleasure of an itch scratched. In most cases it is not necessary to deeply insert the nozzle of the applicator into the ear canal since this can sometimes prove painful if the ear is very inflamed. Sometimes vets will ask you to use ear cleaners on your dog. Often, the aim here is to break-up and disperse discharge that is clogging the ear canal. For this, follow the same method but use generous volumes of the cleaning solution and do this out-of-doors because, as sure as eggs are eggs, once you have massaged a big volume of liquid into an ear, your dog will almost immediately vigorously shake their head to get the fluid out. Oh, I should've said – be prepared to be splattered!

When you want to examine the skin of the underside of your dog, or to look and feel closely at the mammary glands, the axillae ('armpits'), or the penis, then the best way is to get your dog to lie down on their side. For small dogs, again this often is best done with the dog on a table, but for larger dogs it should be done on the floor. This usually takes two, or, for very large strong dogs, three people.

It can be challenging to get dogs to lie down for examination unless they have been trained to do this. I find this usually works well: Figures 10.9a and 10.9b show restaint of a small and medium-sized dog respectively, on a table, whereas larger dogs (Figure 10.9c) require stronger handlers and may have to be done on the floor. To begin, the handlers stand either side of the table with the dog on the table. One handler clasps the dog to their chest and rolls her onto her side on the tabletop. This action can be slightly alarming for the dog, but provided the handlers give reassurance, and adopt firm but gentle, controlled, definite and con-fident actions, in most cases dogs accept this. The second handler leans over the dog from the opposite side of the table, with one forearm across the shoulders/neck to grasp the dog's forelimbs. Their second forearm crosses the back of the abdomen or the flank with the hand grasping the dog's hind-limbs. If the dog is very big or strong and wriggly so that it's difficult to grasp both fore and both hind legs, it is often easiest to concentrate on grasping those legs closest to the table. By applying firm but gentle pressure with the forearms this second handler restrains the dog. Once a dog is in this lying posture they usually will become calm. If the dog is restless, gently slide the forearm forwards so that the dog's upper neck and head are held down close to the table. When the head is prevented from being lifted off the table it is far more difficult for a dog to wriggle free. The first handler is then usually free to examine the dog. Often, the whole of the lower

(a)

(b)

(c)

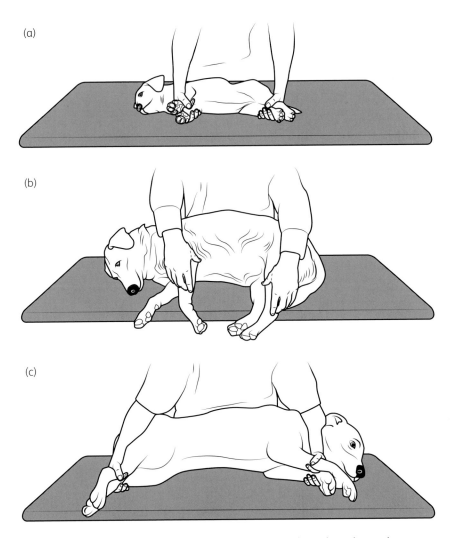

Figure 10.9. Holding a (a) small, (b) medium and (c) large dog in lateral recumbency.

trunk area can be examined from one side. On occasion, the dog must be repositioned to lie on their other side. To examine the lower abdomen, the mammary glands, the penis or the scrotum alter your position slightly (see Figure 10.10).

Occasionally, a dog might become dangerous, either because of severe pain, or some form of behavioural disturbance. In that instance, there might be a necessity to disarm the dog by fashioning a muzzle so that further actions can be taken without people being seriously injured. This should not be done lightly. Don't put

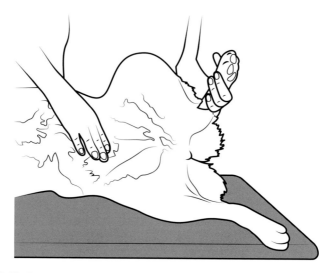

Figure 10.10. Exposing the skin of the ventrum (underside) to allow examination and/or the application of medication.

yourself in serious danger! Also, know that this technique is not safe or applicable to very flat-faced dogs such as bulldogs or pugs. It should also be avoided if there is serious respiratory distress. An effective muzzle can be made with a piece of rope (or a dog lead, or, even a dressing-gown tie) provided it is at least four or five feet in length. First, create a single thumb knot with a single throw in the middle of the rope. Don't pull this closed (see Figure 10.11a). Second, slip the noose that you have created over the dog's muzzle with the throw of the knot directly over the bridge of the dog's nose (Figure 10.11b) and pull this tight (so that the dog's mouth is closed). For almost all breeds of dog, where the muzzle is long enough to accomplish this, they should be able to breathe without difficulties through their nose with the mouth closed in this way. Now pass either end of the rope to cross under the jaw (Figure 10.11c). Finally, take each end of the rope back over the neck behind the ears. Tie tightly in a bow (Figure 10.11d).

URINE SAMPLES

The ideal urine sample is usually the first urine of the day. It is easiest to get this with two people; one walking the dog on a short lead, the other wielding the receptacle. Samples are best collected into a clean, ideally sterile, container that your vet might provide. We use a nifty device that looks a bit like a kids' plastic

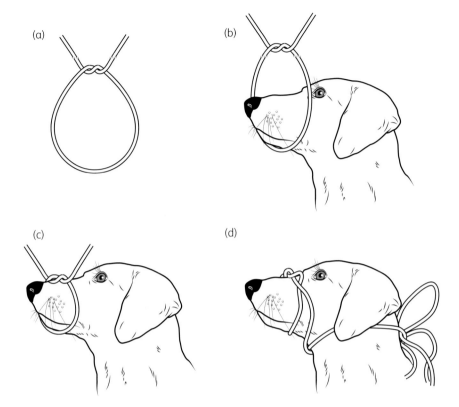

Figure 10.11. How to muzzle a dog when necessary. An improvised muzzle for a dog can easily be made with a length of cord, rope, or even a dressing-gown belt. First, a single throw 'thumb knot' is made in the middle of the cord (a). This is placed over the snout so that it passes under the dog's jaw and over the muzzle (b) and drawn snug with the throw of the knot at the top (c). Finally, the two free ends of the cord are crossed again under the jaw, passed either side of the neck behind the head, and secured at the back of the neck in a bow (d).

shovel in which the 'handle' is a sterile plastic tube (Figure 10.12). This is quite easy to use for both dogs and bitches. However, in a hurry, any clean dry impermeable container would do. For most laboratory work a few teaspoonfuls is all that is required.

For faecal samples, a conventional 'poo bag' is fine. Tie it closed. Deliver samples fresh to your vet.

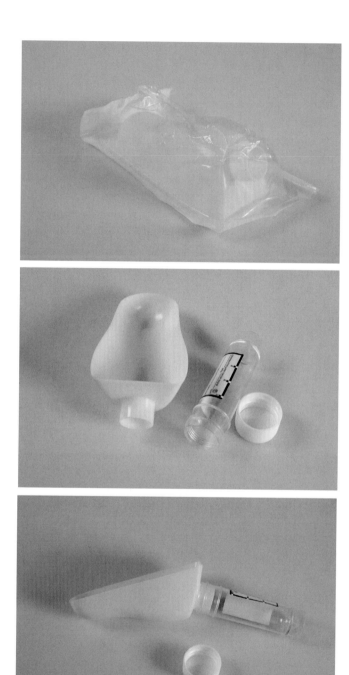

Figure 10.12. A urine sampling device.

FIRST AID

If necessary, at home you can bathe a graze, a wound, a sore ear, a weeping eye, a broken claw, or raw looking skin lesions. In the short term, provided you do this cleanly and gently, you are unlikely to do any serious harm.

Fresh tap or bottled water is acceptable in a first aid situation and should be used in copious amounts to physically flush the wound to remove foreign material such as road grit or mud from a skin abrasion.

In other circumstances, you should ideally use a sterile liquid that has the same concentration of solute particles within it as the cells of the body (an isotonic solution). Sterile saline is ideal in bottles. You might also try sterile saline wound wipes (choose those without alcohol). You can buy both of these from a chemist, without prescription, at low cost.

A simple isotonic solution can be easily made at home if necessary:

1 Boil water in a kettle or on the stove for at least 5 minutes (to render it sterile).

2 Dissolve one level teaspoon of salt (i.e. about 5 grams) in 500 ml (about a pint).

For some indications such a solution can be used warm, NOT HOT, for example, to help to draw infection from an abscess or a bite wound (it should feel very comfortable to your own finger if you dunk it in), but in most situations it should be cool.

A higher salt concentration (two or even three teaspoons per 500 ml) could be used, at a pinch (sorry), if you wanted to make the solution antiseptic, that is, capable of killing bacteria and other microbes. Antiseptics used in human surgical skin preparation, or wound care, such as chlorhexidine, povodine-iodine and TCP are often recommended by vets, provided the appropriate dilutions are used. However, a friend of mine who is a vet specialising in wound management and tissue reconstruction says: 'Antiseptics are to be avoided. They cause pain and potential tissue damage'.

Incidentally, most disinfectants are very toxic to cats. This is not relevant to most dog owners I suppose.

There is evidence to suggest application of sterile hydrogel after flushing is appropriate for most wounds in a first aid situation to suppress bacterial growth and maintain tissue health until assessment by a veterinary professional. Many brands are available, without prescription, from a chemist or online.

DRUGS

> As a general rule, NEVER TREAT YOUR DOG WITH A HUMAN DRUG UNLESS YOU HAVE BEEN SPECIFICALLY TOLD TO DO SO BY A VET. One of the commonest reasons for a dog to be seen by an emergency service is that they have swallowed an unsuitable human drug. This can be fatal.

In this section, I hope to give you some understanding of what different classes of drugs do and how, also disabuse you of what they cannot do. This is far from a complete list.

Antibiotics and anti-fungals (e.g. Penicillin, Amoxycillin, Metronidazole, Miconazole)

Antibiotics and anti-fungals are drugs, generally originally derived from bacteria or yeasts, which themselves are able to kill microorganisms or hinder their growth and reproduction. They are used to treat, or sometimes to prevent, infections. These drugs cannot destroy viruses. All antibiotics and anti-fungals have a limited spectrum of activity, meaning that they can kill some species of microbes at low concentrations, kill, or inhibit, other species at high concentrations, and completely fail against some microbes. So, for instance, miconazole, is able to kill many species of yeasts and some species of bacteria. At first sight, you might think that broad-spectrum antibiotics are better than those with a narrow spectrum but in fact the scatter-gun effects of broad-spectrum drugs cause more side-effects and disruption of the normal commensal microbes in the body, such as those in the gut. It is generally preferable to use narrow-spectrum agents that target the infecting organisms more precisely – an ace assassin, rather than a nail-bomb. Unfortunately, most of these agents used in veterinary medicine must be chosen without knowing the definite identity of the target bugs. So, when a vet chooses an antibiotic or an anti-fungal, they usually do so based on other factors, such as low toxicity, ease of use, and how effective the drug has been shown to be in similar circumstances.

Corticosteroids (e.g. Prednisolone)

The corticosteroids are drugs used to suppress inflammation. They do so mainly by switching off various inflammatory pathways that have been activated during the inflammatory process. They are also immunosuppressants, that is they interfere with the usual immune mechanisms of the body, which can be useful in dealing with situations where the body is attacking itself (auto-immune diseases). Corticosteroids mimic the effects of cortisol, a hormone found within the normal body that has a role in the day–night (diurnal) rhythm of the body. In human medicine, corticosteroids are especially used for asthma, and rheumatoid arthritis, conditions that, thankfully, are uncommon in dogs. When used correctly and for short periods, corticosteroids are excellent drugs. For instance, they are extremely useful in managing inflammation of the ear, otitis, and for itchy skin complaints (see p. 124). However, like almost all potent drugs, corticosteroids have many side effects and other drawbacks, especially when used over periods of more than a few days. So, because they mimic cortisol, they can inhibit the normal diurnal rhythm of this hormone. They cause the body to lose some minerals and hamper the normal immune response to infections, or vaccines. This means that there is a danger that infections take hold when we use these agents. Corticosteroids often make dogs very hungry and thirsty. Thirsty dogs pee more and more often. These drugs can alter the behaviour of some dogs too, making them moody and short-tempered. I could go on and on listing the side effects from this class of drugs, but I'm sure you get my drift. Corticosteroids are a crucial part of our drug repertoire, but we vets try to limit their use.

Non-steroidal anti-inflammatory drugs (e.g. Meloxicam)

Non-steroidal anti-inflammatory drugs, frequently coined NSAIDs, are used for pain relief and to dampen inflammation after surgery or trauma. They help to reduce fevers and are also very widely used in the management of arthritis (see Chapter 7, p. 163). NSAIDs mainly act on a crucial specific inflammatory biochemical cascade in the body known as the arachidonic acid pathway. In a small proportion of dogs these drugs can cause vomiting or diarrhoea. One reason for this is that they can induce ulceration in the stomach. To help prevent this, when the drugs are given by mouth, they are best given with food. NSAIDs must be used with circumspection in dogs with kidney diseases or heart conditions and some dogs just cannot tolerate them; however, the vast majority of dogs can.

Intravenous fluid therapy (e.g. Lactated Ringer's – Hartmann's)

Arguably, intra-venous (IV) fluid therapy has been the most important therapeutic innovation of the last century, in both human and veterinary medicine. In a very broad range of serious disease situations, the patient is compromised because of inadequate blood and tissue fluid volumes, or because the fluid within the body has become imperfect in some way (such as too acidic). Correcting these deficits in fluid balance, with precisely the right fluid in the correct amounts, is often crucial to a patient's survival. This is one reason why intravenous access, through a sterile catheter, is often the first step in managing any seriously ill dog. Patients on IV fluid therapy must be hospitalised and frequently monitored. Twenty or 30 years ago fluids were usually given passively with the aid of gravity, but dogs are not always perfectly compliant, so often the giving sets would kink or otherwise fail. Nowadays fluid pumps are usually used because they are much more reliable, but this has contributed to the increased cost of hospitalisation.

Blood and blood products

Much as I love wine, I must tell you straight; it is not the elixir of life. Blood is. Blood carries oxygen to every corner of the body attached to the red pigment haemoglobin, wrapped up in the red blood cells. When a dog is anaemic, there are too few red blood cells, inadequate amounts of haemoglobin, and so oxygen delivery is compromised. Many different diseases and adversities cause anaemia. When a dog is anaemic, the vet needs to find out why, but in addition, sometimes, when that anaemia is profound, they need to transfuse the patient with supplementary blood. That said, this is not a simple process, because, just as in humans, canine blood for transfusion must be correctly matched to the patient. Most vets do not have facilities to safely store blood. There are also legal constraints around this. So, when a dog needs blood either the practice will have to order that from a blood bank, or they have to find a donor dog, with the correct blood type, to supply the blood fresh.

Blood is composed of other things as well as red corpuscles. There is fluid, called plasma, white blood cells that, amongst other things, guard against infection, many different proteins, and tiny cells called platelets. Platelets are the cells that enable blood to clot. They are very important because they keep the blood vessels intact so that minor bruises and tears do not lead to fatal blood loss. If the platelets numbers fall too low, or they fail to function, haemorrhage occurs. If platelets are over-active this can lead to other problems.

Antihypertensives (e.g. Amlodipine)

Hypertension is high blood pressure, a very common condition in people. This is not common in dogs, although it sometimes does occur, especially in dogs with kidney disease. When a dog has high blood pressure this has knock-on effects on the heart and the rest of the circulation. These dogs are usually given drugs by mouth, which slowly and gently relax the blood vessels to consequently lower that pressure. If the dose of drug given is too high, it can make dogs weak. Finding the right dose of anti-hypertensive drugs for a dog can be quite challenging because the blood pressure found when a dog is at the vets, nervous and excited, might not be a good measure of their blood pressure at home or when they are enjoying a walk.

Immunosuppressant drugs (e.g. Cyclosporin)

Immunosuppressants are particularly used when an exuberant immune response is critical to a problem such as a hypersensitivity of the skin to allergens in the environment, or certain diseases where the body is attacking itself, for example immune-mediated anaemia. Unfortunately, these drugs have side-effects that can increase the likelihood of infection.

Cytotoxic drugs (e.g. Doxirubicin)

Cytotoxic agents kill rapidly dividing cells. They are frequently used in the chemo-therapy of cancer. The drugs must be used very carefully because they are hazardous to people who handle them. Also, sometimes they can be dangerous to the patient because they suppress the white blood cells that fight infection and sometimes have other side-effects. Most dogs who receive these drugs must have their blood frequently assessed to ensure their white blood cell counts are high enough.

Anti-emetics (e.g. Maropitant)

Several different drugs are used by vets to help to prevent vomiting in dogs who have gastroenteritis, or nausea as a result of chemotherapy, an inner ear problem, or travel-sickness. Some of these drugs are also analgesics (they reduce the sensation of pain). These drugs can be so effective that they give a false sense that the underlying problem is resolving when it is not. Consequently, vets rarely use these drugs for more than a few days.

Drugs affecting cell signalling (e.g. Oclacitinib)

All the cells of the body communicate with one another via chemical messengers called cytokines. This messaging between cells has been a subject of scrutiny by physiologists and pathologists for years. Pharmacologists, too, are fascinated. Drugs are just starting to come on stream that target the signalling mechanisms between different cells of the body. These types of drugs are likely to become more and more useful in future. It is hoped that by targeting specific cell messages the treatment of disease can be made more effective and specific to the underlying problem whilst side-effects should be reduced.

Brochodilators (e.g. Theophylline)

Bronchodilators are drugs used in the treatment of chronic bronchitis and other long-standing lung disorders such as asthma and allergic bronchitis. They act, as their name implies, by reducing spasm in the muscles that surround the small airways. If these airways dilate, even slightly, in response to these drugs the clinical effects can be of considerable benefit to the patient. However, bronchodilators tend to have a narrow therapeutic range, meaning that side-effects can be frequent and sometimes mean the drug must be withdrawn. Side-effects can include vomiting, a rapid heart rate, heart rhythm abnormalities, vomiting and excitement.

Diuretics (e.g. Furosemide)

These are agents that make the dog pass more urine than normal. They are most frequently used in dogs with heart disease, especially if the dog is having difficulty breathing or is coughing due to the accumulation of fluid in the lungs ('pulmonary oedema'). For some dogs, diuretics are lifesaving, but as with most drugs, they must be used with caution, especially if kidney function is compromised. If diuretics are used at high doses, the dog could become dehydrated. Diuretics can also sometimes deplete the body of certain salts, especially potassium, which can cause weakness and depress the appetite. In order to use diuretics effectively and safely your vet might need to take lab samples to monitor kidney function and the levels of salts ('electrolytes') in the blood.

Anti-arrhythmics (e.g. Sotalol)

A normal heart rate and rhythm depends on a constant stream of information between the heart, the blood vessels and the brain in which the heart beat is regulated to meet the needs of the whole body during exercise, sleep, excitement, sex, stress, fear and an array of different physiological circumstances. It is rarely necessary for a vet to intrude into this conversation. However, when the heart is diseased, or sometimes when another part of the body is unhealthy, the heart rhythm may become unstable or deranged and this can be fatal. In these cases, it is necessary to establish what exactly is causing this derangement. This requires an electrocardiogram (ECG) or sometimes the use of a time-lapse ECG (a Holter monitor). Once a diagnosis is made, in some instances, drugs that suppress the rhythm disturbance may be useful. Two decades ago, many such drugs were available, but time has shown that many of those drugs were of little lasting value and some actually shortened life. A few of these drugs do seem to be of use but only under the close supervision of a veterinary cardiologist.

Shampoos

For some skin conditions shampoos may be used in the treatment strategy especially for dogs with atopic dermatitis, simply because cleansing of the skin removes allergens, and, where there are surface microbial infections with yeasts or bacteria, antiseptic agents can have a dramatic effect in reducing the microbial load (see p....).

Shampooing itself can help to reduce the sensation of itch, particularly those products based on oatmeal. Read the instructions for use carefully. Remember, that if your dog has been treated with a spot-on drug to kill parasites, this will be washed off if you use a shampoo. Most shampoos must be left on the coat for 10–15 minutes after a lather has been created before washing off. For convenience, this is either best done out of doors, perhaps in a baby bath, or with your dog standing in a bath or the shower. Some dogs seem to revel in this. Others hate it.

Polyunsaturated fatty acids

Strictly speaking, polyunsaturated fatty acids (PUFAs) are not drugs, they are fats, found in the diet, but these are sometimes given as supplements because they can have important biologic effects. Here is some very simple chemistry. Most fats in our diet are triglycerides, which are formed from three fatty acid molecules combined with another chemical, glycerol. You will be aware that saturated fats are often characterised as 'bad fats' and unsaturated fats are said to be 'good fats'. In the saturated fats, the fatty acid parts are formed of long chains of carbon atoms with two hydrogen atoms attached to each carbon atom. Saturated fats are usually solid at room temperature (think lard or butter). Unsaturated fatty acids have some carbon atoms that only have a single hydrogen atom and at this carbon they have a double bond with the neighbouring carbon atom. Unsaturated fatty acids are liquid at room temperature (think cooking oils). When a fatty acid has just one carbon double bond per chain it is classed as monounsaturated (a good example is olive oil). When the chain of carbon atoms forming the fatty acid has more than one carbon double bond it is classed as a PUFA. For omega-3 fatty acids, the first carbon double bond starts at the third carbon atom of the chain, whereas for omega-6 the first double bond begins at the sixth carbon atom of the chain. In the diet, omega-3 PUFAs generally come from fish (especially cod liver oil but sources include salmon and other fish), omega-6 PUFAs typically come from vegetable oils. As a rule of thumb, omega-3 PUFAs seem to have anti-inflammatory effects on the body (in humans and dogs). Fairly good evidence shows that supplementing the diet with omega-3 PUFAs helps dogs with some forms of arthritis. Other problems, including brain diseases, kidney and heart conditions, may also benefit from omega-3 PUFAs. Most diets for humans and dogs are very high in omega-6 PUFAs. However, there are some skin conditions that seem to benefit from supplementation of the diet with omega-6 PUFAs. The ratio between the quantities of omega-6 and omega-3 PUFAs in dogs' diets seems to be important but as yet the precise impli-cations of this for diet are not definitely known. I expect we will learn much more about this in the years ahead.

> This list of drug classes is obviously far from complete. I have simply pro-vided a few examples. At the risk of repeating myself, read the label care-fully. Alongside the drug, you should have been given a datasheet that will give detailed information about the drug including side-effects and possi-ble adverse reactions. If you are confused or anxious about these drugs ask your vet or veterinary nurse for further information.

DIETS

Special diets can contribute to the treatment of several serious diseases that dogs face. These 'prescription' diets are always much more expensive that conventional dog food and are usually available only from vets (although you should look online in case you can find a supplier). My experience is that many people are horrified at the costs of these and assume that vets are making a huge mark-up on the diets. What is rarely understood is that a great deal of scientific research lies behind the development and formulation of these diets, which must ultimately be paid for by the end consumers – dog owners.

Kidney disease

Diets for dogs with serious long-standing kidney disease, chronic renal failure, have been developed through many decades of research. The diets are formu-lated to be low in phosphates, and are supplemented with omega-3 polyunsatu-rated fatty acids (usually from fish) that seem to help control inflammation in the body and are beneficial to intra-renal blood flow. These diets have moderately restricted protein content. The protein in the food is closely matched in amino-acid levels to the theoretical ideal for a dog; in scientific terms, this is protein of 'high biological value'. Much of the toxic waste that the kidneys remove from the body result from protein breakdown; less protein in the diet means a reduced workload for the kidneys.

When choosing a renal diet, it is usually preferable to feed a wet canned diet because dogs with renal disease are highly susceptible to dehydration. Dogs who eat dry foods rarely take in as much fluid as those on wet diets so their risks of deterioration are magnified compared with those dogs on wet food. Above all, the diet given to a dog with kidney disease must be palatable and enjoyed by the dog because no prescription diet will provide any benefit if it isn't eaten. Introduction of a new diet should ideally be done gradually over a few days to improve acceptance and help prevent any dietary upset.

More information on the treatment of kidney disease can be found in Chapter 8.

Bladder stones (urolithiasis)

Dogs sometimes develop signs of pain, irritation, or difficulty when passing, or attempting to pass, urine. This can be due to a variety of diseases, such as inflammation in the bladder (cystitis) or, in male dogs, with prostatic disease. However, one rather important problem is the development of bladder stones, technically called 'uroliths'. Occasionally, this is extremely serious because, if a stone completely obstructs the urethra – the tube leading from the bladder out of the body – the dog will be unable to pass urine, which is very painful and can be fatal if not swiftly relieved. Management of this problem might initially require investigations, such as radiography or ultrasound examination, with surgery to unblock the urethra and remove the bladder stones. Thereafter, these dogs often benefit from being fed wet food, to dilute the urine, and a specific diet to dissolve the uroliths and to prevent recurrence. Although there are dry versions of these diets available, the principal reason these uroliths form in the first place is that the dog's urine is highly concentrated. Feeding a wet diet, possibly with water added to it, can help to prevent recurrence, whereas feeding a dry diet is more likely to lead to recurrence. These diets are often very attractive to dogs because they tend to have a high fat content. They are costly. However, in the majority of cases they need not be fed long-term. In order to choose the precise diet for each case it is often necessary for a sample of the bladder stones to be analysed in detail. This will add to the costs and might delay decisions about the diet.

Gastro-intestinal disease

Dietary intervention can be an essential component of management for dogs with gastrointestinal disease. For acute vomiting and / or diarrhoea, if your vet is comfortable that the cause has been dietary indiscretion, or the signs are mild, their first advice might simply be to withhold food for 12–36 hours, or to feed a very bland diet for a couple of days. However, if the illness seems more serious, then dietary therapy is often recommended, and prescription diets might be advised. Clients also often chose prescription diets for acute vomiting or diarrhoea simply because they are convenient. The precise recommendations will depend on the diagnosis; so, for instance, if it appears that the clinical signs are due to pancreatitis, then a low-fat diet is usually advisable. In such cases, this diet might be recommended for life because it is believed that recurrent pancreatitis can be exacerbated by fatty foods. For recurrent signs of gastrointestinal problems, a chronic inflammatory enteropathy (aka 'inflammatory bowel disease') might be suspected and some form of novel diet or a hypoallergenic foodstuff might be chosen. In these sorts of cases, the diet might be used as a diagnostic test rather than long-term therapy. More information on gastrointestinal diseases can be found in Chapter 8.

Skin diseases

In Chapter 7, I explained that diets can sometimes form part of the management of itchy skin disease when a food sensitivity is suspected to explain the problem. In these cases, novel foods that the dog has never been previously exposed to, or those in which the protein has been partly denatured by hydrolysation, are often utilised, either in a diagnostic or a management role. Very often if these diets are chosen you will be strongly advised that your dog should receive NO OTHER FOODS at all, to prevent recurrent problems. This can be a difficult circle to square.

Diabetes mellitus

The classic diet recommended for dogs with diabetes mellitus has a low glycaemic index, meaning that the carbohydrates in the diet are only rather slowly absorbed into the blood-stream. In this way, diet helps the control of blood sugar, preventing it increasing dramatically soon after feeding. This is achieved partly become a focus of intense medical research but is quite beyond the scope of this book.

HOW COMMON IS CANCER IN DOGS?

Cancer is common in dogs, accounting for perhaps 25–30% of deaths. It seems to be becoming more common, although this claim is disputed. The most likely explanations for this apparent increase are, firstly, that dogs are living longer than they did, say, a generation ago and, secondly, veterinary diagnostic technology has improved and become much more widely used, so the diagnosis is made more frequently. It seems that the lifetime risk of cancer in dogs, is similar to people. Just as in people, we know that some chemicals can act as carcinogens in dogs; for instance, environmental tobacco smoke is a known risk factor, similarly ultraviolet light and other forms of radiation can also cause cancer. However, most cancers arise randomly, so it is usually completely impossible to identify a single cause. Some breeds of dog, including the Bernese Mountain Dog, Boxer, Flat-Coated Retriever and Golden Retriever appear to be predisposed to develop cancer. Contrary to some beliefs, there is no good evidence that vaccinations increase the risk of cancer.

WHEN MIGHT CANCER BE SUSPECTED?

There are no clinical signs that are definite predictors that a dog has cancer. Obviously, if a new mass is discovered on the surface of the body, in the mouth, deforming the mammary glands, a limb or the tail, then this certainly might be a tumour of some kind, but many masses are benign growths. So, for example, the most common lumps found under the surface of the skin in dogs are lipomas, benign fatty tumours, that are generally harmless. Others could be cysts, abscesses, bruises, etc. Any mass that grows quickly, is painful, or becomes ulcerated should be examined by a vet rather urgently. A diagnosis can never be made with certainty from clinical examination alone, further investigation is necessary to disclose the problem.

There are, on the other hand, certain clinical signs that make a good clinician suspect cancer. These include sudden lameness and bony swellings, especially those in large breed dogs close to a joint, spontaneous nosebleeds, particularly if of treatment for many tumours. Chemotherapy for pets is controversial for many people, especially for those who have experienced this themselves. However, as a rule, the approach we use in veterinary medicine is that chemotherapy must never seriously distress a dog or impinge drastically on their quality of life. We aim to prolong quality life rather than necessarily completely eliminating the cancer and curing the patient. So, the protocols and doses of drugs used are devised with this in mind and nasty side-effects from the drugs should not be seen often. Some of the drugs used in chemotherapy are very potent so the vets and nurses handling these drugs need specialist PPE and equipment (such as a fume cupboard). These drugs are often given intravenously, accompanied by fluid therapy, which means the patients must be regularly hospitalised for a few hours or sometimes a day or two. Many protocols for chemotherapy necessitate that additional drugs in tablet or liquid form are given at home. These drugs must be kept securely. Hands should be washed after handling them. For some drug therapy of this sort a dog's urine will contain nasty chemicals after the treatment is given so it needs to be washed away with large volumes of water for the following day or two.

Radiotherapy

Radiation treatment of solid cancerous tumours in dogs has been performed on occasion for many years but is really only in the last two decades that this has become mainstream. This approach to treatment can be particularly appropriate if a cancer cannot be wholly removed by sharp surgery without having very serious consequences for the function and quality of life of the dog. In many cases, this modality is combined with surgery, chemotherapy, or both. Radiation is becoming more commonly used where a large surgery would be debilitating for a patient, and a more conservative surgery combined with radiation can offer a better result. Typically, these are tumours of the nose, the mouth, the brain-case, less frequently the limbs, the heart, or other organs. Radiation is usually delivered very precisely, repeatedly, to minimise radiation damage to normal tissues. The equipment for this is very costly and usually dogs must be anaesthetised each time they are treated. Radiation treatment facilities are limited to a few centres in the UK that are all in specialist referral settings, so the availability varies with geography.

Monitoring and follow-up

Obviously, in the short term, where surgery, intensive chemotherapy or radiation have been used, initial nursing must often take place in hospital for the first few days. Thereafter, most dogs will go home accompanied by detailed instructions for ongoing treatments and follow-up visits. Any dog treated for cancer must be monitored closely to confirm that the treatment is being and has been effective and the dog's quality of life remains acceptable. As far as the vet is concerned this may take the form of clinical re-examination, imaging by radiography, ultrasound or other means, blood tests, etc. The role of observant, caring and committed dog owners is also absolutely crucial in this because they are the ones who are usually most motivated, most able and best equipped to identify how the disease and its treatment is unfolding on a day-to-day trajectory. Good rapport and communication between the dog's family and the veterinary clinicians is key. The frequency of re-examination and follow-up tests depends very much on the original diagnosis, the overall health of the patient, and what treatment(s) have been given. Monitoring does often contribute very substantially to the cost of treatment. It is important that you talk to your vet about this, both at the beginning of any treatment and as that treatment unfolds.

REMISSION

Because cancers are so dangerous and so very likely to recur, vets (and medics) are bound to try to be grounded and realistic. We avoid raising expectations in the families of dogs treated for cancer. In dealing with cancer, even when the outcome seems to be excellent, we rarely use the word 'cure' because it is almost impossible to know that each and every cancer cell has been destroyed. Instead, the term 'remission' is used. When the evidence suggests that the bulk of a tumour has gone, this is termed a 'partial remission'. When the news is more positive and it appears that the tumour has gone completely, the term 'complete remission' is used, meaning that there is no obvious evidence that the tumour remains. If a dog is still alive following several years of apparent complete remission, then the term cure might eventually be used.

RELAPSES

In spite of our best efforts, many tumours do come back, locally or at a distant site from the original. Depending on the tumour type, ongoing treatment can sometimes be rewarding, but often the prognosis for relapsed lesions is considerably worse; for instance, because the recurrence may be much less responsive to the drugs used in the first round of therapy. Even at this point, palliative therapy might be useful, but this could be the time when you have to confront the final question of euthanasia. This subject will be considered more fully in the next chapter.

Pippin, a 13-year-old male Maltese Terrier, frankly had always had a very poor opinion of vets. Larry, who described himself as 'Pippin's mummy', carried Pip into my consulting room, laid his flaccid body on my table, and began to weep. 'Look at my baby!' He's been floppy like this all day. He won't eat a thing, and his wee-wee looks like blood.' Larry can lay it on with a trowel, but these were no empty histrionics. My instant reaction was to think Pippin was at death's door.

Instant reactions are not reliable diagnostic tools. I took a step back. Pippin was certainly dull and weak, so weak he couldn't be bothered to snarl. He was still quite hefty and a good colour, indeed his membranes were really brightly red. Otherwise his vital signs were fairly unremarkable although his body temperature was slightly elevated, 39.7°C. The heart rate was increased to over 150 beats a minute. Pulses were strong.

Larry insisted this illness had appeared suddenly. Until 48 hours before Pippin had been his usual bossy pugnacious self.

I was worried. Platitudes were pointless. I could give no immediate words of comfort to Larry. He gave permission for blood tests, urinalysis and fluid therapy as first steps.

As suspected, the urine was quite bloody, abundant red cells and some protein was present. There was no evidence of an infection. Kidney function itself appeared normal based on the biochemistry, which was a relief given the bloody urine. The most crucial initial findings were in the haematology, which showed that despite the loss of blood Pippin was not anaemic. Rather the contrary. The red cell count and the proportion of red cells in the blood, known as the packed cell volume, was well above normal (72% – a usual value in most dogs is between about 40 and 50%). This is really quite uncommon. Technically, it is called polycythaemia.

Ultrasound examination was the next step. It showed that the anatomy of Pippin's left kidney was very disrupted indeed whereas the other kidney, the bladder and the rest of the urinary system seemed normal. Radiographs of the chest and the skeleton showed no signs of definite metastasis. We could not be sure treatment would help but Larry gave the go-ahead for surgery.

My colleague Ruth undertook the delicate and demanding task to remove the left kidney, which was cancerous. Our pathologist made a diagnosis of renal carcinoma. The high red cell count had occurred because the diseased kidney was spuriously secreting very high levels of erythropoetin, a hormone, which stimulates the bone marrow to manufacture and release red blood cells.

Outlook for this sort of tumour varies. Some dogs do well. With intensive nursing for a few days after surgery Pippin made an excellent recovery. He continued to be vigorous and apparently healthy for more than 15 months afterwards, although he never displayed any gratitude to us. Eventually, Pippin's overall wellbeing began to decline rapidly. Larry decided not to pursue further investigations on this occasion. Pippin was gently put to sleep one afternoon in my consulting room.

12
OLD AGE

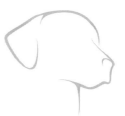

> This chapter is concerned with geriatrics, age-related disease and cognition, organ failure, euthanasia and death. These issues are best dealt with by frank and honest discussions with your vet. You can help your vet and your dog by being open about your worries and discussing the scenarios before you must face them.

People often ask me: 'When does a dog become old?' This is a tough question to give a straight answer to. Firstly, for healthy dogs their breeding has a very considerable impact on their likely lifespan. As you'll know by now, large breeds have shorter lives than small dogs, on average. So, for instance, I would regard an Irish Wolfhound who reached the age of 11 years to be very elderly indeed, whereas for a Jack Russell Terrier the age of 11 would probably equate to late middle age. Also, the old rule of thumb that asserts that one dog year is equivalent to seven human years might seem attractive but in reality, it's fanciful. Dogs, like most carnivores, reach sexual maturity, adult body size and weight quite quickly, often by a year of age, whereas humans spend perhaps a quarter of their lifespan going through this development. There have been several attempts to create more reliable algorithms to equate human and dog growth, youth, maturity and ageing. From these we can say that both species progress through this series of age-related physiological states in the same sequence, but there is no simple linear relationship between dog and human age.

As dogs age after reaching adulthood their likelihood of dying increases, just as it does in people. Also, their chances of developing longstanding diseases increase year on year, so that older dogs often suffer from multiple problems where different diseases and their treatment compound each other. A similar scenario, known as co-morbidity, is very common in older people. Complexities of this sort have not been well studied by my profession. Unfortunately, geriatrics, the specialism that deals with old age in people, does not have a veterinary equivalent, although it certainly should. Detail about the complexities of old age in pet dogs has not been systematically studied. Much of what I am setting down here is derived from a handful of scientific papers, anecdote, discussions with colleagues, or personal experience rather than detailed evidence. A couple of studies have recently begun that aim to investigate in detail how dogs age – namely, the Golden Retriever Lifetime Study (GRLS) and the Dog Ageing Project (DAP). Another is the Old Age Pets Survey (OAPs), which is looking in depth at owners' and vets' experience of geriatric dogs. Long-term projects of this sort should make a serious contribution to veterinary medicine in future. Their findings might have implications for human health too because dogs share our environment closely but live much shorter lives.

We know that diet, exercise and the health of our parents and grandparents has an enormous impact on our own health and the likelihood of when we will die. We also know that abstaining from tobacco, drinking alcohol in moderation, and keeping slim help us to live longer and healthier lives. We know surprisingly little about the effects of diet, exercise, or exposure to environmental factors in dogs. This makes it impossible to give meaningful advice concerning how we might delay ageing or promote long healthy lives for dogs. Although it is sometimes claimed that various super-foods rich in antioxidants, etc., can prolong life there is no compelling evidence that this is the case for dogs. On the other hand, we do know that obesity shortens dogs' lives and the quality of those lives. Also, that conditions such as cancer, arthritis, diabetes, kidney disease, heart failure, etc. do become more prevalent in older dogs. Cognitive decline definitely appears to be common in elderly dogs, but the diagnosis of this is fraught with difficulties and for many dogs as they grow older their owners (and many vets) consider this to be an inevitable part of ageing, so the problem is clouded. Sensory loss accompanies ageing in dogs – certainly their hearing and visual acuity decline. It is likely that their sense of smell deteriorates too, but this is difficult for us to appreciate or to measure.

Determining the difference between normal ageing and age-related disease is rather a tricky problem that vets face every day. Regular health check-ups through the years are certainly very helpful in monitoring the way in which your dog is progressing from maturity onwards. So, for instance, if a dog is weighed regularly, every 6–12 months, the data can be helpful, not only to look for weight gain but also for unexpected weight loss, which is often the first clue that all is not well. We know that evaluating body condition score alongside weight is very helpful (see pp. 95–97, Figure 5.3 for more on this). Inspections of the teeth, counting the heart and pulse rate, listening to the chest, etc., will be part of these checks and will be informative. There is definitely also some merit in additional tests such as urine analysis, blood pressure checks and performing a biochemistry profile as dogs reach the later stages of their life, but, as you might have learned from earlier in the book (Chapter 6), it is important to be a little sceptical because it is easy to become beguiled by any laboratory work. Remember, no test is perfect. There are always some 'false positives' and some 'false negatives'. So, for example, slight to moderate increases in liver enzyme values are found in many older dogs, but these are usually of no serious clinical concern. If these are identified in your older dog, ask your vet whether they think these are really worthy of note, and, if so, what should be done?

What can we do to make the life of an old dog easier? There is no one answer to this. However, if you feel your dog is becoming geriatric, it is an excellent idea to look carefully at your dog's abilities, behaviours, wishes and desires then go to see your vet.

Here are a few things you might want to consider.

Loss of hearing and a diminution of sight are things we associate with ageing in people. Whilst these are not necessarily crucial to systemic health, we know that elderly folk find this can make them unhappy, is frustrating at the least, and often contributes to their sense of social isolation. Dogs rely less on sight than people do, though recognition of movement is very important in hunting as well as ball play. Dogs who become deaf are at greater risk in traffic and crowds. They are less likely to come when called and they tend to sleep more deeply. Elderly deaf dogs are easily startled when they wake, which can mean they become frightened and lash out. A few might show uncharacteristic aggression and become a danger to young children. Except in a few specific cases, we cannot improve the sight or hearing of dogs. So, it might be you have to adjust your behaviour and modify your dog walks.

When I talk to clients about their elderly dogs, they often mention signs that suggest general cognitive decline. Certainly, I've seen this in Tallulah, my long-dog, as she has aged. Things to look out for would be forgetfulness, becoming muddled or disorientated, uncharacteristic behaviours such as failing to recognise family members, and loss of training such as forgetting commands, or suddenly deciding to urinate or defecate indoors. Some dogs will show new behaviours such as barking, growling, unprovoked anger, whining, waking in the night or general restlessness. Obviously, these signs could occur for other reasons such as pain or a neurologic problem. A veterinary consultation might be helpful.

There are some drug therapies that appear to help dogs with cognitive decline, but before resorting to these your vet will want to perform a full neurological examination, assess their hearing, sight and other senses.

Most healthy dogs will greet their owners rather ecstatically when they come home. As your dog gets older, they might be less bothered, perhaps because they are in pain, so that getting to their feet becomes difficult, or simply because old age has reduced their verve. Older dogs might show more general changes in their desire for companionship or isolation. Dogs vary a great deal in this, so the important thing to look for would be a marked change in these behaviours. I had a greyhound, Sheamus, who was very happy to spend hours asleep in his bed, or sunbathing, even when he was a youngster. He did this all his life.

Pain and stiffness are frequent companions to senility; 'old age does not come alone.' Some degree of stiffness is almost universal in older dogs, which might just be manifest first thing in the morning. However, it is really important if you own an older dog to look carefully at their mobility and their gait: Does she want a walk? If so, is she still able to manage her customary 40 minutes or would she rather it was only half an hour, or less? Is she freely mobile, or always a bit stiff? Does she stop for a rest and a really thorough sniff more often than she used to? Does she turn for home rather than tackling that big hill? What about his speed – did he always want to run everywhere and now can only walk? Has the skip in his step disappeared? Can he manage stairs. Can he get into the car? Can she get out? Does he still jump on the couch? Does she need a hand to get down? Frank pain may not always be obvious. Sometimes the only way we can tell that a dog has been suffering is by watching how they behave after starting treatment with analgesic or anti-inflammatory drugs. Look back at Chapter 7, the sections on lameness (p. 155) and osteoarthritis (p. 161) for more on these issues.

It can be challenging to know the difference between the frailty and decline that is simply old age and illness. Many healthy old dogs will have lots of good days and a few bad days. They might sleep a lot more than they did, but still be delighted to go for a short walk, be fed a meal and have a cuddle on the settee. However, if their appetite is seriously depressed, their weight is dropping precipitously, their breathing is noisy or difficult, their toileting habits have changed dramatically, or they seem to be in obvious pain, then you really should see your vet.

There are health questionnaires that vets sometimes use to assess particular aspects of your dog's wellbeing, such as the Liverpool Osteoarthritis in Dogs (LOAD), and the Canine Brief Pain Inventory (CBPI). A new one called the Ageing Canine Toolkit has just been published by the BSAVA. It is easy to use and available free of charge (https://www.bsavalibrary.com/content/cilgrouppetsaversact). It looks to me to be useful. A good policy, if you have an older dog, might be to use this toolkit frequently as a simple hack to monitor their wellbeing. At present there is no one universally accepted tool that has been adopted to assess the overall quality of a dog's life. Perhaps this is a good thing? Every dog is different and the things that profoundly affect the wellbeing of one dog are not precisely the same for the next dog. You almost certainly will know and understand your dog better than other people do. But, on the other hand, the more objective judgement of a veterinary professional can certainly help.

THE END OF LIFE

If you have an old dog who is in declining health it can be really helpful to talk openly with your vet about the future. Planning for a good death might seem morbid but it can help you and your family. We wish our old friend will die peacefully in their sleep. Sadly, this very rarely happens. Death is an inevitable end for all living things but rarely comes quietly.

Time helps people prepare. If you have a dog with a terminal illness, then in the months and weeks before the end you can brace yourself that there will be a decision to face when your dog is too ill to continue with life. I think this opportunity can be a valuable moment to allow you to face the death of a loved one.

For some dogs the end of life comes as a slow decrepitude. If a dog is simply old and frail, often vets can provide medicine to help that animal from day-to-day.

Sometimes we can signpost how things might progress and give guidance to allow you to gauge the decline. Gradually, stuttering, they have more and more bad days. It becomes your duty to weigh up their life. Does it seem worth living? I know this responsibility can be a terrible burden.

There is not one answer. You must decide, but your vet will help you.

Sooner or later, you might have to face the morning when your dog is simply unable to get up, or is forced to defecate where they lie. By then most people are ready and resigned.

For some dogs a sudden and dramatic change in their health occurs. A marked increase in thirst, sudden weight loss, complete loss of appetite, severe protracted coughing, breathing difficulties, vomiting or diarrhoea, collapse, profound lethargy and loss of interest are typical signs. These dogs might have organ failure or some sort of a tumour. Sometimes they might have a perfectly treatable condition. A veterinary examination will be urgently required. In these circumstances, it is usually impossible to know the precise cause, or the future, without tests to show the problem. It might be necessary to give supportive treatments, such as fluid therapy, whilst waiting for these.

Now is the time to think carefully about what you want. Here we all struggle. Should we proceed with test after test to find the diagnosis, so that we know for sure if anything can be done? Should we opt for euthanasia? Sometimes, especially when I have a definitive diagnosis, as a vet I can be sure death is coming, but, when the diagnosis is in doubt, or the patient's condition is deteriorating quickly, then I have to be more speculative and uncertain. We all prefer certainty.

When is it right to say: 'Enough is enough'?

There is not one answer. You must decide, but your vet will help you.

Where it is especially difficult is if the problem is very acute, such as a road accident, or a young dog who was well two days ago but now is found to have an aggressive tumour, or another catastrophic problem. In the absence of any premonition of the issue you might be distraught and angry, sometimes unable to face death at all. As vets, we try to give clients time to phone their partner, their parent or a close friend, and perhaps spend a cherished final hour with the dog.

Euthanasia means 'well death'. It is never a routine procedure. Some young vets consider euthanasia to represent failure. I think they are mistaken. All lives must end. Some lives are just not worth living. For me, euthanasia can be the best end to a good life. I think it is better to end a life this way, than to let it end in pain. I have made up my mind that what I do, when I deliberately give an anaesthetic overdose to 'put a dog to sleep', is to run the clock forwards quickly to hasten their inevitable death, and believe doing that is almost always justifiable because the alternative is worse. There are occasions where I know that the dog might rally for a short while, but the owners are unable to provide the care for that to happen. In the vast majority of cases where we euthanase a pet it is because the alternative would be a painful death.

If you decide your dog should be euthanased, you will be given the opportunity to be there when it happens. A short form must be signed. Some vets will first give your dog a sedative and put a catheter into a vein, usually in a front leg. The anaesthetic, which is given into the bloodstream, is a barbiturate at a very high dose. Your dog will quietly breathe more shallowly for a few breaths, perhaps sigh, stop breathing and then go limp. Their heart will stop. Sometimes they will pass urine or poo. Occasionally, a moment later they might make a final gasp. Their eyes do not close.

I always like to leave grieving owners alone with the body for a few minutes after their dog has died to allow them to say goodbye. My clients seem to appreciate this.

After your dog has died, you can take the body home to bury if you want. There are many ways you can commemorate your dog; for instance, an ink paw-print can be made, or a lock of their hair can be cut as a keep-sake. Most often the body is cremated afterwards by a firm specialising in this. This is usually a communal cremation but individual cremations are increasingly done and the ashes returned. People often choose to have these returned in a special container.

GRIEF

As a Scot brought up in the 1960s and 1970s, I was taught to believe that emotions should be held in check and a grown man should never cry. What tosh! Love cannot be cured. The price we pay for love is grief. Anyone who's ever had a dog will know that their death can be a grievous injury. Cut yourself some slack. Cry if you want to. Unfortunately, some people around you may not appreciate how you are feeling. Don't let them make you feel weak or guilty. Pity them. They have probably never experienced the special precious joy of dog ownership. We have.

'Dogs' lives are too short. Their only fault, really.'

Agnes Sligh Turnbull

LITTLE DOG'S RHAPSODY IN THE NIGHT

He puts his cheek against mine

and makes small, expressive sounds.

And when I'm awake, or awake enough

he turns upside down, his four paws

in the air

and his eyes dark and fervent.

'Tell me you love me,' he says.

'Tell me again.'

Could there be a sweeter arrangement? Over and over

he gets to ask.

I get to tell.

Part III

FREQUENTLY ASKED QUESTIONS AND RELATED ISSUES

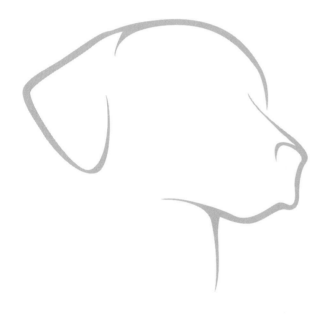

13

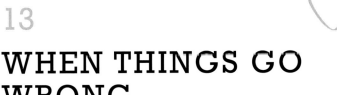

WHEN THINGS GO WRONG

This chapter is designed to help you when things seem to be going wrong. What should you do if you can't afford the tests and treatments? How to go about changing your vet when the need arises. How to ask for a referral to a specialist. What to expect from a specialist referral. How to make a complaint to, or about, your vet when you feel things have been badly handled, and how that complaint may be dealt with.

WHAT SHOULD YOU DO IF YOU CAN'T AFFORD THE TESTS AND TREATMENTS?

Veterinary medicine is expensive. I wish it were cheaper, but vets have to run profitable businesses and there is no NHS for animals. When choosing a pet, it is wise to consider your budget before getting a dog (see Chapter 2). If you are out of work or in receipt of benefits you might be able to sign on with the PDSA (People's Dispensary for Sick Animals) who will often be able to provide help towards the cost of veterinary care, though usually only for one pet per household. Occasionally, you can find other local charities that might be able to offer you some support.

If you take your dog to the vet and it turns out to need expensive tests or treatments that you cannot afford the best policy is to immediately explain your financial position. You don't need to go into details. Vets are used to this dilemma and usually very willing to try to find a practical solution.

The first thing you need is to understand what is being proposed by the vet and why. Sometimes, the problem your dog has will not justify the expense at all. Often, symptomatic treatment of a problem, treating the most likely condition in a way that is most likely to be successful, is appropriate and an economic way forward. In many other instances, the vet might be able to adapt the investigations and treatments in ways that lessen the costs substantially; for example, some tests might be proposed that are not strictly essential, or which can be postponed, for further down the line, if symptomatic treatment fails to solve the problem. In some instances, a cheap drug can be substituted for the more expensive, gold standard treatment. The outcome might not be quite as good, or side-effects more likely, so you should ask about that. However, you also need to be aware that vets are obliged, by law, to use licensed veterinary drugs where they are available, even where there might be cheaper human generic versions of these drugs (see The Prescribing Cascade, p. 301).

Sometimes it is possible to obtain the appropriate drugs from an online veterinary pharmacy at a price far below the one your own vet would charge you. To do so you will need a written prescription, signed and validated by your vet (who will charge a small fee for this). The option of a written prescription and use of an online supplier can be particularly economic for drugs that are being used long-term, for example for arthritis, skin allergies, or heart disease. Most vets privately admit they find it galling that these online pharmacies often can sell the drugs far cheaper than we can get them from our own wholesale suppliers.

If these strategies are not an option, your vet might be able to work out a payment plan where you pay in instalments. However, vets are not licensed as moneylenders and to protect the public the rules on credit have been tightened up over the past few decades to ensure that this is not the usual way we do business.

WHAT SHOULD I DO IF THE INSURANCE PREMIUMS FOR MY DOG SEEM TO HAVE BECOME EXORBITANT?

As dogs age, their health insurance costs tend to increase and/or the benefits might become more limited. This tends to be true even if the policy you have is labelled as 'Lifetime Cover'. Obviously, as dogs get older, they are increasingly likely to eventually develop chronic diseases that require continuous treatments. They are also at increased risk of developing a life-threatening illness. Many clients are horrified and angry when they find that year-on-year the cost of veterinary insurance for their ageing companion increases much faster than inflation. If this applies to you and you are tempted to switch insurers, think twice or three times before doing so. When you switch insurers for an older dog, or one who has any longstanding medical problems that require frequent or expensive treatment, it is almost inevitable that you will get a worse deal from the new insurers. Don't act in haste. Read the small print.

If you do decide to cease paying for insurance it would be very wise to squirrel away some cash every month to cover future veterinary fees.

HOW TO GO ABOUT CHANGING YOUR VET WHEN THE NEED ARISES?

If you move house, change circumstance, or are simply not completely satisfied with the vet you have, how do you change practices?

Switching veterinary practice can be a wrench or a relief – depending on your experiences in the past. It is not something you need to feel embarrassed about. All vets expect to lose and to gain some clients at intervals. The process is easy. First decide which vet practice you want to move to. For advice on this, see Chapter 3. Next, inform both practices that you want to do this. Usually, within a day or two, the new practice should receive a complete case record of your dog's health from the previous practice.

If you are asked why you are changing vets then give honest answers. It might help other clients and if you've been dissatisfied it can feel liberating to get this off your chest.

HOW TO ASK FOR A REFERRAL TO A SPECIALIST?

Vets in companion practice tend to be generalists. Many will have some particular special interests and skills. All regularly have post-graduate training. Nevertheless, it is impossible for any vet to be a complete master of the entire subject.

Also, some conditions call for highly specialised procedures and equipment. So, inevitably, there are times when your vet will not be able to provide the best possible care for your dog's particular problems. When this stage is reached you might like your dog to be seen by an Advanced Veterinary Practitioner or by a Specialist.

The UK boasts one of the best further education programmes for vets in the world, led by the Royal College of Veterinary Surgeons (RCVS) and the British Small Animal Veterinary Association (BSAVA). Some vets will have passed post-graduate certificates in certain domains, but very few will be specialists. Experienced small animal practitioners who have obtained post-graduate expertise and RCVS certificates may be designated as Advanced Veterinary Practitioners. Those who claim Specialist Status have to have additional training, experience, qualifications and regular peer review.

If your vet realises that they have reached the limits of their own expertise with a particular case, they should offer to refer you to someone with more expertise. If this is not offered, but you are concerned that your vet is getting out of their depth, you can bring this up yourself. Often, the vet will be delighted to hand-over the responsibility for a challenging case to a more experienced colleague. The RCVS has a register of Veterinary Specialists that you can find online at: https://findavet.rcvs.org.uk. Beware. It is important to be a little bit picky about this. Your vet might be tempted, for commercial or political reasons, to refer you to a colleague in the same practice or one who works for the same corporate veterinary group. Sometimes they might be tempted to send you to a specialist a long distance away, despite the fact that there is one within a few miles. That might not always be the best choice, so you should ask why exactly they suggest you see a certain person, rather than another, and then make up your own mind.

It is always more expensive to see a specialist than a generalist vet. This is because the Specialist will usually be able and willing to spend much more time with each case and will have the expertise, experience and facilities for more rigorous investigations and more effective treatments. In the long-term, the outcomes should be better, but, just as in human medicine, specialist vets tend to see the most severely compromised animals, which means they are more likely to see those which cannot be completely cured.

WHAT TO EXPECT FROM A SPECIALIST REFERRAL

There are limited numbers of Veterinary Specialists and Advanced Veterinary Practitioners, so it is very likely you will have to travel some distance to see one. Ahead of time, you should be given full details of how to get there, how long you are likely to be there, and some idea of the likely costs involved. If your dog is insured it would be usual for specialist referral costs to be covered by your insurers, although there are some sneaky insurers who find ways around this. If in any doubt contact your insurers before you go.

When you see an Advanced Veterinary Practitioner or a Veterinary Specialist you will usually have an extended appointment with them at which your dog's history is explored, a detailed examination is performed, and the further investigation and treatment of your dog is planned. Your primary vet should have forwarded their notes and a copy of any laboratory tests that have already been done. You should also have been given the opportunity to provide supplemental data yourself, such as relevant video clips of behaviour, or questions you'd like to be addressed at the appointment.

In my own experience, I find it a challenge to give accurate estimates of the costs likely to be incurred with any particular case until I see the dog and their owner face-to-face and make my own examination. Having said that, once I have a good understanding of the case from this initial meeting, usually it becomes much easier, so I expect to be able to provide a fairly detailed estimate of the expenses at that point, but this does vary. So, for example, sometimes testing for certain problems must be done as a package, whilst for other issues, some lab results must come in before another range of tests are done. This means some dogs can be dealt with at a single visit in an hour or two, or a day, whereas others need to come back and forth several times. It is rarely possible for you to be with your dog for the complete referral visit, because many procedures must be done in operating theatres, or for reasons of safety the public must be excluded (e.g. for X-rays). This was especially true during the Covid-19 pandemic.

Most specialists will provide a report to the referring vet soon after seeing a referral. Interim reports will be provided if the process involves several visits. Personally, I like to get a report out within 48 hours. Reports may be written in highly technical language that is often baffling to the general public. Ask the Specialist vet for a lay translation of technical terms. I like to copy my report to you, the dog's owners; but not all specialists will do this, so I would ask.

DRUG SIDE-EFFECTS AND ADVERSE REACTIONS TO DRUGS

All potent and useful drugs can have side-effects, which are inherent to the way that drugs work. Antibiotics are liable to impact the normal microbiological ecology of the body, which can mean that the bacterial flora of the gut is upset and diarrhoea results. Corticosteroids – which are potent and highly effective anti-inflammatory agents – suppress the immune system, which is often why they are used, but will tend to impair the response to vaccination. They also have a gamut of other side-effects, such as a tendency to cause an increase in appetite and thirst. I am giving only two examples here but some side-effects from drugs are almost universal. Very often your vet will warn you of the most likely side-effects from the drugs they prescribe. They should always also provide a package insert with the prescriptions that, amongst other things, list side effects. It is a good idea to read this leaflet. Don't throw it away.

Adverse effects are more idiosyncratic than side-effects; that is to say, only a small proportion of the treated animals will display these, but again they are fairly frequent. So, for instance, non-steroidal anti-inflammatory agents, which are frequently prescribed for acute or chronic pain, especially arthritis, sometimes cause vomiting or diarrhoea. These gut signs rarely are accompanied by bleeding. If your dog seems to exhibit obvious adverse effects to a drug, inform your vet immediately. Withdrawal of that drug is often necessary and will frequently solve the problem. Often, another drug can be used instead.

SURGICAL COMPLICATIONS

All surgery involves wounding, which is of course an insult to the body. Surgical acumen demands profound anatomical knowledge, great spatial awareness, dexterity and an ability to make clear and quick decisions, even in the face of inadequate information. Surgery requires excellent anaesthesia and sterility as well as good surgical tools and a clear head. 'Be quick, be clean, be careful' is the surgeon's motto.

Sometimes the effects of surgical injury inevitably lead to complications such as wound infections or more pain for the patient than had been anticipated. An artery might be inadvertently cut, a nerve severed, or healthy tissue might be damaged in the course of trying to close a laceration or remove a tumour. So, after we operate, in the hours and days following surgery, we like to re-assess our patients to ensure that complications are absent or at least recognised early in the dog's recovery. After surgery many patients are sent home with pain-killing drugs. Dressings or bandages may have been applied. Often, your dog will come home wearing a head-collar so that they are unable to lick or chew the wound or remove a bandage. Please follow the instructions you are given when your dog is discharged to you. The advice is intended to help prevent complications. It is a great shame when a dog has to endure another anaesthetic or the complex and costly treatment of a wound infection because the client has removed a bandage or a head-collar in the mistaken belief that their dog does not need these. If you are concerned that a surgical wound is angry and red, painful, discharging or smelly, contact your vet promptly.

MISTAKES

A few years into my career I made an error during routine surgery that killed a cat. After I realised what I'd done I was overcome with guilt and self-loathing. I also wanted to annul the event, to pretend it had never happened. I have gone over this in my mind many, many times since. Even now I feel shame and disgust as I write this. But the truth is I am not alone. All vets, however conscientious, however experienced and dedicated, make mistakes.

There are currently no reliable data to quantify how often mistakes happen during veterinary care. In human medicine in the UK, it is said that errors of patient care kill more people each year than breast cancer. Veterinary practice is unlikely to be any safer. Deliberate neglect and intentional or plainly inadequate care are probably very infrequent. On the other hand, misdiagnoses seem to be common, especially when limited funds, inadequate equipment or time-pressure mean that short-cuts are taken. Many other mistakes are lapses or slips that occur when vets or nurses are distracted whilst doing routine procedures, especially if they are over-burdened, tired or working at the limits of their abilities. Another common source of error is when the responsibility for a case is handed over from one clinician to another, especially if there is no formal handover procedure with time devoted specifically to that. Finally, there is no doubt that sometimes a vet will simply be out of their depth and might not even be aware that they are floundering.

For years vets have been held up as paragons by the public and the media; indeed, many vets set themselves impossible standards believing that they should be able to achieve perfection. This is not helpful, it fosters a situation where mistakes are more likely to be hidden than properly investigated, and where some vets become depressed or suicidal because they cannot deal with their feeling of failure when things go wrong. The suicide rate for vets is extremely high.

As a profession, vets do need to improve. We know that. But sometimes we have failed to fully comprehend what that means in practice or how that can be achieved. Many vets focus on technical and clinical aspects of the job, but most mistakes seem to arise from elsewhere; human factors, communication with clients and within veterinary teams, and other non-technical skills such as drug dispensing or time-management.

Things are changing. In the last decade there has been increased emphasis on understanding how mistakes arise and how these can be prevented, often by simple measures such as the introduction of checklists. The RCVS, the governing body of the veterinary profession in the UK, actively encourages vets to hold regular meetings within their practices to discuss 'near-misses' and cases where the outcome fell below expectations, where the aim is to learn from mistakes without apportioning blame. Blaming a vet for an error will seldom prevent further errors, but by analysing these mistakes it might be possible to understand why they happened and prevent them being repeated. As an example, a couple of months ago, I drew up a drug into a syringe then realised it was completely the wrong drug. I had drawn up butorphanol when I meant to administer buprenorphine. This happened because the two different drugs have similar names, are found in vials that look very similar, and were stored close to each other in our pharmacy. We changed where the two drugs are kept as a result.

When a mistake happens, it can be helpful for the clinician to disclose this to others, including the client, but many vets fear doing so because they anticipate a complaint or litigation will follow. The Veterinary Defence Society (VDS), who provide indemnity insurance for vets, advises that when something goes wrong the vet should not immediately admit liability without first investigating a case carefully, because this would put their insurance in jeopardy. The rationale behind this is clear and sensible but I think the waters are muddied and clients can be furious if they think their concerns are being ignored or fobbed off. One unintended consequence of this is that some vets have developed a sort of clinical paranoia;

they become very risk averse and would rather refer a complex or difficult case than deal with that dog's problem themselves. This is a difficult circle to square. Openness and honesty between the vet and the client do help but can only be achieved in the context of mutual trust.

COMPLAINTS: HOW TO MAKE THEM AND HOW THEY ARE DEALT WITH

No vet is infallible. If you suspect that a mistake has been, or is being, made in the care of your dog, speak up. If you are constructive, you should expect a constructive response.

Most problems can be resolved by speaking up to the vet or nurse, or perhaps their senior, promptly, when a problem arises. If a simple error has been made this can often swiftly be settled. Where the vet, or the practice, agree they are at fault they will be apologetic and keen to make amends. When informal resolution cannot be reached in this way then a more rigorous and documented complaints procedure will be available.

If you feel you have a grievance that has not been promptly and informally settled, the first thing to do is ask for a copy of your vet's records for your dog. The vet practice is legally obliged to provide this. This will help you set-out your complaint. You should make your complaint in writing, clearly and dispassionately if possible, explaining exactly your concerns and how you feel this can be resolved. I would expect the practice to acknowledge receipt of this formal complaint within a few days, explain how they will investigate, and to provide you with a timeline saying when to expect a written response or a meeting to discuss the problem. For practices that belong to a corporate group: if a complaint cannot be settled at a local level then the complaint can be escalated further up the chain of command and investigated again at a regional or national level.

In cases where you remain dissatisfied, there is another tier to this ladder via:

The Veterinary Client Mediation Service, VCMS.
6 Market Square
Bishop's Stortford
Hertfordshire

CM23 3UZ
Phone 0345 0405834
www.vetmediation.co.uk

The VCMS claims to provide a cost-effective opportunity for pet owners and their vets to resolve complaints quickly, fairly and effectively. Both the vet and pet owner must voluntarily agree to use the VCMS. They do not require you to have face to face meetings with your vet. On the contrary, they tend to discuss the problem separately with each party with the aim of gaining a holistic view of the nub of the issue. They will not provide you, or the practice, with legal advice, but they will try to provide you with a realistic understanding of your consumer rights and whether the professional conduct of the vet might be relevant.

Most of the complaints taken to the VCMS result in some sort of conclusion or resolution that might involve explanations and apologies from the vet as well as a formal recognition of your grievance. A proportion of cases do lead to a financial settlement, but this is not the majority.

For a few of the most serious concerns only, it is appropriate to approach the Disciplinary Board of the Royal College of Veterinary Surgeons (RCVS). This can be done through the RCVS website (rcvs.org.uk). This service has a limited remit and can only deal with cases where the veterinary surgeon or nurse is accused of:

- very poor performance

- fraud / dishonesty

- criminal behaviour or convictions

- physical or mental health problems that have, or could, impair their abilities.

APPENDICES

This takes the form of some addenda that address specific issues such as: The Law relating to dogs and dog ownership, The Royal College of Veterinary Surgeons (RCVS), and other useful contacts, web locations, etc.

ORGANISATIONS

Here are some organisations that you will find useful to know as a dog owner. The sites also have useful information supplementary to that which I have given in this book, covering much of the same territory, from their own perspective.

Animal Poison Line: https://www.animalpoisonline.co.uk; phone: 01202 509000
This is a dedicated 24/7 amenity run by vets and toxicologists from the Veterinary Poisons Information Service.

Assistance Dogs: https://www.assistancedogs.org.uk
Assistance Dogs UK (ADUK) was established in 1995 and is an umbrella organisation and hub for assistance dog-related information and good practice.

It is formed of 11 member organisations accredited by Assistance Dogs International (ADI) and / or The International Guide Dog Federation (IGDF), together with six organisations (candidates) that are working towards the same accreditation. Some of these organisations are well known, such as Guide Dogs and Hearing Dogs for Deaf People, and some are less well known, such as Service Dogs UK and Medical Detection Dogs.

British Veterinary Association (BVA): https://www.bva.co.uk
This organisation is run by and for vets. It acts as a kind of professional trade union and publishes some important journals, most notably the *Veterinary Record*. The BVA runs certain health screening schemes, via vets, such as the Hip Dysplasia Scheme. The BVA also has a charitable arm, The Animal Welfare Foundation (AWF), which is focused on animal welfare for both agricultural animals and companions, including dogs. The AWF funds research, supports veterinary education, provides pet care advice and encourages debate on key animal welfare issues. The puppy contract, which I discussed in Chapter 2, was jointly created by AWF and The Royal Society for the Protection of Animals (RSPCA) (puppycontract. org.uk).

British Small Animal Veterinary Association (BSAVA): https://www.bsava.com
The BSAVA represents vets and nurses involved in companion animal practice. It organises a large annual congress as well as many smaller professional development events. BSAVA publishes several books and journals, specifically the *Journal of Small Animal Practice*, and has local branches throughout the country. It also funds some veterinary research through a charity: Petsavers.

Dogs Trust: dogstrust.org.uk
The Dogs Trust is the charity who coined the famous slogan: 'A Dog is for life, not just for Christmas.' It is principally involved in rehoming dogs, rehabilitating dogs who have behavioural problems and in dog training. They provide veterinary care to their own dogs.

Guide Dogs for the Blind: guidedogs.org.uk
The Guide Dogs Charity, formed in 1931, was created to breed and train dogs as guides for people with visual impairments. They have several dedicated centres throughout the UK. They also sponsor veterinary research into some important dog diseases.

Kennel Club: https://www.thekennelclub.org.uk
Another charity. The Kennel Club is principally involved with pedigree dogs, sets breed standards and runs dog shows, most notably Crufts. More recently, this organisation has diversified to some extent, becoming involved with dog health and public education. The Kennel Club also provides some funding for important veterinary research. It administers the Assured Breeders Scheme.

PDSA: pdsa.org.uk

The People's Dispensary for Sick Animals (PDSA) has many veterinary hospitals throughout the country. They are a charity funded by public donations, including from those receiving help, which provides low-cost veterinary care to people on certain benefits, usually only one pet per household. You must be able to provide proof of eligibility. They have details and an eligibility checker on their website.

Pet Blood Bank UK: petbloodbankuk.org

This charity was set up about 15 years ago to provide blood and blood products to vets to give to dogs who are in a crisis. Managing a blood bank is complex and costly but a unit of blood can often save more than one dog's life. The service, which is based in Loughborough, is invaluable. They also run a blood collection service and are always delighted to organise dogs to give donations. If you have a healthy, vaccinated, young dog of a large breed and would like it to become a donor they will be interested (phone: 01509 232 222).

The Royal College of Veterinary Surgeons (RCVS): info@rcvs.org.uk
The Cursitor, 38 Chancery Lane, London, WC2A 1EN; phone: 020 7222 2001.

This is the governing body of the veterinary profession in the UK that licenses vets to practice and sets standards. Here is their mission statement:

> We aim to enhance society through improved animal health and welfare. We do this by setting, upholding and advancing the educational, ethical and clinical standards of veterinary surgeons and veterinary nurses.

The Veterinary Client Mediation Service, VCMS: www.vetmediation.co.uk
6 Market Square, Bishop's Stortford, Hertfordshire, CM23 3UZ; phone: 03450 405834.

DOGS, OWNERS AND THE LAW

Many laws apply to dog owners. These laws tend to differ slightly between the different countries of the UK.

Briefly: If you buy a puppy, under the age of six months, the seller should either be a rehoming centre or be the breeder, and, if they breed more than an occasional litter they should be licensed by their local authority.

A few breeds of dog are prohibited, meaning you must not possess, sell, abandon or give away these dogs: The Pit Bull Terrier, The Japanese Tosa, Dogo Argentino American Bully and Fila Brasileiro. This law was introduced because these breeds are considered to be dangerous. Many animal charities and most vets consider this to be an idiotic law backed by little good evidence. On the other hand these dogs and others certainly can be very dangerous if the dogs are not properly handled (see below).

A dog is considered to be a possession. Ownership disputes are relatively common during divorces.

The Animal Welfare Act stipulates that if you own a dog you must cater for their needs and provide the following:

- a suitable environment

- a suitable diet

- opportunities for the dog to exhibit normal behaviours such as exercise and play

- suitable housing apart from, or with, other animals

- protection from pain, suffering, injury and disease.

Codes of practice for the welfare of dogs can be obtained from governmental websites.

All dogs aged eight weeks or more should be microchipped. Several different microchip databases exist but they share data. It is your responsibility to ensure the microchip data for your dog held on the microchip database is kept up to date.

In addition to a microchip, dogs must wear a collar and tag that identify you as the owner.

When in a public place, you are obliged to pick up your dog's poo. It is wise to always carry several poo bags.

All dogs will bark occasionally but 'unreasonable barking' is prohibited. You should try to prevent your dog barking during unsociable hours or persistently to the annoyance of your neighbours.

Dogs should never be allowed to be dangerously out of control anywhere where they could injure someone or cause serious alarm – in a public place, in your own home, or another private place, such as a neighbour's garden.

In addition to this, further restrictions are applied to some public places by Public Space Protection Orders (PSPOs). The additional restrictions will be specified but can include limiting the number of dogs under the control of an adult, and keeping those dogs on lead.

If you travel with a dog in a car they must be adequately restrained; for instance, by the use of a harness, so that they don't distract or injure you whilst you are driving.

If your dog worries, kills or injures farm livestock, this is an offence for which you are responsible.

AUTHORISED VETERINARY MEDICINES AND THE PRESCRIBING CASCADE

A recurring theme of this book has been that many veterinary medicines are expensive and I know that clients are often quite shocked by the prices of drugs. There have been huge advances in the drugs available to treat dogs in the last 40 years which are due largely to the fact that pharmaceutical companies have found that veterinary drugs research and development can be a profitable business. Moreover, there has been a sustained and concerted effort by clinicians to better understand canine diseases and the effective treatment of these through randomised and controlled drug trials, which (believe you me) are enormously complex and expensive to run.

In the UK, vets are usually legally obliged to only use drugs for dogs that have been through a very strict authorisation process in which the drug has been proven to be safe and effective in dogs for the disease which has been diagnosed. This law is enshrined in the Veterinary Medicines Regulations (2013). The law recognises that there are some circumstances where the benefits of treating a dog with an unauthorised drug outweigh the risks of doing so. Vets are permitted in exceptional circumstances to use drugs outside the terms of the original authorisation following a protocol known as the prescribing cascade.

If there are no drugs that are authorised for a particular condition in dogs, then a drug that has been licensed for another condition in dogs can be used. However, there are many conditions where effective drug regimens have not been definitively established and in other scenarios there may be drugs that have been thoroughly studied and authorised for a related condition in another species. Some drugs that are safe in one species are less safe in another, so there are potential risks to this strategy. Furthermore, sometimes a drug has been identified elsewhere in the world for a condition infrequently seen in the UK, where that drug has been proven to be safe and effective, but no similar drug is authorised here. In circumstances such as these, a vet is permitted to use drugs for which the evidence has not been approved by the licensing authorities. These cases are described as or 'off label' use.

When a vet proposes to use a drug for which no authorisation has been granted, such 'off-label' use must be explained to the client and the potential risks explained. A client's permission must be obtained orally or in writing.

USEFUL BOOKS

Here are a few texts that I have found immensely useful while writing this book

Bowman, D.D. (ed.) (2021) *Georgis' Parasitology for Veterinarians* (11th edn). Elsevier, St. Louis, MO, USA.

Bradshaw, J. (2011) *In Defence of Dogs*. Penguin Books, London, UK.

Case, L., Daristotle, L., Hayek, M.G. and Foess Raasch, M. (2011) *Canine and Feline Nutrition* (3rd edn). Mosby Elsevier, Maryland Heights, MO, USA.

Gawande, A. (2010) *The Checklist Manifesto: How to Get Things Right*. Profile Books, London, UK.

Hill, P., Warman, S. and Shawcross, G. (2011) *100 Top Consultations in Small Animal General Practice*. Wiley-Blackwell, Chichester, UK.

Horowitz, A. (2012) *Inside of a Dog*. Scribner, New York, USA.

Hutchinson, T. and Robinson, K. (2015) *BSAVA Manual of Canine Practice*. BSAVA, Gloucester, UK.

Maddison, J., Volk, H. and Church, D. (2015) *Clinical Reasoning in Small Animal Practice*. Wiley-Blackwell, Chichester, UK.

Mattinson, P. (2014) *The Happy Puppy Handbook: Your Definitive Guide to Puppy Care and Early Training*. Ebury Press, London, UK.

Miklosi, A. (2016) *Dog Behaviour, Evolution and Cognition*. Oxford University Press, Oxford, UK.

Miklosi, A. (ed.) (2018) *The Dog: A Natural History*. Ivy Press, London, UK.

Montgomery, K. (2006) *How Doctors Think*. Oxford University Press, Oxford, UK.

Mukherjee, S. (2015) *The Laws of Medicine: Field Notes from an Uncertain Science*. TED Books, Simon and Schuster, London, UK.

Packer, R.M.A. and O'Neill, D.G. (eds) (2022) *Health and Welfare of Brachycephalic (Flat-faced) Companion Animals: A Complete Guide for Veterinary and Animal Professionals*. CRC Press, Boca Raton, FL, USA.

Schon, D.A. (1982) *The Reflective Practitioner: How Professionals Think in Action*. Basic Books, New York, USA.

Serpell, J. (ed.) (1995) *The Domestic Dog*. Cambridge University Press, Cambridge, UK.

Whitehead, S. (2012) *Clever Dog*. Collins, London, UK.

ACKNOWLEDGEMENTS

I've spent my whole professional life as a vet. I've been tutored by, and collaborated with, many different people from whom I have learnt much about dogs, canine medicine, surgery, nutrition and welfare. This book has taken the best part of four years to write but is the fruit of a much longer journey.

It would be impossible to list everyone who has helped me. However, I'd like to formally acknowledge a few. Jo Tristram put the idea in my head. Friends and veterinary colleagues Dan Shaw, Mark Morton, Mark Hurst, Stephen Hanvidge, Nazaret Marechal, Helen Groves, Niall Connell (past president of the RCVS), Nicola Robinson (from the Veterinary Poisons Information Service), David Argyll (Dean and Head of School at the R(D)SVS Vet School in Edinburgh) and Phillipa Yam (Senior Lecturer at Glasgow University Veterinary School GUVS) read large parts of this book. Their critical feedback and advice have been enormously helpful. Phil Carter and Rachel Groarke from the Dogs Trust provided a great sounding board when I was writing the early chapters of this text, especially concerning puppy farms, and rescue and rehoming of indigenous and imported dogs. Carri Westgarth, Professor of Human–Animal Interaction at Liverpool Veterinary School was especially encouraging to me, particularly about the need for a book like this and the process of getting published. Gemma Crossley, head of the professional conduct department of the RCVS, and Jennie Jones, of the Veterinary Client Mediation Service, gave me sterling advice about complaints and complain complaint procedures.

I am enormously grateful to a few select friends, clients, dog owners and potential owners who were willing to plough through much of the text and provide encouraging feedback, namely: Alan Rollo, Paul Wookey, Lucy Boutwood,

David and Jo Pick, and the author and personal friend Pippa Marland. My sister Ros, my brother Simon, Emily my daughter and Denise my wife have also provided a wonderful cocktail of straight-talking criticism and enthusiastic encouragement. I'd like to believe the final product was worth their while. Finally, I want to thank the team at 5m Books: Adrienne Bayley, Sarah Hulbert, Alessandro Passini and Jeremy Toynbee together with the illustrator Elaine Leggett who transformed my sketches and photographs into the final drawings.

GLOSSARY

acetabulum	the socket joint of the hip located in the pelvis
Addison's disease	a condition of the adrenal glands in which they are virtually inactive
adipsia	failure to drink
amino acids	the building blocks of protein
anaemia	inadequate numbers of red cells and/or haemoglobin in the blood
anaesthesia	lack of perception mimicking sleep, due to the administration of drugs.
analgesia	reduced perception of pain due to the administration of drugs
analgesics	drugs which dampen the sensation of pain
anti-emetics	drugs which prevent vomiting and/or reduce nausea
arachidonic acid cascade (or pathway)	a key chemical pathway in the body in which inflammatory chemicals are synthetised.
atrophy	shrinkage (usually applied to muscles, caused by disuse)
auto-immune disease or disorder	an inflammatory condition in which the body is reacting against its own tissue
axillae	the 'arm-pits', where the shoulder joints meets the body wall
blepharospasm	screwing-up of the eyes
brachycephalic	flat-faced / short snouted
cachexia	generalised weight loss and withering of the tissues (usually caused by serious disease).
carpus	the wrist joint of the foreleg. the joint below the elbow.

cataract	clouding of the lens of the eye
chemotherapy	drug therapy to kill cancer cells
cleft palate	a defect in the roof of the mouth
congenital disorder(s)	disease(s) which an animal has been born with
contagious disease(s)	disease(s) which spread rapidly within a species
cytokines	chemical messenger signal molecules produced by cells of the body
cytotoxic agent	a drug used to kill cells, most often used in the chemotherapy of cancer.
disseminated lymphadenopathy	a disorder of the lymph nodes of the body which affects a large number of these
dysplasia	abnormal growth
dyspnoea	difficult and / or painful breathing
dysphonia	altered voice
electrolytes	salts within the body (such as sodium, potassium, chloride and bicarbonate) and fluids containing these given as therapy
Eliza test	enzyme-linked immunoassay; a common type of blood test
electrocardiogram (ECG)	an electronic recording of the heart showing the rate, rhythm and behaviour of the heart muscle
erythrocytes	the red blood cells which contain haemoglobin and transport oxygen
erythropoetin	a home produced by the kidneys which stimulates the bone marrow to produce red blood cells
haematology	the study of cells in the blood. a crucial blood test
herd immunity	a population effect where such a large proportion of a population are immune to a disease that the disease is unable to spread because very few individuals are susceptible
hip dysplasia	a common anatomic disorder of the hip of the dog
histiocytoma	a skin tumour which often resolves spontaneously
hock	the joint below the stifle in the hind-leg, equivalent to the human ankle
Holter monitor	an instrument used to record a time-lapse electrocardiogram
hyper...	excessive level or behaviour of ... e.g. hyperthermia is high body temperature

hypo...	inadequate level or behaviour of ... e.g. hypothyroidism is deficiency in thyroid function
immunoglobulins	unique specialised proteins synthesised by the immune system to protect against invaders (also called antibodies)
insulin	a hormone synthesised in the pancreas released to reduce blood glucose and permit glucose to cross into cells
intestinal lymphoma	a cancer of the immune system localised to the gut
keratitis	inflammation of the cornea - the 'window' of the eye
laparotomy	surgical procedure opening into the abdomen
leukaemia	a cancer of the circulating white blood cells
lymphoma	a cancer of the immune system
mast cell tumour	a cancer, most usually found in the skin, with a very variable outcome
melaena	altered blood present in the poo giving it a tarry appearance
melanoma	a cancer of pigment producing cells usually located in the skin, the mouth or the eye
nor-adrenalin	a hormone produced in the adrenal glands and the heart which raises the heart rate and blood pressure.
neutering	de-sexing. in males the term 'castration' is often used. for females the operation has several different terms such as 'ovariohysterectomy' or 'speying'
osteomyelitis	infection of the bone(s)
otitis	inflammation of the ear
paratenic host	an animal which has become accidentally host to a parasite
plasmacytoma	a rapidly developing soft-tissue tumour usually found in the skin
pulmonary bullae	air-filled defects within the lung which can rupture
pulmonary oedema	fluid build-up within the lungs, sometimes caused by heart failure
pupae	an immature and inactive phase of an insect between the larval stage and adulthood e.g. a chrysalis
pyo...	pertaining to pus e.g. pyoderma is pus in the skin, pyometra is pus in the womb

radiographs	x-ray pictures
sarcopaenia	muscle wastage (often seen with severe disease or accompanying old age
soft-tissue sarcoma	a cancerous tumour of the connective tissue
squamous-cell carcinoma	a skin tumour which is often locally aggressive
stem-cell therapy	a novel therapeutic method with uses immature cells
syncope	fainting or transient loss of consciousness
tapetum	reflective membrane found at the back of the eye in dogs, cats and many other mammals but not in people
thiols	strong-smelling sulphur containing compounds
trachea	the windpipe
triage	literally 'sorting-out'; preliminary assessment of a patient to determine urgency
ultrasonography	visualisation and examination of the body using high-frequency sound waves. the same technique is used to see babies in the womb
uveitis	inflammation of the posterior chamber of the eye
vasodilators	drugs used to reduce blood pressure and in the treatment of heart disease
vestibular syndrome	a common but poorly understood sudden derangement of balance which often improves spontaneously
vestibular system	the balancing mechanism of the body

BIBLIOGRAPHY

CHAPTER 1

Archer, J. (1997) Why do people love their pets? *Evolution and Human Behavior* 18, 237–259. https://doi.org/10.1016/S0162-3095(99)80001-4.

Barker, S.B. and Wolen, A.R. (2008) The benefits of human–companion animal interaction: A review. *Journal of Veterinary Medical Education* 35, 487–495. https://doi.org/10.3138/jvme.35.4.487.

Caya, S. (2015) The importance of house pets in emotional development. *Procedia – Social and Behavioral Sciences* 185, 411–416. https://doi.org/10.1016/j.sbspro.2015.03.388.

Dotson, M.J. and Hyatt, E.M. (2008) Understanding dog–human companionship. *Journal of Business Research* 61, 457–466. https://doi.org/10.1016/j.jbusres.2007.07.019.

Friedmann, E. and Thomas, S.A. (1995) Pet ownership, social support, and one year survival after acute myocardial infarction in the Cardiac Arrhythmia Suppression Trial (CAST). *American Journal of Cardiology* 76, 1213–1217. https://doi.org/10.1016/S0002-9149(99)80343-9.

Gácsi, M., Maros, K., Sernkvist, S., Faragó, T. and Miklósi, A. (2013) Human analogue safe haven effect of the owner: Behavioural and heart rate response to stressful social stimuli in dogs. *PLOS ONE* 8, e58475. https://doi.org/10.1371/journal.pone.0058475.

Gee, N.R., Mueller, M.K. and Curl, A.L. (2017) Human–animal interaction and older adults: An overview. *Frontiers in Psychology* 8, 1416. https://doi.org/10.3389/fpsyg.2017.01416.

Hart, L.A. (1995), Chapter 12 Dogs as human companions: A review of the relationship. In: Serpell, J. (ed.) *The Domestic Dog: Its Evolution,*

Behaviour, and Interactions with People. Cambridge University Press, Cambridge.

Horowitz, A. (2012) *Inside of a Dog.* Scribner, New York, USA.

Kazi, D.S. (2019) Who is rescuing whom? Dog ownership and cardiovascular health circulation. *Circulation. Cardiovascular Quality and Outcomes* 12, e005887. https://doi.org/10.1161/CIRCOUTCOMES.119.005887.

Kramer, C.K., Mehmood, S. and Suen, R.S. (2019) Dog ownership and survival: A systematic review and meta-analysis. *Circulation. Cardiovascular Quality and Outcomes* 12, e005554. https://doi.org/10.1161/CIRCOUTCOMES.119.005554.

Lodge, C.J., Allen, K.J., Lowe, A.J., et al. (2012) Perinatal cat and dog exposure and the risk of asthma and allergy in the urban environment: A systematic review of longitudinal studies. *Clinical and Developmental Immunology* 2012, 176484. https://doi.org/10.1155/2012/176484.

Lødrup Carlsen, K.C., Roll, S., Carlsen, K.H., et al. (2012) Does pet ownership in infancy lead to asthma or allergy at school age? Pooled analysis of individual participant data from 11 European birth cohorts. *PLOS ONE* 7, e43214. https://doi.org/10.1371/journal.pone.0043214.

Lundqvist, M., Carlsson, P., Sjödahl, R., Theodorsson, E. and Levin, L.Å. (2017) Patient benefit of dog-assisted interventions in health care: A systematic review. *BMC Complementary and Alternative Medicine* 17, 358. https://doi.org/10.1186/s12906-017-1844-7.

McNicholas, J., Gilbey, A., Rennie, A. et al. (2005) Pet ownership and human health: A brief review of evidence and issues. *BMJ* 331, 1252–1254. https://doi.org/10.1136/bmj.331.7527.1252.

Mills, D. and Hall, S. (2014) Animal-assisted interventions: Making better use of the human-animal bond. *Veterinary Record* 174, 269–273. http://doi.org/10.1136/vr.g1929.

Mubanga, M., Byberg, L., Egenvall, A., Ingelsson, E. and Fall, T. (2019) Dog ownership and survival after a major cardiovascular event: A register-based prospective study. *Circulation. Cardiovascular Quality and Outcomes* 12, e005342. https://doi.org/10.1161/CIRCOUTCOMES.118.005342.

Okada, H., Kuhn, C., Feillet, H. and Bach, J.F. (2010) The 'hygiene hypothesis' for autoimmune and allergic diseases: An update. *Clinical and Experimental Immunology* 160, 1–9. https://doi.org/10.1111/j.1365-2249.2010.04139.x.

Ownby, D.R., Johnson, C.C. and Peterson, E.L. (2002) Exposure to dogs and cats in the first year of life and risk of allergic sensitization at 6 to 7 years of age. *JAMA* 288, 963–972. https://doi.org/10.1001/jama.288.8.963.

Stanley, I.H., Conwell, Y., Bowen, C. and Van Orden, K.A. (2014) Pet ownership may attenuate loneliness among older adult primary care patients who live alone. *Aging and Mental Health* 18, 394–399. https://doi.org/10.1080/13607863.2 013.837147.

Tun, H.M., Konya, T., Takaro, T.K., et al. (2017) Exposure to household furry pets influences the gut microbiota of infants at 3–4 months following various birth scenarios. *Microbiome* 5, 40. https://doi.org/10.1186/s40168-017-0254-x.

Van Houtte, B.A. and Jarvis, P.A. (1995) The role of pets in preadolescent psychosocial development. *Journal of Applied Developmental Psychology* 16, 463–479. https://doi.org/10.1016/0193-3973(95)90030-6.

Walsh, F. (2009) Human–animal bonds I: The relational significance of companion animals. *Family Process* 48, 462–480. https://doi.org/10.1111/j.1545-5300.2009.01296.x.

Wells, D.L. (2007) Domestic dogs and human health: An overview. *British Journal of Health Psychology* 12, 145–156. https://doi.org/10.1348/135910706X103284.

CHAPTER 2

Asher, L., Diesel, G., Summers, J.F., McGreevy, P.D. and Collins, L.M. (2009) Inherited defects in pedigree dogs. Part 1: Disorders related to breed standards. *Veterinary Journal* 182, 402–411. https://doi.org/10.1016/j.tvjl.2009.08.033.

Bray, E.E. et al. (2021) Early-emerging and highly heritable sensitivity to human communication in dogs. *Current Biology* 31, 3132-3136. https://doi.org/10.1016/j.cub.2021.04.055.

Duffy, D.L., Hsu, Y. and Serpell, J.A. (2008) Breed differences in canine aggression. *Applied Animal Behaviour Science* 114, 441–460. https://doi.org/10.1016/j.applanim.2008.04.006.

Ekenstedt, K.J., Crosse, K.R. and Risselada, M. (2020) Canine brachycephaly: Anatomy, pathology, genetics and welfare. *Journal of Comparative Pathology* 176, 109–115. https://doi.org/10.1016/j.jcpa.2020.02.008.

Elegans, C. (2012) 100 years of breed 'improvement'. https://dogbehaviorscience.wordpress.com/2012/09/29/100-years-of-breed-improvement/.

Institute of Canine Biology. https://www.instituteofcaninebiology.org/blog/coi-faqs-understanding-the-coefficient-of-inbreeding.

McGreevy, P.D., Wilson, B.J., Mansfield, C.S. et al. (2018) Labrador retrievers under primary veterinary care in the UK: Demography, mortality and disorders.

Canine Genetics and Epidemiology 5, 8. https://doi.org/10.1186/s40575-018-0064-x.

O'Neill, D.G., Church, D.B., McGreevy, P.D., Thomson, P.C. and Brodbelt, D.C. (2013) Longevity and mortality of owned dogs in England. *Veterinary Journal* 198, 638–643. https://doi.org/10.1016/j.tvjl.2013.09.020.

PAW (2019) PDSA Animal Wellbeing Report. http://www.pdsa.org.uk/paw-2019.

PAW (2020) PDSA Animal Wellbeing Report. http://www.pdsa.org.uk/paw-2020.

Rooney, N.J. (2009) The welfare of pedigree dogs: Cause for concern. *Journal of Veterinary Behavior* 4, 180–186. https://doi.org/10.1016/j.jveb.2009.06.002.

CHAPTER 3

Blue, C. Choosing the right vet practice. https://www.bluecross.org.uk/advice/pets/choosing-the-right-vet-practice.

Elliot, P., et al How to choose a Vet. wikiHow.com.

Royal College of Veterinary Surgeons. Find a Vet. findavet.rcvs.org.uk.

CHAPTER 4

American Veterinary Society of Animal Behavior (2008) AVSAB Position Statement on Puppy Socialization.

Caron-Lormier, G., Harvey, N.D., England, G.C. and Asher, L. (2016) Using the incidence and impact of behavioural conditions in guide dogs to investigate patterns in undesirable behaviour in dogs. *Scientific Reports* 6, 23860. https://doi.org/10.1038/srep23860.

Creevy, K.E., Grady, J., Little, S.E. et al. (2019) 2019 AAHA canine life stage guidelines. *Journal of the American Animal Hospital Association* 55, 267–290. https://doi.org/10.5326/JAAHA-MS-6999.

Day, M.J., Horzinek, M.C., Schultz, R.D. and Squires, R.A. (2016) WSAVA Guidelines for the vaccination of dogs and cats. *Journal of Small Animal Practice* 57, E1–E45. https://doi.org/10.1111/jsap.2_12431.

Guide dogs. Puppy socialisation. https://www.guidedogs.org.uk/.../dog-care-and-welfare/puppy-socialisation.

Hammerle, M., Horst, C., Levine, E. et al. (2015) 2015 AAHA canine and feline behavior management guidelines. *Journal of the American Animal Hospital Association* 51, 205–221. https://doi.org/10.5326/JAAHA-MS-6527.

Hutchinson, T. (2019). Chapter 15 *BSAVA Manual of Canine Practice: A Foundation Manual*, p. 181.

Lopes Fagundes, A.L., Hewison, L., McPeake, K.J., Zulch, H. and Mills, D.S. (2018) Noise sensitivities in dogs: An exploration of signs in dogs with and without musculoskeletal pain using qualitative content analysis. *Frontiers in Veterinary Science* 5, 17. https://doi.org/10.3389/fvets.2018.00017.

Mattinson, P. https://thehappypuppysite.com/puppy-development-stages.

Mattinson, P. (2014) *The Happy Puppy Handbook: Your Definitive Guide to Puppy Care and Early Training*. Ebury Press.

Nijsse, R., Ploeger, H.W., Wagenaar, J.A. and Mughini-Gras, L. (2015) Toxocara canis in household dogs: Prevalence, risk factors and owners' attitude towards deworming. *Parasitology Research* 114, 561–569. https://doi.org/10.1007/s00436-014-4218-9.

Seksel, K., Mazurski, E.J. and Taylor, A. (1999) Puppy socialisation programs: Short and long term behavioural effects. *Applied Animal Behaviour Science* 62, 335–349. https://doi.org/10.1016/S0168-1591(98)00232-9.

Smith, T. (2016) Leadchanges: Puppy development and socialisation. https://leadchanges.net/puppy-development-and-socialisation-its-effects-on-behaviour/.

Young, L.M., Wiseman, S., Crawley, E., et al. (2021) Effectiveness of Credelio® Plus, a novel chewable tablet containing milbemycin oxime and lotilaner for the treatment of larval and immature adult stages of Toxocara canis in experimentally infected dogs. *Parasites and Vectors* 14, 14 May, 256. https://doi.org/10.1186/s13071-021-04762-x.

CHAPTER 5

Arnold, S., Hubler, M. and Reichler, I. (2009) Urinary incontinence in spayed bitches: New insights into the pathophysiology and options for medical treatment. *Reproduction in Domestic Animals* 44(Suppl 2), 190–192. https://doi.org/10.1111/j.1439-0531.2009.01407.x.

Axelsson, E., Ratnakumar, A., Arendt, M.L., et al. (2013) The genomic signature of dog domestication reveals adaptation to a starch-rich diet. *Nature* 495, 360–364. https://doi.org/10.1038/nature11837.

Beauvais, W., Cardwell, J.M. and Brodbelt, D.C. (2012) The effect of neutering on the risk of mammary tumours in dogs – A systematic review. *Journal of Small Animal Practice* 53, 314–322. https://doi.org/10.1111/j.1748-5827.2011.01220.x.

Blake, A.B. and Suchodolski, J.S. (2016) Importance of gut microbiota for the health and disease of dogs and cats. *Animal Frontiers* 6, 37–42. https://doi.org/10.2527/af.2016-0032.

Böhm, M., Thompson, H., Weir, A. et al. (2004) Serum antibody titres to canine parvovirus, adenovirus and distemper virus in dogs in the UK which had not been vaccinated for at least three years. *Veterinary Record* 154, 457–463. http://doi.org/10.1136/vr.154.15.457.

Bosch, G., Hagen-Plantinga, E.A. and Hendriks, W.H. (2015) Dietary nutrient profiles of wild wolves: Insights for optimal dog nutrition? *British Journal of Nutrition* 113(Suppl), S40–S54. https://doi.org/10.1017/S000711451400 2311.

Brown, W.Y. and McGenity, P. (2005) Effective periodontal disease control using dental hygiene chews. *Journal of Veterinary Dentistry* 22, 16–19. https://doi.org/10.1177/089875640502200102.

Buff, P.R., Carter, R.A., Bauer, J.E. and Kersey, J.H. (2014) Natural pet food: A review of natural diets and their impact on canine and feline physiology. *Journal of Animal Science* 92, 3781–3791. https://doi.org/10.2527/jas.2014-7789.

Byron, J.K., Taylor, K.H., Phillips, G.S. and Stahl, M.S. (2017) Urethral sphincter mechanism incompetence in 163 neutered female dogs: Diagnosis, treatment, and relationship of weight and age at neuter to development of disease. *Journal of Veterinary Internal Medicine* 31, 442–448. https://doi.org/10.1111/jvim.14678.

Cooley, D.M., Beranek, B.C., Schlittler, D.L., et al. (2002) Endogenous gonadal hormone exposure and bone sarcoma risk. *Cancer Epidemiology, Biomarkers and Prevention* 11, 1434–1440.

Coren, S. (2011) How good is your dog's sense of taste? In a taste sensitivity contest with dogs, humans clearly win. *Psychology Today*, 19 April 2011.

Courcier, E.A., Mellor, D.J., Thomson, R.M. and Yam, P.S. (2011) A cross sectional study of the prevalence and risk factors for owner misperception of canine body shape in first opinion practice in Glasgow. *Preventive Veterinary Medicine* 102, 66–74. https://doi.org/10.1016/j.prevetmed.2011.06.010.

Culp, W.T., Mayhew, P.D. and Brown, D.C. (2009) The effect of laparoscopic versus open ovariectomy on postsurgical activity in small dogs. *Veterinary Surgery* 38, 811–817. https://doi.org/10.1111/j.1532-950X.2009.00572.x.

de Bleser, B., Brodbelt, D.C., Gregory, N.G. and Martinez, T.A. (2011) The association between acquired urinary sphincter mechanism incompetence in bitches and early spaying: A case-control study. *Veterinary Journal* 187, 42–47. https://doi.org/10.1016/j.tvjl.2009.11.004.

Enlund, K.B., Brunius, C., Hanson, J., et al. (2020) Dental home care in dogs – A questionnaire study among Swedish dog owners, veterinarians and veterinary nurses. *BMC Veterinary Research* 16, 90. https://doi.org/10.1186/s12917-020-02281-y.

Finch, D., Schofield, H., Floate, K.D., Kubasiewicz, L.M. and Mathews, F. (2020) Implications of endectocide residues on the survival of aphodiine dung beetles: A meta-analysis. *Environmental Toxicology and Chemistry* 39, 863–872. https://doi.org/10.1002/etc.4671.

Gawor, J., Jank, M., Jodkowska, K., Klim, E. and Svensson, U.K. (2018) Effects of edible treats containing Ascophyllum nodosum on the oral health of dogs: A double-blind, randomized, placebo-controlled single-center study. *Frontiers in Veterinary Science*, 27 July 2018. https://doi.org/10.3389/fvets.2018.00168.

German, A.J., Ryan, V.H., German, A.C., Wood, I.S. and Trayhurn, P. (2010) Obesity, its associated disorders and the role of inflammatory adipokines in companion animals. *Veterinary Journal* 185, 4–9. https://doi.org/10.1016/j.tvjl.2010.04.004.

German, A.J., Holden, S.L., Wiseman-Orr, M.L., et al. (2012) Quality of life is reduced in obese dogs but improves after successful weight loss. *Veterinary Journal* 192, 428–434. https://doi.org/10.1016/j.tvjl.2011.09.015.

Gibson, A., Dean, R., Yates, D. and Stavisky, J. (2013) A retrospective study of pyometra at five RSPCA hospitals in the UK: 1728 cases from 2006 to 2011. *Veterinary Record* 173, 396. https://doi.org/10.1136/vr.101514.

Glickman, L.T., Glickman, N.W., Moore, G.E., Goldstein, G.S. and Lewis, H.B. (2009) Evaluation of the risk of endocarditis and other cardiovascular events on the basis of the severity of periodontal disease in dogs. *Journal of the American Veterinary Medical Association* 234, 486–494. https://doi.org/10.2460/javma.234.4.486.

Goulson, D. (2013) Review: An overview of the environmental risks posed by neonicotinoid insecticides. *Journal of Applied Ecology* 50, 977–987. http://doi.org/10.1111/1365-2664.12111.

Grüntzig, K., Graf, R., Boo, G., et al. (2016) Swiss canine cancer registry 1955–2008: Occurrence of the most common tumour diagnoses and influence of age, breed, body size, sex and neutering status on tumour development. *Journal of Comparative Pathology* 155, 156–170. https://doi.org/10.1016/j.jcpa.2016.05.011.

Hallmann, C.A., Sorg, M., Jongejans, E., et al. (2017) More than 75% decline in 27 years in total flying insect biomass in protected areas. *PLOS ONE* 12, e0185809. https://doi.org/10.1371/journal.pone.0185809.

Hart, B.L., Hart, L.A., Thigpen, A.P. and Willits, N.H. (2014) Long-term health effects of neutering dogs: Comparison of Labrador retrievers with golden retrievers. *PLOS ONE* 9, e102241. https://doi.org/10.1371/journal.pone.0102241.

Hart, B.L., Hart, L.A., Thigpen, A.P. and Willits, N.H. (2016) Neutering of German Shepherd dogs: Associated joint disorders, cancers and urinary incontinence. *Veterinary Medicine and Science* 2, 191–199. https://doi.org/10.1002/vms3.34.

Hart, B.L., Hart, L.A., Thigpen, A.P. and Willits, N.H. (2020) Assisting decision-making on age of neutering for 35 breeds of dogs: Associated joint disorders, cancers, and urinary incontinence. *Frontiers in Veterinary Science* 7, 388. https://doi.org/10.3389/fvets.2020.00388.

Harvey, C.E., Shofer, F.S. and Laster, L. (1996) Correlation of diet, other chewing activities and periodontal disease in North American client-owned dogs. *Journal of Veterinary Dentistry* 13, 101–105. https://doi.org/10.1177/0898 75649601300304.

Harvey, C.E., Serfilippi, L. and Barnvos, D. (2015) Effect of frequency of brushing teeth on plaque and calculus accumulation and gingivitis in dogs. *Journal of Veterinary Dentistry* 32, 16–21. https://doi.org/10.1177/089875641503200102.

Hussein, H.S., Flickinger, E.A. and Fahey, G.C., Jr. (1999) Petfood applications of inulin and oligofructose. *The Journal of Nutrition* 129(Suppl), 1454S–1456S. https://doi.org/10.1093/jn/129.7.1454S.

Ishangulyyev, R., Kim, S. and Lee, S.H. (2019) Understanding food loss and waste – Why are we losing and wasting food? *Foods* 8, 297. https://doi.org/10.3390/foods8080297.

Jitpean, S., Hagman, R., Ström Holst, B. et al. (2012) Breed variations in the incidence of pyometra and mammary tumours in Swedish dogs. *Reproduction in Domestic Animals* 47(Suppl 6), 347–350. https://doi.org/10.1111/rda.12103.

Kealy, R.D., Lawler, D.F., Ballam, J.M., et al. (2002) Effects of diet restriction on life span and age-related changes in dogs. *Journal of the American Veterinary Medical Association* 220, 1315–1320. https://doi.org/10.2460/javma.2002.220.1315.

Killey, R., Mynors, C., Pearce, R., et al. (2018) Long-lived immunity to canine core vaccine antigens in UK dogs as assessed by an in-practice test kit. *Journal of Small Animal Practice* 59, 27–31. https://doi.org/10.1111/jsap.12775.

Kortegaard, H.E., Eriksen, T. and Baelum, V. (2008) Periodontal disease in research beagle dogs – An epidemiological study. *Journal of Small Animal Practice* 49, 610–616. https://doi.org/10.1111/j.1748-5827.2008.00609.x.

Kustritz, M.V.R., Slater, M.R., Weedon, G.R. and Bushby, P.A. (2017) Determining optimal age for gonadectomy in the dog: A critical review of the literature to guide decision making. *Clinical Theriogenology* 9, 167–211.

Logan, E.I. (2006) Dietary influences on periodontal health in dogs and cats. *Veterinary Clinics of North America. Small Animal Practice* 36, 1385–1401. https://doi.org/10.1016/j.cvsm.2006.09.002.

Marx, F.R., Machado, G.S., Pezzali, J.G., et al. (2016) Raw beef bones as chewing items to reduce dental calculus in Beagle dogs. *Australian Veterinary Journal* 94, 18–23. https://doi.org/10.1111/avj.12394.

Miller, B.R. and Harvey, C.E. (1994) Compliance with oral hygiene recommendations following periodontal treatment in client owned dogs. *Journal of Veterinary Dentistry* 11, 18–19. https://doi.org/10.1177/0898756494011 00103.

Muraro, L. and White, R.S. (2014) Complications of ovariohysterectomy procedures performed in 1880 dogs. *Tierarztliche Praxis. Ausgabe K, Kleintiere/Heimtiere* 42, 297–302. https://doi.org/10.1055/s-0038-1623776.

Okin, G.S. (2017) Environmental impacts of food consumption by dogs and cats. *PLOS ONE* 12, e0181301. https://doi.org/10.1371/journal.pone.0181301.

Okkens, A.C., Kooistra, H.S. and Nickel, R.F. (1997) Comparison of long-term effects of ovariectomy versus ovariohysterectomy in bitches. *Journal of Reproduction and Fertility. Supplement* 51(Suppl), 227–231.

Pavlica, Z., Petelin, M., Juntes, P., et al. (2008) Periodontal disease burden and pathological changes in organs of dogs. *Journal of Veterinary Dentistry* 25, 97–105. https://doi.org/10.1177/089875640802500210.

Perkins, R. (2020) Are pet parasite products harming the environment more than we think? *Veterinary Record* 187, 197. http://doi.org/10.1136/vr.m3453.

Perkins, R., Whitehead, M., Civil, W. and Goulson, D. (2021) Potential role of veterinary flea products in widespread pesticide contamination of English rivers. *Science of the Total Environment* 755, 143560. https://doi.org/10.1016/j.scitotenv.2020.143560.

Raubenheimer, D., Machovsky-Capuska, G.E., Gosby, A.K. and Simpson, S. (2015) Nutritional ecology of obesity: From humans to companion animals. *British Journal of Nutrition* 113(Suppl), S26–S39. https://doi.org/10.1017/S0007114514002323.

Roberts, M.T., Bermingham, E.N., Cave, N.J., et al. (2018) Macronutrient intake of dogs, self-selecting diets varying in composition offered ad libitum. *Journal of Animal Physiology and Animal Nutrition* 102, 568–575. https://doi.org/10.1111/jpn.12794.

Salt, C., Morris, P.J., German, A.J. et al. (2017) Growth standard charts for monitoring bodyweight in dogs of different sizes. *PLOS ONE* 12, e0182064. https://doi.org/10.1371/journal.pone.0182064.

Schneider, R., Dorn, C.R. and Taylor, D.O. (1969) Factors influencing canine mammary cancer development and postsurgical survival. *Journal of the National Cancer Institute* 43, 1249–1261.

Schultz, R.D., Thiel, B., Mukhtar, E., Sharp, P. and Larson, L.J. (2010) Age and long-term protective immunity in Dogs and Cats. *Journal of Comparative Pathology* 142(Suppl 1), S102–S108. https://doi.org/10.1016/j.jcpa.2009.10.009.

Shariati, E., Bakhtiari, J., Khalaj, A. and Niasari-Naslaji, A. (2014) Comparison between two portal laparoscopy and open surgery for ovariectomy in dogs. *Veterinary Research Forum* 5, 219–223.

Simonet, P. (2005) Dog-laughter: Recorded playback reduces stress related behaviour in shelter dogs. In: Proceedings of the 7th international conference on environmental enrichment.

Simpson, M., Albright, S., Wolfe, B., et al. (2019) Age at gonadectomy and risk of overweight/obesity and orthopaedic injury in a cohort of Golden Retrievers. *PLOS ONE* 14, e0209131. https://doi.org/10.1371/journal.pone.0209131.

Trevejo, R., Yang, M. and Lund, E.M. (2011) Epidemiology of surgical castration of dogs and cats in the United States. *Journal of the American Veterinary Medical Association* 238, 898–904. https://doi.org/10.2460/javma.238.7.898.

Urfer, S.R. and Kaeberlein, M. (2019) Desexing dogs: A review of the current literature. *Animals (Basel)* 9, 1086. https://doi.org/10.3390/ani9121086.

Vale, R. and Vale, B. (2009) *"Time to Eat the Dog?": The Real Guide to Sustainable Living*. Thames and Hudson.

Waters, D.J., Kengeri, S.S., Maras, A.H., Suckow, C.L. and Chiang, E.C. (2017) Life course analysis of the impact of mammary cancer and pyometra on age-anchored life expectancy in female rottweilers: Implications for envisioning ovary conservation as a strategy to promote healthy longevity in pet dogs. *Veterinary Journal* 224, 25–37. https://doi.org/10.1016/j.tvjl.2017.05.006.

Witter, R.E. (1949) Diseases of the external ear of the dog. *Cornell Veterinarian* 39, 11–31.

Yam, P.S., Butowski, C.F., Chitty, J.L., et al. (2016) Impact of canine overweight and obesity on health-related quality of life. *Preventive Veterinary Medicine* 127, 64–69. https://doi.org/10.1016/j.prevetmed.2016.03.013.

Yamamuro, M., Komuro, T., Kamiya, H., et al. (2019) Neonicotinoids disrupt aquatic food webs and decrease fishery yields. *Science* 366, 620–623. https://doi.org/10.1126/science.aax3442.

Yavor, K.M., Lehmann, A. and Finkbeiner, M. (2020) Environmental impacts of a pet dog: An LCA case study. *Sustainability* 12, 3394. https://doi.org/10.3390/su12083394.

Zink, M.C., Farhoody, P., Elser, S.E., et al. (2014) Evaluation of the risk and age of onset of cancer and behavioral disorders in gonadectomized vizslas. *Journal of the American Veterinary Medical Association* 244, 309–319. https://doi.org/10.2460/javma.244.3.309.

CHAPTER 6

Alves, J.C., Santos, A., Jorge, P., Lavrador, C. and Carreira, L.M. (2022) Evaluation of four clinical metrology instruments for the assessment of osteoarthritis in dogs. *Animals: An Open Access Journal from MDPI* 12, 2808. https://doi.org/10.3390/ani12202808.

Armstrong, N. and Hilton, P. (2014) Doing diagnosis: Whether and how clinicians use a diagnostic tool of uncertain clinical utility. *Social Science and Medicine* 120, 208–214. https://doi.org/10.1016/j.socscimed.2014.09.032.

Brown, C.R., Garrett, L.D., Giles, W.K., et al. (2021) Spectrum of care; more than treatment options. *Journal of the American Veterinary Medical Association* 221, 12–17. https://doi.org/10.2460/javma.259.7.712.

Croskerry, P. (2003) The importance of cognitive errors in diagnosis and strategies to minimise them. *Academic Medicine* 78, 775–780. https://doi.org/10.1097/00001888-200308000-00003.

Croskerry, P. (2013) From mindless to mindful practice – Cognitive bias and clinical decision making. *New England Journal of Medicine* 368, 2445–2448. https://doi.org/10.1056/NEJMp1303712.

Elwyn, G., Frosch, D., Thomson, R., et al. (2012) Shared decision making: A model for clinical practice. *Journal of General Internal Medicine* 27, 1361–1367. https://doi.org/10.1007/s11606-012-2077-6.

Han, P.K.J., Klein, W.M.P. and Arora, N.K. (2011) Varieties of uncertainty in health care: A conceptual taxonomy. *Medical Decision Making* 31, 828–838. https://doi.org/10.1177/0272989x11393976.

Hilbig, B.E., Scholl, S.G. and Pohl, R.F. (2010) Think or blink – Is the recognition heuristic and 'intuitive' strategy. *Judgment and Decision Making*. Society for Judgement and Decision Making 5, 300–309. https://doi.org/10.1017/S1930297500003533.

Jones, D.S. and Podolsky, S.H. (2015) The history and fate of the gold standard. *Lancet* 385, 1502–1503. https://doi.org/10.1016/S0140-6736(15)60742-5.

Klein, J.G. (2005) Five pitfalls in decisions about diagnosis and prescribing. *BMJ* 330, 781–783. https://doi.org/10.1136/bmj.330.7494.781.

McKenzie, B.A. (2014) Veterinary clinical decision-making: Cognitive biases, external constraints, and strategies for improvement. *Journal of the American Veterinary Medical Association* 244, 271–276. https://doi.org/10.2460/javma.244.3.271.

McKenzie, B.A. (2016) Overdiagnosis. *Journal of the American Veterinary Medical Association* 249, 884–889. https://doi.org/10.2460/javma.249.8.884.

Maddison, J., Volk, H. and Church, D. (2015) *Clinical Reasoning in Small Animal Practice*. Wiley-Blackwell, Chichester, UK.

Montgomery, K. (2006) *How Doctors Think*. Oxford University Press, Oxford, UK.

Mukherjee, S. (2015) *The Laws of Medicine: Field Notes from an Uncertain Science*. TED Books, Simon & Schuster.

Saposnik, G., Redelmeier, D., Ruff, C.C. and Tobler, P.N. (2016) Cognitive biases associated with medical decisions: A systematic review. *BMC Medical Informatics and Decision Making* 16, 138. https://doi.org/10.1186/s12911-016-0377-1.

Schon, D.A. (1982) *The Reflective Practitioner: How Professionals Think in Action*. Basic Books.

Skipper, A., Gray, C., Serlin, R., et al. (2021) "*Gold standard care*" is an unhelpful term. *Veterinary Record* 23/30 October, 189, 331.

Smith, C.S., Hill, W., Francovich, C. et al. (2014) Diagnostic reasoning across the medical education continuum. *Healthcare* 2, 253–271. https://doi.org/10.3390/healthcare2030253.

CHAPTER 7

Abercromby, R., Innes, J. and May, C. (2018) Arthritis. *BSAVA Manual of Musculoskeletal Disease*, 81–109. https://doi.org/10.22233/9781910443286.6.

Anderson, K.L., Zulch, H., O'Neill, D.G., Meeson, R.L. and Collins, L.M. (2020) Risk factors for canine osteoarthritis and its predisposing arthropathies: A systematic review. *Frontiers in Veterinary Science* 7, 220. https://doi.org/10.3389/fvets.2020.00220.

Bellows, J., Berg, M.L., Dennis, S. et al. (2019) 2019 AAHA Dental care guidelines for dogs and *cats*. *Journal of the American Animal Hospital Association* 55, 49–69. https://doi.org/10.5326/JAAHA-MS-6933.

Belshaw, Z., Asher, L., Harvey, N.D. and Dean, R.S. (2015) Quality of life assessment in domestic dogs: An evidence-based rapid review. *Veterinary Journal* 206, 203–212. https://doi.org/10.1016/j.tvjl.2015.07.016.

Botto, R., Riccio, V., Galosi, L., et al. (2022) Effects of intra-articular autologous adipose micrograft for the treatment of osteoarthritis in dogs: A prospective, randomized, controlled study. *Animals (Basel)* 12, 1844. https://doi.org/10.3390/ani12141844.

Brown, D.C., Boston, R.C., Coyne, J.C. and Farrar, J.T. (2008) Ability of the canine brief pain inventory to detect response to treatment in dogs with osteoarthritis. *Journal of the American Veterinary Medical Association* 233, 1278–1283. https://doi.org/10.2460/javma.233.8.1278.

Bui, L.M. and Bierer, T.L. (2003) Influence of green lipped mussels (Perna canaliculus) in alleviating signs of arthritis in dogs. *Veterinary Therapeutics: Research in Applied Veterinary Medicine* 4, 397–407.

Canine Brief Pain Inventory. http://www.CanineBPI.com.

Chesney, C.J. (2002) Food sensitivity in the dog: A quantitative study. *Journal of Small Animal Practice* 43, 203–207. https://doi.org/10.1111/j.1748-5827.2002.tb00058.x.

Enomoto, M., Mantyh, P.W., Murrell, J., Innes, J.F. and Lascelles, B.D.X. (2019) Anti-nerve growth factor monoclonal antibodies for the control of pain in dogs and cats. review. *Veterinary Record*. https://doi.org:10.1136/vr.104590.

Favrot, C., Steffan, J., Seewald, W. and Picco, F. (2010) A prospective study on the clinical features of chronic canine atopic dermatitis and its diagnosis. *Veterinary Dermatology* 21, 23–31. https://doi.org/10.1111/j.1365-3164.2009.00758.x.

Fischer, N., Spielhofer, L., Martini, F., Rostaher, A. and Favrot, C. (2021) Sensitivity and specificity of a shortened elimination diet protocol for the diagnosis of food-induced atopic dermatitis (FIAD). *Veterinary Dermatology* 32, 247–e65. https://doi.org/10.1111/vde.12940.

Gould, D. and McLelllan, G. (2014) *BSAVA Manual of Canine and Feline Ophthalmology* (3rd edn). BSAVA.

Harvey, H.J. (1990) Complications of small intestinal biopsy in hypoalbuminemic dogs. *Veterinary Surgery* 19, 289–292. https://doi.org/10.1111/j.1532-950X.1990.tb01188.x.

Harvey, R. (2022) A review of recent developments in veterinary otology. *Veterinary Sciences* 9, 161. https://doi.org/10.3390/vetsci9040161.

Harvey, R., Harari, J. and Delauche, A.J. (2001) *Ear Disease of the Dog and Cat*. Manson Publishing Ltd.

Hercock, C.A., Pinchbeck, G., Giejda, A., Clegg, P.D. and Innes, J.F. (2009) Validation of a client-based clinical metrology instrument for the evaluation of canine elbow osteoarthritis. *Journal of Small Animal Practice* 50, 266–271. https://doi.org/10.1111/j.1748-5827.2009.00765.x.

Hillier, A., Lloyd, D.H., Weese, J.S., et al. (2014) Guidelines for the diagnosis and antimicrobial therapy of canine superficial bacterial folliculitis (antimicrobial Guidelines Working Group of the International Society for Companion Animal Infectious Diseases). *Veterinary Dermatology* 25, 163–e43. https://doi.org/10.1111/vde.12118.

Lascelles, B.D.X., Gaynor, J.S., Smith, E.S., et al. (2008) Amantidine in a multi-modal analgesic regimen for alleviation of refractory osteoarthritis pain in dogs. *Journal of Veterinary Internal Medicine* 22, 53–59. https://doi.org/10.1111/j.1939-1676.2007.0014.x.

Little, C.J.L., McNeil, P.E. and Robb, J. (1991) Hepatopathy and dermatitis in a dog associated with the ingestion of mycotoxins. *Journal of Small Animal Practice* 32, 23–26. https://doi.org/10.1111/j.1748-5827.1991.tb00853.x.

Lundberg, A., Koch, S.N. and Torres, S.M.F. (2022) Local treatment for canine anal sacculitis: A retrospective study of 33 dogs. *Veterinary Dermatology* 33, 426–434. https://doi.org/10.1111/vde.13102.

Malek, S., Sample, S.J., Schwartz, Z., et al. (2012) Effect of analgesic therapy on clinical outcome measures in a randomised controlled trial using client-owned dogs with hip osteoarthritis. *BMC Veterinary Research* 8, 185. https://doi.org/10.1186/1746-6148-8-185.

Marcellin-Little, D.J. (2009) Medical treatment of coxofemoral joint disease. In: John Bonagura, D. and Twedt, D.C. (eds) *Current Veterinary Therapy XIV*, p. 1120–1125.

Marignac, G., Petit, J.Y. and Jamet, J.F. (2019) double blinded, randomized and controlled comparative study evaluating the cleaning activity of two ear cleaners in client-owned dogs with spontaneous otitis externa. *Open Journal of Veterinary Medicine* 9, 93460. https://doi.org/10.4236/ojvm.2019.96006.

Meeson, R.L., Todhunter, R.J., Blunn, G., Nuki, G. and Pitsillides, A.A. (2019) Spontaneous dog osteoarthritis – A One Medicine vision. *Nature Reviews. Rheumatology* 15, 273–287. https://doi.org/10.1038/s41584-019-0202-1.

Muller, C., Gaines, B., Gruen, M. et al. (2016) Evaluation of clinical metrology instrument in dogs with osteoarthritis. *Journal of Veterinary Internal Medicine* 30, 836–846. https://doi.org/10.1111/jvim.13923.

Olivry, T., DeBoer, D.J., Favrot, C., et al. (2010) Treatment of canine atopic dermatitis: Clinical practice guidelines from the International Task Force on Canine Atopic Dermatitis. *Veterinary Dermatology* 21, 233–248. https://doi.org/10.1111/j.1365-3164.2010.00889.x.

O'Neill, D.G., Corah, C.H., Church, D.B., Brodbelt, D.C. and Rutherford, L. (2018) Lipoma in dogs under primary veterinary care in the UK: Prevalence and breed associations. *Canine Genetics and Epidemiology* 5, 9. https://doi.org/10.1186/s40575-018-0065-9.

O'Neill, D.G., Lee, Y.H., Brodbelt, D.C., et al. (2021) Reporting the epidemiology of aural haematoma in dogs and proposing a novel aetiopathogenetic pathway. *Scientific Reports* 11, 21670. https://doi.org/10.1038/s41598-021-00352-0.

O'Neill, D.G., Volk, A.V., Soares, T., et al. (2021) Frequency and predisposing factors for canine otitis externa in the UK – A primary veterinary care epidemiological view. *Canine Medicine and Genetics* 8, 7. https://doi.org/10.1186/s40575-021-00106-1.

Paterson, S. (2016) Topical ear treatment – Options, indications and limitations of current therapy. *Journal of Small Animal Practice* 57, 668–678. https://doi.org/10.1111/jsap.12583.

Pettitt, R.A. and German, A.J. (2015) Investigation and management of canine osteoarthritis. *In Practice* 37(Suppl 1), 1–8. http://doi.org/10.1136/inp.h5763.

Reid, J., Wiseman-Orr, M.L., Scott, E.M. and Nolan, A.M. (2013) Development, validation and reliability of a web-based questionnaire to measure health-related quality of life on dogs. *Journal of Small Animal Practice* 54, 227–233. https://doi.org/10.1111/jsap.12059.

Roberts, C., Armson, B., Bartram, D., et al. (2021) Construction of a conceptual framework for assessment of health-related quality of life in dogs with osteoarthritis. *Frontiers in Veterinary Science* 8, 741864. https://doi.org/10.3389/fvets.2021.741864.

Sanderson, R.O., Beata, C., Flipo, R.M., et al. (2009) Systematic review of the management of canine osteoarthritis. *The Veterinary Record* 164, 418–424. http://doi.org/10.1136/vr.164.14.418.

Shales, C.J., Warren, J., Anderson, D.M., Baines, S.J. and White, R.A. (2005) Complications following full–thickness small intestinal biopsy in 66 dogs: A retrospective study. *Journal of Small Animal Practice* 46, 317–321. https://doi.org/10.1111/j.1748-5827.2005.tb00326.x.

Vandeweerd, J.M., Coisnon, C., Clegg, P., et al. (2012) Systematic review of efficacy of nutraceuticals to alleviate clinical signs of osteoarthritis. *Journal of Veterinary Internal Medicine* 26, 448–456. https://doi.org/10.1111/j.1939-1676.2012.00901.x.

White, A., Foster, N., Cummings, M. and Barlas, P. (2006) The effectiveness of acupuncture for osteoarthritis of the knee – A systematic review. *Acupuncture in Medicine* 24, 40–48. https://doi.org/10.1136/aim.24.Suppl.40.

Wright, A., Amodie, D.M., Cernicchiaro, N., et al. (2022) Identification of canine osteoarthritis using an owner-reported questionnaire and treatment monitoring using functional mobility tests. *Journal of Small Animal Practice* 63, 609–618. https://doi.org/10.1111/jsap.13500.

CHAPTER 8

Harris, G.L., Brodbelt, D., Church, D., et al. (2018) Epidemiology, clinical management, and outcomes of dogs involved in road traffic accidents in the United Kingdom (2009–2014). *Journal of Veterinary Emergency and Critical Care* 28, 140–148. https://doi.org/10.1111/vec.12704.

King, L.G. and Boag, A. (2018) *BSAVA Manual of Canine and Feline Emergency and Critical Care* (3rd edn).

Little, C.J.L., McNeil, P.E. and Robb, J. (1991) Hepatopathy and dermatitis in a dog associated with the ingestion of mycotoxins. *Journal of Small Animal Practice* 32, 23–26. https://doi.org/10.1111/j.1748-5827.1991.tb00853.x.

O'Neill, D.G., Lee, M.M., Brodbelt, D.C., Church, D.B. and Sanchez, R.F. (2017) Corneal ulcerative disease in dogs under primary veterinary care in England: Epidemiology and clinical management. *Canine Genetics and Epidemiology* 4, 5. https://doi.org/10.1186/s40575-017-0045-5.

CHAPTER 9

Foth, S., Meller, S., Kenward, H., et al. (2021) The use of ondansetron for the treatment of nausea in dogs with vestibular syndrome. *BMC Veterinary Research* 17, 222. https://doi.org/10.1186/s12917-021-02931-9.

Henze, L., Foth, S., Meller, S., et al. (2022) Ondansetron in dogs with nausea associated with vestibular disease: A double-blinded, randomized placebo-controlled crossover study. *Journal of Veterinary Internal Medicine* 36, 1726–1732. https://doi.org/10.1111/jvim.16504.

Hulsebosch, S.E., Pires, J., Bannasch, M.J. et al. (2022) Ultra-long-acting recombinant insulin for the treatment of diabetes mellitus in dogs. *Journal of Veterinary Internal Medicine* 36, 1211–1219. https://doi.org/10.1111/jvim.16449.

Li, Q., Heaney, A., Langenfeld-McCoy, N., Boler, B.V. and Laflamme, D.P. (2019) Dietary intervention reduces left atrial enlargement in dogs with early preclinical myxomatous mitral valve disease: A blinded randomised controlled study in 36 dogs. *BMC Veterinary Research* 15, 425. https://doi.org/10.1186/s12917-019-2169-1.

Mattin, M.J., Boswood, A., Church, D.B., et al (2015) Prevalence of and risk factors for degenerative mitral valve disease in dogs attending primary-care veterinary practices in England. *Journal of Veterinary Internal Medicine* 29, 847–854. https://doi.org/10.1111/jvim.12591.

Mattin, M., O'Neill, D., Church, D. et al. (2014) An epidemiological study of diabetes mellitus in dogs attending first opinion practice in the UK. *Veterinary Record* 174, 349. https://doi.org/10.1136/vr.101950.

O'Neill, D.G., Elliott, J., Church, D.B., et al. (2013) Chronic kidney disease in dogs in UK veterinary practices: Prevalence, risk factors, and survival. *Journal of Veterinary Internal Medicine* 27, 814–821. https://doi.org/10.1111/jvim.12090.

O'Neill, D.G., Brodbelt, D.C., Keddy, A., Church, D.B. and Sanchez, R.F. (2021) Keratoconjunctivitis sicca in dogs under primary veterinary care in the UK: An epidemiological study. *Journal of Small Animal Practice* 62, 636–645. https://doi.org/10.1111/jsap.13382.

O'Neill, D.G., Scudder, C., Faire, J.M., et al. (2016) Epidemiology of hyperadrenocorticism among 210,824 dogs attending primary-care veterinary practices in the UK from 2009 to 2014. *Journal of Small Animal Practice* 57, 365–373. https://doi.org/10.1111/jsap.12523.

Orlandi, R., Gutierrez-Quintana, R., Carletti, B., et al. (2020) Clinical signs, MRI findings and outcome in dogs with peripheral vestibular disease: A retrospective study. *BMC Veterinary Research* 16, 159. https://doi.org/10.1186/s12917-020-02366-8.

Radulescu, S.M., Humm, K., Eramanis, L.M. et al. (2020) Vestibular disease in dogs under UK primary veterinary care: Epidemiology and Clinical management. *Journal of Veterinary Internal Medicine* 34, 1993–2004. https://doi.org/10.1111/jvim.15869.

Schofield, I., Brodbelt, D.C., Niessen, S.J.M., et al. (2020) Development and internal validation of a prediction tool to aid the diagnosis of Cushing's syndrome in dogs attending primary-care practice. *Journal of Veterinary Internal Medicine* 34, 2306–2318. https://doi.org/10.1111/jvim.15851.

Schofield, I., O'Neill, D.G., Brodbelt, D.C., et al. (2019) Development and evaluation of a health-related quality-of-life tool for dogs with Cushing's syndrome. *Journal of Veterinary Internal Medicine* 33, 2595–2604. https://doi.org/10.1111/jvim.15639.

Troxel, M.T., Drobatz, K.J. and Vite, C.H. (2005) Signs of neurologic dysfunction in dogs with central versus peripheral vestibular disease. *Journal of the American Veterinary Medical Association* 227, 570–574. https://doi.org/10.2460/javma.2005.227.570.

CHAPTER 10

https://www.bristol.ac.uk/media-library/sites/vetscience/documents/clinical-skills.
Restraining a dog in standing. https://youtu.be/RI8ulDFLgQc.

Canine restrain in lateral recumbency. https://youtu.be/sOIHjSZyVNw.

Veterinary technician and assistant training: handling and restraining dogs. https://youtu.be/ULFwjoZoRt8.

Li, Q., Heaney, A., Langenfeld-McCoy, N., Boler, B.V. and Laflamme, D.P. (2019) Dietary intervention reduces left atrial enlargement in dogs with early preclinical myxomatous mitral valve disease: A blinded randomised controlled study in 36 dogs. *BMC Veterinary Research* 15, 425. https://doi.org/10.1186/s12917-019-2169-1.

CHAPTER 11

Bellows, J., Colitz, C.M.H., Daristotole, L., et al. (2011) Defining healthy aging in older dogs and differentiating healthy aging from disease. *Journal of the American Veterinary Medical Association* 246, 77–89. https://doi.org/10.2460/javma.246.1.77h17.

Butterwick, R.F. (2015) Impact of nutrition on ageing the process. Bridging the Gap: The animal perspective. *British Journal of Nutrition* 113 (Suppl), S23–S25. https://doi.org/10.1017/S0007114514003900.

Creevy, K.E., Austad, S.N., Hoffman, J.M., O'Neill, D.G. and Promislow, D.E.L. (2016) The companion dog as a model for the longevity dividend. In: Olshansky, S.J., Kirkland, J.L. and Martin, G.M. (eds) *Aging: The Longevity Dividend.* Cold Spring Harbor Laboratory Press, Cold Spring Harbor, New York, pp. 107–120. https://doi.org/10.1101/cshperspect.a026633.

Dobson, J.M. (2013) Breed-predispositions to cancer in pedigree dogs. *ISRN Veterinary Science*, 17 Jan 2013 2013, 941275. https://doi.org/10.1155/2013/941275.

Dobson, J.M., Samuel, S., Milstein, H., Rogers, K. and Wood, J.L. (2002) Canine neoplasia in the UK: Estimates of incidence rates from a population of insured dogs. *Journal of Small Animal Practice* 43, 240–246. https://doi.org/10.1111/j.1748-5827.2002.tb00066.x.

Egenvall, A., Bonnett, B.N., Öhagen, P. et al. (2005) Incidence of and survival after mammary tumors in a population of over 80,000 insured female dogs in Sweden from 1995 to 2002. *Preventive Veterinary Medicine* 69, 109–127. https://doi.org/10.1016/j.prevetmed.2005.01.014.

Guy, M.K., Page, R.L., Jensen, W.A., et al. (2015) The Golden Retriever lifetime study: Establishing an observational cohort study with translational relevance for human health. *Philosophical Transactions of the Royal Society of London. Series B, Biological Sciences* 370. https://doi.org/20140230.10.1098/rstb.2014.0230.

Hoffman, J.M., Creevy, K.E. and Promislow, D.E.L. (2013) Reproductive capability is associated with lifespan and cause of death in companion dogs. *PLOS ONE* 8, e61082. https://doi.org/10.1371/journal.pone.0061082.

Jin, K., Hoffman, J.M., Creevy, K.E., O'Neill, D.G. and Promislow, D.E. (2016) Multiple morbidities in companion dogs: A novel model for investigating age-related disease. *Pathobiology of Aging and Age Related Diseases* 6, 33276. https://doi.org/10.3402/pba.v6.33276.

Kaeberlein, M., Creevy, K.E. and Promislow, D.E. (2016) The dog ageing project: Translational geroscience in companion animals. *Mammalian Genome* 27, 279–288. https://doi.org/10.1007/s00335-016-9638-7.

Landsberg, G. and Araujo, J.A. (2005) Behavior problems in geriatric pets. *Veterinary Clinics of North America. Small Animal Practice* 35, 675–698. https://doi.org/10.1016/j.cvsm.2004.12.008.

Landsberg, G.M., Deporter, T. and Araujo, J.A. (2011) Clinical signs and management of anxiety sleeplessness and cognitive dysfunction in the senior pet. *Veterinary Clinics of North America. Small Animal Practice* 41, 565–590. https://doi.org/10.1016/j.cvsm.2011.03.017.

Merlo, D.F., Rossi, L., Pellegrino, C., et al (2008) Cancer incidence in pet dogs: Findings of the animal tumor registry of Genoa, Italy. *Journal of Veterinary Internal Medicine* 22, 976–984. https://doi.org/10.1111/j.1939-1676.2008.0133.x.

Michell, A.R. (1999) Longevity of British breeds of dog and its relationships with sex, size, cardiovascular variables and disease. *The Veterinary Record* 145, 626–629. https://doi.org/10.1136/vr.145.22.625.

Patronek, G.J., Waters, D.J. and Glickman, L.T. (1997) Comparative longevity of pet dogs and humans: Implications for gerontology research. *Journals of Gerontology. Series A, Biological Sciences and Medical Sciences* 52, B171–B178. https://doi.org/10.1093/gerona/52A.3.B171.

Rosenberger, J.A., Pablo, N.V. and Crawford, P.C. (2007) Prevalence of and intrinsic risk factors for appendicular osteosarcoma in dogs: 179 cases (1996–2005). *Journal of the American Veterinary Medical Association* 231, 1076–1080. https://doi.org/10.2460/javma.231.7.1076.

Selman, C., Nussey, D.H. and Monaghan, P. (2013) Ageing: It's a dog's life. *Current Biology* 23, R451–R453. https://doi.org/10.1016/j.cub.2013.04.005.

Shoop, S.J., Marlow, S., Church, D.B., et al. (2015) Prevalence and risk factors for mast cell tumours in dogs in England. *Canine Genetics and Epidemiology* 2, (1). https://doi.org/10.1186/2052-6687-2-1.

Teske, E., Naan, E.C., van Dijk, E.M., Van Garderen, E. and Schalken, J.A. (2002) Canine prostate carcinoma: Epidemiological evidence of an increased risk in castrated dogs. *Molecular and Cellular Endocrinology* 197, 251–255. https://doi.org/10.1016/S0303-7207(02)00261-7.

Torres de la Riva, G.T., Hart, B.L., Farver, T.B., et al. (2013) Neutering dogs: Effects on joint disorders and cancers in golden retrievers. *PLOS ONE* 8, e55937. https://doi.org/10.1371/journal.pone.0055937.

Wang, T., Ma, J., Hogan, A.N. et al. (2020) Quantitative translation of dog-to-human aging by conserved remodelling of the DNA methylome. *Cell Systems* 11, 185. https://doi.org/10.1016/j.cels.2020.06.006.

CHAPTER 12

Oxtoby, C., Ferguson, E., White, K. and Mossop, L. (2015) We need to talk about error: Causes and types of error in veterinary practice. *The Veterinary Record* 177, 438. https://doi.org/10.1136/vr.103331.

INDEX

NOTES